logical and Clinical Aspects of Hematology

Pathological and Clinical Aspects of Hematology

Edited by **Brian Jenkins**

FOSTER ACADEMICS

New Jersey

Published by Foster Academics,
61 Van Reypen Street,
Jersey City, NJ 07306, USA
www.fosteracademics.com

Pathological and Clinical Aspects of Hematology
Edited by Brian Jenkins

International Standard Book Number: 978-1-63242-313-9 (Hardback)

Printed in the United States of America.

Contents

Preface

The purpose of the book is to provide a glimpse into the dynamics and to present opinions and studies of some of the scientists engaged in the development of new ideas in the field from very different standpoints. This book will prove useful to students and researchers owing to its high content quality.

Hematology encircles the physiology and pathology of blood and of the blood-forming organs. In similar areas of medicine, the pace of improvements in hematology has been rapid over the recent years. Now various treatment options are available to the modern hematologist and a great advanced outlook for the broad majority of patients with blood disorders. Developments in the clinic depict, and in various aspects are driven by, improvements in scientific grasping of hematological procedures under normal as well as in disease conditions. This book has two important sections: hematological pathologies and hematology in the clinic. It will serve as an important source of reference for both experts and amateur readers about some of the latest developments in hematology, in both laboratory and clinic.

At the end, I would like to appreciate all the efforts made by the authors in completing their chapters professionally. I express my deepest gratitude to all of them for contributing to this book by sharing their valuable works. A special thanks to my family and friends for their constant support in this journey.

Editor

Part 1

Hematological Pathologies

1

Translational Control in Myeloid Disease

Nirmalee Abayasekara and Arati Khanna-Gupta
*Brigham and Women's Hospital,
Harvard Medical School, Boston, MA,
USA*

1. Introduction

Over the years a wealth of information on the role played by transcription factors in myeloid biology has contributed to our understanding of both normal and abnormal myeloid development. However, the regulation of mRNA translation in myeloid cell maturation has, in comparison, been a neglected area of study. A better understanding of the translational control of myeloid gene expression will undoubtedly provide important insights into both normal and abnormal myeloid maturation. This chapter summarizes our current understanding of the regulation of myeloid gene expression at the mRNA translational level and delineates levels of disruption in myeloid disease, with an emphasis on leukemias.

2. Myeloid differentiation and neutrophil development

During hematopoiesis, granulocytes and monocytes arise from a common progenitor cell in the bone marrow and differentiate in response to cytokines and transcription factors ultimately giving rise to mature neutrophils and monocytes in the circulation. The granulocyte progenitor cells pass through several identifiable maturational stages, during which they acquire the morphologic appearance and granule contents that characterize the mature granulocyte(Rev in(Berliner, 1998)). The earliest identifiable granulocyte precursor is the myeloblast, which is characterized by very few granules, little cytoplasm and a prominent nucleolus. Transition to the promyelocyte stage is associated with the acquisition of primary granules. Primary granules are found in both granulocytes and monocytes and contain many of the proteins necessary for intracellular microbicidal activity (Bainton, 1975). The transition to the myelocyte stage is associated with the acquisition of secondary or "specific" granules(Bainton, 1971). Myelocytes further mature to give rise to bands and mature neutrophils. The appearance of secondary granules and their content proteins, provides a unique marker of commitment to terminal neutrophil differentiation (reviewed in (Borregaard *et al.*, 2001)). Several lines of evidence from our laboratory have established that the expression of the secondary granule protein (SGP) genes, which are functionally diverse and physically unlinked, is coordinately regulated at the level of mRNA transcription (reviewed in(Berliner, 1998)). Absence of SGP gene expression is a consistent abnormality in Myelodysplastic syndrome (MDS) and acute myeloid leukemia (AML).

2.1 Transcriptional control of myeloid maturation

Maturation of myeloid progenitor cells into specialized blood cells that play a vital role in innate immunity, is regulated by a well-orchestrated interplay of transcription factors (Tenen, 2003). Recent studies have delineated transcription factors that contribute to the process of maturation. These include a category of factors termed "master regulators" of lineage development and include PU.1, and CCAAT enhancer-binding protein-α (C/EBPα) (Tenen, 2003). These factors not only promote lineage-specific gene expression but also suppress alternative lineage pathways. For example, Laslo et al (Laslo *et al.*, 2006) elegantly demonstrated that cell fate determination is dependent upon subtle changes in expression levels of transcription factors, which regulate differential lineage maturation. Levels of PU.1 expression are increased by Egr-1/Nab-2 in developing monocytes/macrophages; while Egr-1 simultaneously represses the expression of the neutrophil specific Gfi-1 transcription factor (see below), thereby repressing the neutrophil development program.

2.1.1 C/EBPα

C/EBPα has been recognized to be a master regulator of the granulopoietic developmental program. It is expressed at high levels throughout myeloid differentiation (Tsukada *et al.*, 2011). C/EBPα binds to the promoters of multiple myeloid-specific genes, thereby regulating gene expression at many different stages of myeloid maturation. C/EBPα$^{-/-}$ mice die perinatally due to defects in gluconeogenesis that result in fatal hypoglycemia, and demonstrate an early block in the differentiation of granulocytes without affecting either monocyte/macrophage maturation or the differentiation of other hematopoietic lineages. The expression of C/EBPα is associated with growth arrest and differentiation of granulocyte precursor cells. This block in proliferation is thought to occur via the interaction of C/EBPα with cyclin-dependent protein kinases (cdk2 and cdk4), resulting in a block in cell proliferation. In addition, C/EBPα inhibits E2F-dependent transcription, which also contributes to inhibition of cell proliferation and induction of differentiation associated with C/EBPα-induced granulopoiesis (Timchenko *et al.*, 1997; Timchenko *et al.*, 1999)

2.1.2 PU.1

A second master myeloid regulator PU.1, is a member of the Ets family of transcription factors and is expressed in both B cells and monocyte/macrophages (Chen *et al.*, 1995). PU.1 is also expressed at lower levels in granulocytes and eosinophils as well as in CD34^{+} hematopoietic progenitor cells. High levels of PU.1 expression in fetal livers of mice preferentially directs monocyte/macrophage development, whereas low levels of PU.1 result in B-cell development (DeKoter and Singh, 2000). Studies have revealed that downregulation of c-Jun, a coactivator of PU.1, by C/EBPα is necessary for granulocytic maturation and is the mechanism through which C/EBPα blocks macrophage development (Rangatia *et al.*, 2002). Gene knockout studies of PU.1 in mice resulted in perinatal lethality accompanied by the absence of mature monocytes/macrophages, B cells as well as and delayed and reduced granulopoiesis (Scott *et al.*, 1994). Following *in vitro* differentiation, embryonic stem (ES) cells derived from PU.1$^{-/-}$ blastocysts fail to express mature myeloid cell markers, suggesting that PU.1 is not essential for the initial events associated with myeloid lineage commitment but is necessary for the later stages of development.

2.1.3 Growth Factor Independence-1 (Gfi-1)

Gfi-1 is a highly conserved transcriptional repressor that encodes a 55kD nuclear proto-oncogene that is composed of six zinc finger domains at the carboxy terminus and a N-terminal SNAG or repression domain (rev in (van der Meer *et al.*, 2010). Gfi-1 is expressed at high levels in the thymus and bone marrow, while its paralog Gfi1B, is expressed in the bone marrow and spleen. An essential role of Gfi-1 in neutrophil differentiation became apparent following reports of gene disruption in mice (Hock *et al.*, 2003). Gfi1-null mice are severely neutropenic and eventually succumb to bacterial infections. These mice lack mature neutrophils and their granulocyte precursors are unable to differentiate into mature neutrophils and also lack expression of specific granule proteins (SGPs). In addition, Gfi-1–/– bone marrow expresses atypical $Gr1^{+}Mac1^{+}$ myeloid precursor cells that appear to have characteristics of both granulocyte and macrophage precursors. These observations confirm a critical role for Gfi-1 in the neutrophil maturation program. Work from our laboratory has shown that Gfi-1 synergizes with another member of the CCAAT enhancer binding protein family of transcription factors, C/EBPε to transactivate the promoters of late myeloid genes. This synergy is lost in a patient with specific granule deficiency (SGD), who has a heterozygous substitution mutation in the C/EBPε gene as well as decreased levels of Gfi-1 in the bone marrow (Khanna-Gupta *et al.*, 2007). Heterozygous dominant negative mutations in the Gfi-1 gene have been described in two patients with severe congenital neutropenia (SCN) (Person *et al.*, 2003), thus emphasizing the role of Gfi-1 in the neutrophil maturation pathway.

Over the years a great deal of information pertaining to the transcriptional regulation of myeloid development has become available and has aided in our understanding of the process of granulopoiesis and how it goes awry in myeloid leukemias. In contrast, as outlined below, the role of mRNA translation in the process of normal myeloid development is only just beginning to be understood (rev in (Khanna-Gupta, 2011))

3. An overview of the process of mRNA translation in eukaryotic cells

Eukaryotic protein synthesis involves the coordinated interplay of hundreds of macromolecules such as mRNAs, tRNAs, activating enzymes, protein factors and ribosomes. Ribosomes are the protein synthetic factories upon which protein synthesis proceeds and are composed of a large (60S) and a small (40S) subunit. Each of these subunits is composed of two-thirds RNA and one-third protein. Protein synthesis occurs on the ribosome in three phases: translation initiation, elongation and termination. Regulation of gene expression takes place primarily at the initiation stage which therefore is the rate-limiting step in protein synthesis. The delicate balance of events leading to protein expression is critical for cellular growth, proliferation, differentiation and apoptosis (Rev in (Van Der Kelen *et al.*, 2009)). In eukaryotes, translation initiation factors (eIFs) play a crucial role in the dissociation of 40S and 60S ribosomal subunits thus enabling recruitment of mRNA and initiator tRNAs to the 40S subunit followed by interaction with the 60S subunit resulting in the reformation of the 80S ribosome allowing for elongation and termination of the polypeptide chain to ensue (rev in (Van Der Kelen *et al.*, 2009)).

3.1 Control of translation initiation

The first step in the translation of mRNA in eukaryotic cells begins with the binding of the 40S small ribosomal subunit to the 5′ end of the mRNA to be translated in the process of 5′

cap-dependent translation. Cap-binding protein eukaryotic initiation factor 4E (eIF4E) recognizes and binds to the m^{7}GpppN cap (where m is a methyl group and N any nucleotide) structure at the 5′end of the mRNA to be translated. Under normal physiologic conditions, eIF4E strongly associates with 4E-binding proteins (4E-BPs) thus preventing eIF4E from initiating protein synthesis, this represents the first rate limiting step in the process of protein synthesis. This inhibition is overcome by the phosphorylation of 4E-BPs via signal transduction pathways (involving PI3K and mTOR among others, see below) that are regulated by growth factors and nutrient status of the cell, thus causing 4E-BPs to be phosphorylated and to dissociate from eIF4E (Figure 1). This enables a competing adapter molecule eIF4G, to bind to eIF4E. eIF4G then recruits the ATP-dependent RNA helicase eIF4A (eIF4E, 4G and 4A are collectively referred to as eIF4F in the literature), the ubiquitously expressed cofactor eIF4B as well as eIF3, a multisubunit initiation factor, all of which bind to the 5′ cap region of the mRNA, thus setting the stage for mRNA translation to begin (rev in(Sonenberg and AG., 2009)).

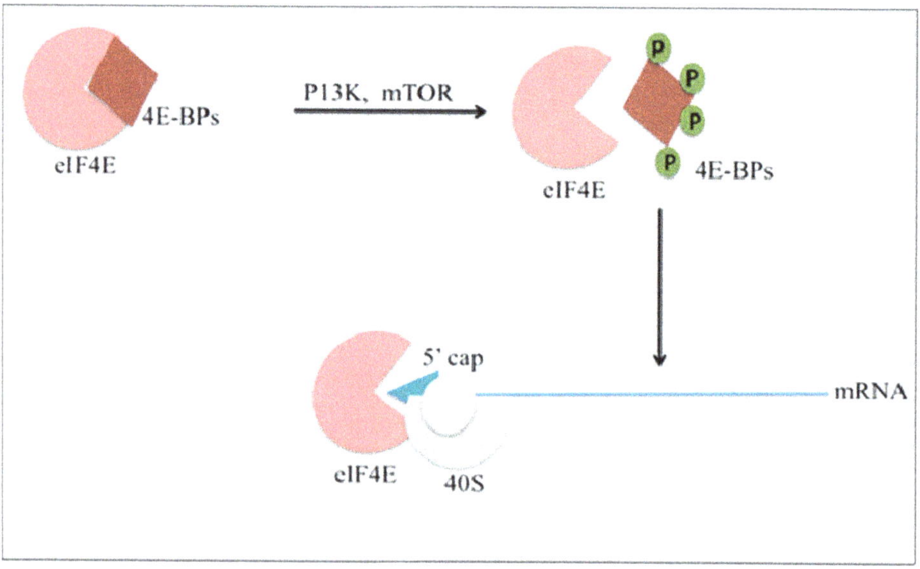

Fig. 1. Under basal conditions eIF4E is tightly bound to 4E-BPs. When cells are under stress or nutrient deprived, Phosphorylation of 4E-BPs is triggered by P13K (Phospho-inositol Kinase) and mTOR, which causes the 4E-BPs to be phosphorylated and/or to have reduced affinity for eIF4E. eIF4E is now free to bind eIF4G to initiate mRNA translation.

Translation initiation however requires the small ribosomal subunit 40S to be complexed with the so called ternary complex before it associates with the mRNA (Figure 2). The assembly of the ternary complex, consisting of the G protein eIF2B, eIF2, the initiator tRNA, tRNAi ^{met} and GTP, is the second rate-limiting step in mRNA translation. Recognition of the first AUG codon in the mRNA to be translated followed by initiation of protein synthesis is dependent on this process. Upon recognition of the first in-frame AUG, eIF2-GTP is hydrolyzed and the resulting eIF2-GDP is restored to eIF2-GTP by the guanine-nucleotide-exchange factor known as eIF2B to continue another round of translation initiation (Figure

2). This process is inbibited when the α subunit (S51 residue) of eIF2 is phosphorylated. This is brought about by the activation of a number of eIF2α kinases which are activated under conditions of cellular stress and aid in the reduction of protein synthesis until the stressful circumstance has passed (Figure 2). If stress remains unabated, apoptosis ensues. EIF2α kinases include the Heme-regulated inhibitor kinase (HRI), RNA-dependent protein kinase (PKR), PKR-like endoplasmic-reticulum kinase (PERK) and mGCN2(mammalian general control non-derepressing) (rev in (Raven and AE., 2008) and (Chen, 2007) and references therein). Since phosphorylated eIF2α has a higher affinity for eIF2B than eIF2α, phosphorylation of even a small percentage of eIF2α can lead to a reduction in protein synthesis. Phosphorylation of eIF2α can be reversed upon removal of the phosphate group by specific phosphatases thus restoring the cell to homeostasis (Harding *et al.*, 2009).

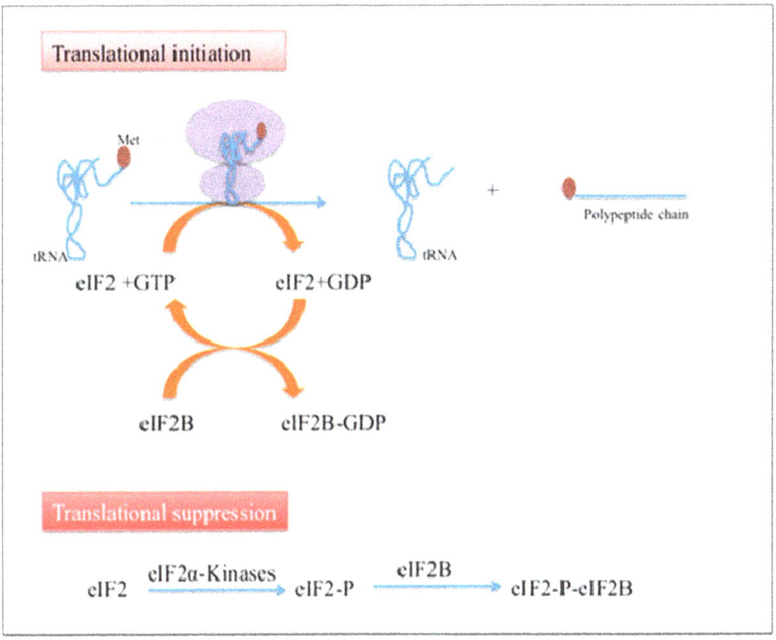

Fig. 2. During initiation, a GTP molecule is hydrolyzed to GDP which is then recycled by eIF2B, making eIF2α-GTP available for the continuation of the synthesis cycle. However, under cellular stress conditions, alterations in nutrient status, growth factors, mitogens and inducers of differentiation a variety of a eIF2α kinases are activated which causes the phosphorylation of eIF2α which has an increased affinity towards eIF2B. This traps available eIF2α and eIF2B resulting in a block in protein synthesis.

Formation of the 43S preinitiation complex occurs once the ternary complex binds to the 40S subunit complexed with eIF3 and eIF1A. The pre-initiation complex further associates with the mRNA through eIF3 and eIF4G, thus forming the 48S initiation complex. mRNA scanning begins when the 40S subunit moves along the mRNA in a 5′ to 3′ direction. Upon encountering the first in-frame translation initiation codon AUG, a codon (mRNA) - anticodon (tRNA) recognition is established resulting in the dissociation of initiation factors from the 40S subunit. This enables the binding of the 60S subunit resulting in the assembly of the functional ribosome (80S) and for peptide elongation to proceed.

The 3′ end of the mRNA together with a number of the initiation factors ensure the stabilization of ribosome-mRNA interaction. Poly (A) tail and polyA binding protein (PABP) interact with eIF4G to form a pseudo-circular mRNA. This structure is thought to reduce the translational error rate as translation from intact RNAs alone would be permitted. This mRNA configuration also gives the initiation factors the necessary spatial proximity that ensures efficient dissociation and re-association capabilities to permit another round of protein synthesis to occur.

3.2 The mTOR pathway

mTOR (mammalian/mechanistic target of rapamycin) is involved in an evolutionarily conserved pathway that is critical for cellular responses to environmental cues. mTOR is a serine/threonine protein kinase belonging to the phospho inositide 3-kinase (PI3K)-related protein kinases (PIKK) family of protein kinases, which consists of a protein complex that enable organisms to cope with metabolic, environmental and genetic stresses (rev in (Sengupta *et al.*, 2010)). Mammalian TOR forms two structurally and functionally distinct multiprotein complexes, mTORC1: in which mTOR is complexed with Raptor (the regulatory protein of mTOR), LST8 (also called GβL) and PRAS40 (proline-rich Akt/PKB substrate 40kDa), and mTORC2, harboring both LST8 and Rictor (rapamycin-insensitive companion of mTOR). Only mTORC1 is responsive to the inhibitory effects of the antibiotic rapamycin (Figure 3) (Wullschieger *et al.*, 2006). When activated, mTORC1 functions to regulate protein synthetic pathways in response to nutritional, environmental and growth factor mediated signals. The TCS1 and TCS2 (tuberous sclerosis 1 and 2) proteins form a tumor suppressor complex that transmits signals to mTORC1 by regulating the activation of Rheb (Ras homolog enriched in brain; a GTP-GDP exchange protein). The TCS1 and TSC2 complex regulates the GTP-loading state of Rheb. GTP-bound Rheb interacts with mTORC1 and renders it active. The two major targets of mTOR are the 4E-BPs (see Figure 1) and the 40S ribosomal protein S6 kinase (S6K1), both important components of the translational machinery (Figure 3).

Upon activation, mTORC1 regulates the phosphorylation/activation of p70 S6 kinase (S6K1) and the phosphorylation/deactivation of 4E-BP1(Platanias, 2005). Activation of S6 kinase modulates ribosome biogenesis through the activation of ribosomal protein S6 (rpS6)(Lee-Fruman *et al.*, 1999) (Figure 3). S6K1 also phosphorylates eIF2B, SKAR (S6K1 Aly/REF-like target) and eukaryotic elongation factor 2 kinase, thus affecting both the initiation and elongation stages of mRNA translation.

As described above, hypo-phosphorylation of the 4E-BPs increases their affinity for eIF4E, thus blocking the interaction of eIF4G and eIF4A thereby hampering translation initiation of mRNA from proceeding (Figure 1). However, phosphorylation of the 4E-BPs by activation of the mTORC1 signaling pathway (Figure 3) results in lowered affinity of these proteins for eIF4E, thus allowing for the formation of the competing eIF4E-eIF4G-eIF4A (eIF4F)-mRNA complex that permits mRNA translation to proceed(Gingras *et al.*, 2001). Thus inhibition of mTORC1 activity results in the down regulation of the activity of several components of the translational machinery resulting in a block in cell proliferation and eventually to cell death.

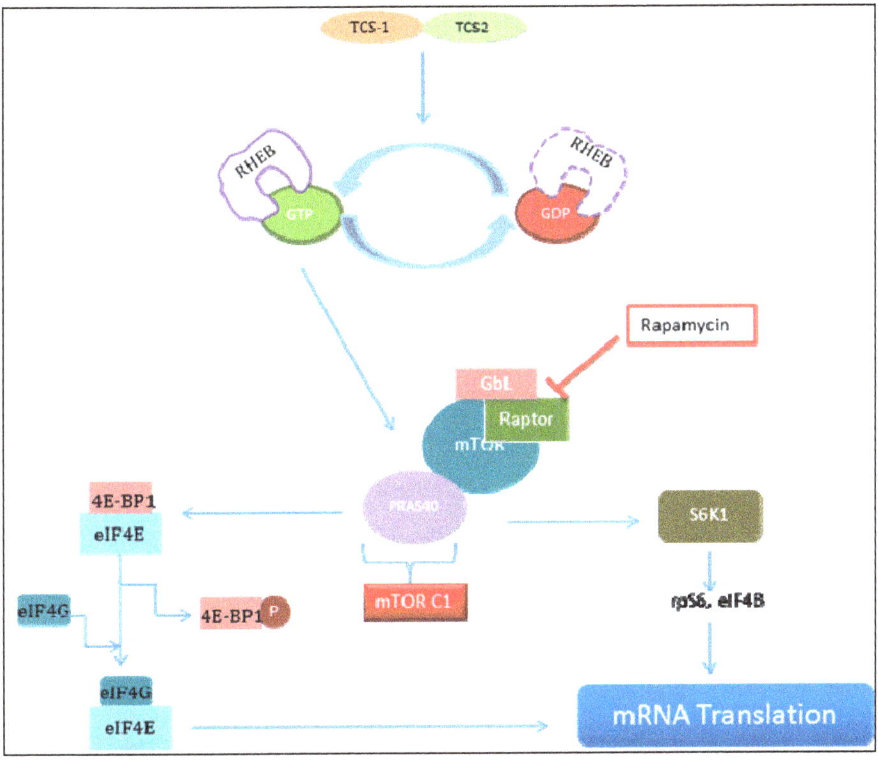

Fig. 3. mTOR pathway. See text for details

4. Translation control in Myeloid cells

While the general principles of mRNA translation hold in myeloid cells, it has been shown that when *4E-BP1* and *4E-BP2* genes were knocked out in mice an impairment of myelopoiesis was observed with no obvious effect on thymocyte maturation(Olson *et al.*, 2008). An increase in the number of immature granulocytic precursors and a decrease in the numbers of mature granulocytes was observed in these mice compared to their wild type littermates. Other studies have shown that expression of the 4E-BPs is significantly increased during granulopoiesis(Grolleau *et al.*, 1999). It was thus concluded that 4E-BP1 and 4E-BP2 play an important role in the early phases of granulo-monocytic differentiation thereby highlighting a critical role for translation initiation during granulopoiesis. It should be noted that 4E-BP1 has been shown to be constitutively phosphorylated in both chronic myeloid leukemia (CML) and in acute myeloid leukemia (AML) due to the constitutive activation of mTOR and Bcr-Abl in CML(Ly *et al.*, 2003) and PI3K-Akt in AML(Xu *et al.*, 2003).

4.1 Translational defects in myeloid leukemias

Activation of aberrant transcriptional and signaling pathways leading to enhanced survival and proliferation of leukemic progenitors is a hallmark of acute myeloid leukemia (AML)

(Scholl *et al.*, 2008; Tenen, 2003). The recent past has seen marked changes for the better in our understanding of the biology underlying AML. Based on these advances, targeting overactive signaling pathways in transformed cells has become an active area of research with the ultimate goal of finding molecules that specifically target only the transformed cell.

4.1.1 mTOR

The mTOR pathway has been shown to be activated in a number of cancers including AML (rev in (Tamburini *et al.*, 2009a)). In fact, mTORC1 has been shown to be activated in over 90% of primary AML samples (Tamburini *et al.*, 2009b). There has thus been a great effort to demonstrate the efficacy and use of Rapalogs, a class of drugs that include the mTORC1 inhibitor Rapamycin (see Figure 3) and RAD001, as anti-cancer agents. However, despite the anticipated cell death that blocking the mTORC1 pathway should result in, it has been demonstrated that the anti-leukemic effects of rapalogs are merely cytostatic. This is likely due to the fact that mTORC1 inhibition by rapalogs results in the activation of a number of feedback loops involving leukemogenic kinases such as P13K and ERK, thus limiting the anti-leukemic effects of this class of drugs.(Wang *et al.*, 2008)

4.1.2 Oncogenic mRNAs

The translation efficiencies of different mRNAs are dependent partly on the structural complexity of their 5'UTR (untranslated region). mRNAs with simple or short 5'UTRs, such as in the actin mRNA, are translated with high efficiency even in untransformed cells. However, mRNAs harboring long and complex 5'UTRs are generally translated with low efficiency and are referred to as "weak" mRNAs because of weak interactions with the eIF4F translation initiation complex (see above). In transformed cells on the other hand, this interaction improves due to the increased activity of eIF4F leading to increased translation of the weak mRNAs. It is noteworthy that a number of these weak mRNAs have oncogenic potential because they encode proteins involved in cell cycle regulation (e.g. cyclin D1) DNA replication (ornithine decarboxylase) and other pathways (c-myc, VEGF, Bcl-2, survin), all of which contribute to cell survival and proliferation. Expression of such mRNAs is regulated at the translational level and their overexpression likely contributes to the transformation process in AML ((Tamburini *et al.*, 2009a) and references therein). Since these "oncogenic" mRNAs have been found to be more sensitive to translation inhibition, there has been an effort to identify compounds that block mRNA translation. An example of such a compound is 4EGI-1 which is a 4E-BP1 mimetic and potently blocks the interaction of eIF4E and eIF4G during translation initiation (see above). 4EGI-1 has been shown to abrogate the expression of c-Myc and Bcl-x_L, both proteins with oncogenic potential. Additionally, this compound has shown therapeutic potential as it induces selective apoptosis in AML blast while allowing normal CD34+ hematopoietic progenitors to survive (Tamburini *et al.*, 2009b).

Overexpression of the initiation factor eIF4E has been described in primary cells derived from M4/M5 AML compared to bone marrow mononuclear cells (Topisirovic *et al.*, 2003). EIF4E expression has been known to increase protein synthesis and to transform cells (Wendel *et al.*, 2007). It should be noted that the antiviral compound ribavarin has been shown to inhibit the activity of eIF4E (Kentsis *et al.*, 2004). In a small study involving 11 M4/M5 AML patients who were given ribavarin, three patients responded with one in complete remission and two in partial remission (Assouline *et al.*, 2009). This study demonstrates that blocking the translational engine could prove to be a very important tool in the development of future AML therapeutics.

5. Translational control of the myeloid master regulator C/EBPα

C/EBPα is the founding member of a family of basic region/leucine zipper (bzip) transcription factors many of which contribute to granulopoiesis and are regulated at the translation level. (Rev in(Fuchs, 2007; Koschmieder *et al.*, 2009; Muller and Pabst, 2006; Schuster and Porse, 2006)). For the sake of simplicity only the translational control of the master myeloid regulator C/EBPα will be discussed here.

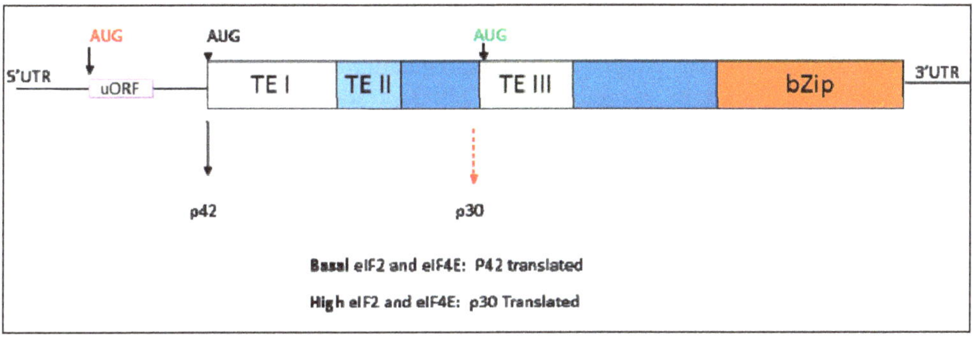

Fig. 4. Structure of the C/EBPα mRNA. TE I, II and III are activation domains. bZip is the basic leucine-zipper DNA binding domain.

Profound hematopoietic abnormalities have been reported for mice in which C/EBPα is ablated(Zhang *et al.*, 1997). The C/EBPα gene is intronless and generates two isoforms as a result of the differential utilization of alternate translation start codons. The resultant p42kD (full length) and p30kD (truncated) C/EBPα proteins differ from each other at the N-terminus, which is shorter in the p30kD protein (Figure 4). Translational control of C/EBPα-isoform expression occurs via a conserved cis-regulatory uORF (upstream open reading frame) in the 5'UTR (untranslated region) that is out of frame with the coding region of C/EBPα and is thought to be responsive to the activities of the translation initiation factors eIF4E and eIF2 (Figure 4 and see above). Thus, an increase in the activity of eIF2 or eIF4E, results in the increase in expression of the shorter p30 isoform (rev in(Calkhoven *et al.*, 2000)). An uORF monitors the site of translation initiation by sensing the activity of the eIF2 and eIF4E. When levels of these factors are high, the out-of-frame uORF (Figure 4, red AUG) is translated, but termination of its translation very close to the translational start site (black AUG) for p42 is thought to prevent reinitiation at the p42 AUG. Instead, ribosomes continue to scan and reinitiate at a downstream AUG (Figure 4, green AUG), resulting in the expression of C/EBPα p30. In contrast, under basal conditions, when levels of the initiation factors are relatively low, most ribosomes do not initiate translation at the uORF but instead initiate translation at the p42 AUG by a process involving "leaky ribosome scanning", resulting in translation of the full length C/EBPα p42 isoform(Calkhoven *et al.*, 2000). This mechanism of translational control appears to be conserved among key regulatory proteins which govern differentiation and proliferation (rev in (Khanna-Gupta, 2011)).

High levels of expression of the p30 C/EBPα protein have been shown to interfere with the DNA binding ability of the full length p42 C/EBPα, thus inhibiting transactivation of key granulocytic target genes in a dominant-negative manner (Pabst *et al.*, 2001), In addition, p30 transactivates the expression of a distinct subset of target genes different from that of the full length p42 C/EBPα thereby altering their expression (Geletu *et al.*, 2007). Mice engineered to express only the p30 C/EBPα isoform resulted in the development of AML with complete penetrance (Kirstetter *et al.*, 2008). Thus changes in the ratio of p42:p30 isoforms of C/EBPα play a critical role in contributing to AML(Fu *et al.*, 2010).

Suppression of C/EBPα translation has also been observed in the leukemic blasts of patients with CML (chronic myelogenous leukemia). This occurs via an RNA binding protein, hnRNP-E2, which binds to the uORF of the C/EBPα mRNA, thereby inhibiting translation. Expression of hnRNP-E2 is thought to be upregulated by the activity of the oncogenic BCR-ABL fusion protein in CML patients, and downregulation of hnRNP-E2 by the BCR-ABL inhibitor Imatinib results in restoration of C/EBPα protein expression and granulocytic differentiation of the CML blasts(Perrotti *et al.*, 2002).

6. Role of microRNAs in translation control

6.1 General principles

MicroRNAs (miRNAs) are 18-24 nucleotides long non-coding RNAs that regulate eukaryotic gene expression influencing cellular functions as diverse as cell proliferation, differentiation and apoptosis. miRNAs are non-coding RNAs which silence target genes post-transcriptionally by binding to complementary sequences in the 3′UTR (untranslated region) of the target mRNA resulting in either mRNA degradation or translation repression (rev in (Ambros, 2004)). More than 100 miRNAs are expressed in the hematopoieteic compartment (rev in (Gazzar and McCall, 2011)). MiRNAs are encoded in the genome and are initially transcribed by RNA polymerase II as long primary transcripts referred to as primary miRNAs (pri-miRNAs). These hairpin transcripts are recognized and processed by RNase III enzymes called Drosha and DGCR8 into 60-80 nucleotide intermediates called precursor miRNAs (pre-miRNAs) which are then exported to the cytoplasm by Exportin 5 where a second ribonuclease termed Dicer cleaves the pre-miRNAs to generate double stranded 18-24 nucleotide long miRNAs. One strand of the miRNA is next destroyed and the remaining strand, the guide strand, is then incorporated into the RNA-induced silencing complex or RISC, a large protein complex that also contains the Argonaute 2 or mRNA cleaving proteins. The miRNA guides the RISC complex to target complementary regions in the 3′UTRs of mRNAs, leading to repression of translation or destabilization of the mRNA by deadenylation. (rev in (Manikandan *et al.*, 2008)). In mammalian cells, 6-8 nucleotides of the miRNA (known as the seed region) base pair with the cognate recognition sequence in the 3′UTR of the target mRNA. In general, a perfectly matched sequence between the seed region and mRNA target results in degradation of the mRNA target. An imperfect match however, results in translation repression (rev in (Gazzar and McCall, 2011)). MiRNAs are thought to repress translation by blocking translation initiation of the target mRNA (Filipowicz *et al.*, 2008).

6.2 miRNAs in myeloid biology

An increasing body of evidence implicates miRNA activity in mediating both normal and abmormal myelopoiesis (rev in (Pelosi *et al.*, 2009) and (Gazzar and McCall, 2011)).

Granulocytes arise from the GMPs (granulocyte monocyte progenitors) which are capable of developing into granulocytes or monocytes as a result of cytokines and thus transcription factor activation (Dahl R *et al.*, 2003). MiRNAs have been shown to activate or be activated by myeloid specific transcription factors such as PU.1, C/EBPα and Gfi-1. Mir-223, for example, is thought to be a direct target of C/EBPα and its expression increases during granulopoiesis. C/EBPα is a master regulator of granulopoiesis (Tenen, 2003). Complete loss of mir-223 in mice results in the expansion of granulocyte precursor cells resulting from a cell autonomous increase in the number of granulocytic progenitors (Johnnidis *et al.*, 2008). In contrast, overexpression of mir-223 in acute promyelocytic leukemia (APL) cells results in an enhanced capacity for granulocytic differentiation (Fazi *et al.*, 2005). Mir-223 is thus thought to be a positive regulator of granulopoietic differentiation. It has also been shown that mir-223 targets E2F1, a master cell cycle regulator, by inhibiting translation of its mRNA. Thus, granulopoiesis appears to be regulated by a C/EBPα–miR-223–E2F1 axis, where miR-223 functions as a key regulator of myeloid cell proliferation associated with E2F1 in a negative feedback loop(Pulikkan *et al.*, 2010).

In a recent study, Eiring et al demonstrated a new "decoy" role for miRNAs involving the master reugator C/EBPα. They showed that mir-328 is down regulated in myeloid cells of chronic myelogenous leukemia (CML) patients in blast crisis. Restoration of mir-328 expression however rekindles differentiation in the CML blast cells by a mechanism involving the simultaneous interaction of mir-328 with the C/EBPα translational inhibitor hnRNP-E2 (see above), as well as with the mRNA for PIM1, a survival factor. Since, the interaction with hnRNP-E2 occurs independently of mir-328's seed sequence, this miRNA acts as a "sink" for hnRNA-E2 binding allowing for the release of C/EBPα mRNA from the negative effects of hnRNA-E2-mediated translational inhibition. Thus mir-328 appears to control cell fate by its ability to base pair with the 3'UTR of target mRNAs (PIM1) as well as by acting as a decoy for hnRNP binding resulting in the release of C/EBPα from translational inhibition, thereby altering cell fate(Eiring *et al.*, 2010).

Gfi-1 (growth factor independence-1), a transcriptional repressor that promotes granulocytic differention, has been shown to regulate the expression of mir-196b (Velu *et al.*, 2009). The expression of mir-196b is high in the common myeloid progenitors (CMPs) which can differentiate either along the granulocytic or monocytic lineages. Gfi-1 has been shown to bind to the promoter of mir-196b thereby repressing its expression and promoting granulopoiesis. Additionally, overexpression of mir-196b was shown to block granulopoieis, confirming the importance of low level expression of this miRNA in contributing to granulopoietic maturation (Hock *et al.*, 2003) .

PU.1, a master transcriptional regulator of monocyte/macrophage differentiation, regulates the expression of mir-424, which in turn inhibits the expression of the transcription factor NFI-A. Mir-424 expression has been shown to promote monocyte/macrophage differentiation. Thus the two primary transcriptional determinants of myeloid differentiation, PU.1 and C/EBPα, both involve the activity of microRNAs for lineage maturation (Rosa *et al.*, 2007). Thus, miRNAs and myeloid specific transcription factors play a critical role in lineage maturation pathways by forming lineage-specific regulatory loops (rev in (Gazzar and McCall, 2011)), which if disrupted can lead to the development of leukemias.

Numerous studies have analyzed the expression of miRNAs in acute myeloid leukemias and the resulting miR signatures generated have proved to be helpful in classifying sub-types of AML and hence the choice of treatment options to be used, as well as in determining the efficacy of targeted therapies against AML. For example, Pelosi et al analyzed the expression of 12 selected granulocytic signature miRNAs and the impact of all *trans*-retinoic acid (ATRA)-based therapy in a cohort of acute promyelocytic leukemia (APL) patients (Pelosi *et al.*, 2009). APL is a subtype of acute leukemia and is characterized by the accumulation of promyelocytes as a result of a chromosomal translocation, most commonly involving the retinoic acid alpha receptor and the PML gene in a t(15;17) configuration. APL patients respond well to treatment with retinoic acid, a vitamin A derivative. The authors demonstrated using a quantitative real time PCR approach, that 9 miRNAs were overexpressed while three (mir-107, -342 and Let-7c) were downregulated in the blasts of APL patients, compared to normal promyelocytes. They showed in addition, that patients successfully treated with ATRA showed down regulation of mir-181b and upregulation of mir-15b, -16,-107, -223, -342 and let-7c. Thus, a small subset of miRNAs appeared to be differentially regulated in APL and could be modulated by treatment with ATRA. This approach is fast becoming a paradigm in diagnosing and determining the efficacy of treatment regimens used in acute myeloid leukemias.

7. Concluding remarks and perspectives

Inspite of the fact that there has been a surge of interest in the role of mRNA translational regulation in mediating gene expression in myeloid cells in recent times, a great deal of work has yet to be done. A general interest in this subject derives its source from the fact that cellular pathways commonly deregulated in AML including cell cycle progression, proliferation and differentiation are mechanistically tied to mRNA translation. For example, several upstream (AKT, TSC1/2) and downstream (eIF4E) mediators of the mTORC1 pathway are either mutated or activated in AML. Although there has been an intense search for therapeutic strategies targeting the mTOR pathway in myeloid cells, much work is yet to be done to gain a fundamental understanding of the role of the key players that contribute to translation initiation and control in normal and abnormal myeloid cells.

8. References

Ambros V (2004). The functions of animal microRNAs. *Nature* 431: 350-55.

Assouline S, Culjkovic B, Cocolakis E, Rousseau C, Beslu N, Amri A *et al* (2009). Molecular targeting of the oncogene eIF4E in AML: a proof-of-principle clinical trial with ribavarin. *Blood* 114: 257-60.

Bainton D (1975). Neutrophil granules. *Br. J Hematol* 29: 19.

Bainton D, Ullyot, JL, Farquhar, MG (1971). The development of the neutrophil secondary granule. *J Exp Med* 134: 907.

Berliner N (1998). Molecular biology of neutrophil differentiation. *Curr Opin Hematol* 5: 49-53.

Borregaard N, Theilgaard-Monch K, Sorensen O, Cowland J (2001). Regulation of human neutrophil granule protein expression. *Curr. Opin. Hematol* 8: 23-27.

Calkhoven C, Müller C, A. L (2000). Translational control of C/EBPalpha and C/EBPbeta isoform expression. *Gene Dev* 14: 1920-32.

Chen HM, Zhang P, Voso MT, Hohaus S, Gonzalez DA, Glass CK *et al* (1995). Neutrophils and monocytes express high levels of PU.1 (Spi-1) but not Spi-B. *Blood* 85: 2918-28.

Chen J (2007). Regulation of protein synthesis by the heme-regulated eIF2 kinase: relevance to anemias. *Blood* 109: 2693-2699.

Dahl R, Walsh JC, Lancki D, Laslo P, Iyer SR, Singh H *et al* (2003). Regulation of macrophage and neutrophil cell fates by the PU.1:C/EBPalpha ratio and granulocyte colony-stimulating factor.

DeKoter RP, Singh H (2000). Regulation of B- lymphocyte and macrophage development by graded expression of PU.1. *Science* 288: 1439-41.

Eiring A, Harb JG, Neviani P, Garton C, Oaks JJ, Spizzo R *et al* (2010). miR-328 functions as an RNA decoy to modulate hnRNP E2 regulation of mRNA translation in leukemic blasts. *Cell* 140: 652-65.

Fazi F, Rosa A, Fatica A, Gelmetti V, De Marchis ML, Nervi C *et al* (2005). Aminicircuitry comprised of microRNA-223 and transcription factors NFI-A and C/EBPalpha regulates human granulopoiesis. *Cell* 123: 819-31.

Filipowicz A, Bhattacharyya S, Sonenberg N (2008). Mechanisms of post transcriptional regulation by microRNAs: are the answers in sight? *Nat Rev Genet* 9: 102-114.

Fu C-T, Zhu K-Y, Mi J-Q, Liu Y, ST M, Fu Y-F *et al* (2010). An evolutionarily conserved PTEN-C/EBPα-CTNNA1 axis controls myeloid development and transformation. *Blood* ePublication April 6th.

Fuchs O (2007). Growth-inhibiting activity of transcription factor C/EBPa, its role in hematopoiesis and its tumour suppressor or oncogenic properties in leukaemias. *Folia Biologica (Praha)* 53: 97-108.

Gazzar M, McCall C (2011). MicroRNAs regulatory network in myeloid lineage development and differentiation: regulators of the regulators. *Immunology Cell Biol*: 1-7.

Geletu M, Balkhi M, Peer Zada A, Christopeit M, J, Pulikkan J, Trivedi A *et al* (2007). Target proteins of C/EBPalphap30 in AML: C/EBPalphap30 enhances sumoylation of C/EBPalphap42 via up-regulation of Ubc9. *Blood* 110: 3301-9.

Gingras A-C, Raught B, Sonenberg N (2001). Regulation of translation initiation by FRAP/mTOR. *Gene Dev* 15: 807-26.

Grolleau A, Sonenberg N, J W, L B (1999). Differential regulation of 4E-BP1 and 4E-BP2, two repressors of translation initiation, during human myeloid cell differentiation. *J Immunol.* 162: 3491-7.

Harding H, Zhang Y, D S, JJ C, RJ K, D R (2009). Ppp1r15 gene knockout reveals an essential role for translation initiation factor 2 alpha (eIf2a) dephosphorylation in mammalian delvelopment. *Proc Natl Acad Sci USA* 106: 1832-37.

Hock H, Hamblen M, Rooke H, Traver D, Bronson R, Cameron S *et al* (2003). Intrinsic requirement for zinc finger transcription factor Gfi-1 in neutrophil differentiation. *Immunity* 18: 109-120.

Johnnidis J, Harris MH, Wheeler RT, Stehling-Sun S, Lam MH, Kirak O *et al* (2008). Regulation of progenitor cell proliferation and granulocyte function by microRNA-223. *Nature* 451: 1125-29.

Kentsis A, Topisirovic I, Culjkovic B, Shao L, Borden K (2004). Ribavarin supresses eIF4E-mediated oncogenic transfornation by physical mimicry of the 7-methyl guanosine mRNA cap. *Proc Natl Acad Sci USA* 101: 18105-10.

Khanna-Gupta A (2011). Regulation and deregulation of mRNA translation during myeloid maturation. *Exp Hematol* 39: 133-41.

Khanna-Gupta A, Sun H, Zibello T, Lee H, Dahl R, Boxer L *et al* (2007). Growth factor independence-1 (Gfi-1) plays a role in mediating specific granule deficiency (SGD) in a patient lacking a gene-inactivating mutation in the C/EBPepsilon gene. *Blood* 15;109.: 4181-90.

Kirstetter P, Schuster MB, Bereshchenko O, Moore S, Dvinge H, Kurz E *et al* (2008). Modeling of C/EBPalpha mutant acute myeloid leukemia reveals a common expression signature of committed myeloid leukemia-initiating cells. *Cancer Cell* 13: 299-310.

Koschmieder S, Halmos B, Levantini E, DG. T (2009). Dysregulation of the C/EBPalpha differentiation pathway in human cancer. *J.Clin. Oncol.* 27: 619-28.

Laslo P, Spooner CJ, Warmflash A, Lancki DW, Lee HJ, Sciammas R *et al* (2006). Multilineage transcriptional priming and determination of alternate hematopoietic cell fates. *Cell* 126.

Lee-Fruman K, CJ K, J L, N T, J B (1999). Characterization of S6K2, a novel kinase homologous to S6K1. *Oncogene* 18: 5108-114.

Ly C, Arechiga AF, Melo JV, Walsh CM, Ong CM (2003) Bcr-Abl kinase modulates translation regulators ribosomal protein S6 and 4E-BP1 in chronic myelogenous leukemia via the mammalian targtet of rapamycin. Cancer Res. 63, 5716-22

Manikandan J, Aarthi JJ, Kumar SD, PN P (2008). Oncomirs: The potential role of non-coding microRNAs in understanding cancer. *Bioinformation* 8: 330-4.

Muller B, Pabst T (2006). C/EBPα and the pathophysiology of acute myeloid leukemia. *Curr Opin Hematol* 13: 7-14.

Olson K, GC B, F P, Sonenberg N, L B (2008). Impaired myelopoiesis in mice lacking the repressors of translation initiation, 4E-BP1 and 4E-BP2. *Immunology* 128: e379-e384.

Pabst T, Muller B, Zhang P (2001). Dominant negative mutations of CEBPA encoding CCAAT/enhancer binding protein-α (C/EBPα), in acute myeloid leukemia. *Nat Genet* 27: 263-270.

Pelosi E, Labbaye C, U. T (2009). MicroRNAs in normal and malignant myelopoiesis. *Lukemia Res* 33: 1584-93.

Perrotti D, Cesi V, Trotta R, Guerzoni C, Santilli G, Campbell K *et al* (2002). BCR-ABL suppresses C/EBPalpha expression through inhibitory action of hnRNP E2. *Nat Genet.* 30: 48-58.

Person R, Li F, Duan Z, Benson K, Wechsler J, Papadaki H *et al* (2003). Mutations in protooncogene Gfi1 cause human neutropenia and target ELA2. *Nat. Genet.* 34: 308-312.

Platanias L (2005). Mechaisms of type-1 and type-II interferon-mediated signaling. *Nat Rev Immunol* 5: 375-86.

Pulikkan J, Dengler V, Peramangalam PS, Peer Zada AA, Müller-Tidow C, Bohlander SK *et al* (2010). Cell-cycle regulator E2F1 and microRNA-223 comprise an autoregulatory negative feedback loop in acute myeloid leukemia. *Blood* 115: 1768-78.

Rangatia J, Vangala R, Treiber N, Zhang P, Radomska H, Tenen D *et al* (2002). Downregulation of c-Jun expression by transcription factor C/EBPalpha is critical for granulocytic lineage commitment. *Mol. Cell.Biol* 22: 8681-94.

Raven J, AE. K (2008). PERK and PKR: old kinases learn new tricks. *Cell Cycle* 7: 1146-50.

Rosa A, Ballarino M, Sorrentino A, Sthandier O, De Angelis F, Marchioni M *et al* (2007). The interplay between the master transcription factor PU1 and mir-424 regulates human monocyte/macrophage differentiation. *Proc Natl Acad Sci USA* 104: 19849-54.

Scholl C, Gilliland D, Frohling S (2008). Deregulation of signaling pathways in acute myeloid leukemia. *Semin Oncol* 35: 336-45.

Schuster M, Porse B (2006). C/EBPa: a tumour suppressor in multiple tissues? *Biochim. Biophys. Acta* 1766: 88-103.

Scott EW, Simon MC, Anastasi J, Singh H (1994). Requirement of transcription factor PU.1 in the development of multiple hematopoietic lineages. *Science* 265: 1573-1577.

Sengupta S, Peterson T, Sabatini D (2010). Regulation of the mTOR Complex 1 Pathway by Nutrients, Growth Factors, and Stress. *Mol Cell* 40: 310-22.

Sonenberg N and Hinnebucsh AG (2009) Regulation of translation initiation in eukaryotes: mechanisms and biological targets. Cell 136, 731-45.

Tamburini J, Green A, Chapuis N, Bardet V, Lacombe C, Mayeux P *et al* (2009a). Targeting translation in acute myeloid leukemia. A new paradigm for therapy. *Cell Cycle* 23: 3893-99.

Tamburini J, Green AS, Bardet V, Chapuis N, Park S, Willems L *et al* (2009b). Protein synthesis is resistant to rapamycin and constitutes a promising therapeutic target in acute myeloid leukemia. *Blood* 114.

Tenen D (2003). Disruption of differentiation in human cancer: AML shows the way. *Nature Rev: Cancer* 3: 89-101.

Timchenko N, Harris T, Wilde M, al. e (1997). CCAAT/enhancer binding protein alpha regulates p21 protein and hepatocyte proliferation in newborn mice. *Mol Cell Biol* 17: 7353-61.

Timchenko N, Wilde M, Darlington G (1999). C/EBPalpha regulates formation of S-phase-specific E2F-p107 complexes in livers of newborn mice. *Mol Cell Biol* 19: 2936-45.

Topisirovic I, Guzman ML, McConnell MJ, Licht JD, Culjkovic B, Neering SJ *et al* (2003). Aberrant eukaryotic translation initiation factor 4E-dependent mRNA transport impedes hematopoietic differentiation and contributes to leukemogenesis. *Mol Cell Biol* 23: 8992-9002.

Tsukada J, Yoshida Y, Kominato Y, Auron P (2011). The CCAAT/enhancer (C/EBP) family of basic-leucine zipper (bZIP) transcription factors is a multifaceted highly regulated system for gene regulation. *Cytokine* 54: 6-19.

Van Der Kelen K, Beyaert R, Inzé D, L. DV (2009). Translational control of eukaryotic gene expression. *Crit Rev Biochem Mol Biol.* 44: 143-68.

van der Meer L, Jansen JH, BA. vdR (2010). Gfi1 and Gfi1b: key regulators of hematopoiesis. . *Leukemia* 24: 1834-43.

Velu C, Baktula AM, HL. G (2009). Gfi1 regulates miR-21 and miR-196b to control myelopoiesis. *Blood* 113: 4720-8. .

Wang X, Hawk N, Yue P, Kauh J, Ramalingam S, Fu H *et al* (2008). mTOR inhibition induced paradoxical activation of survival signalling pathways enhances mTOR inhibitors' anti-cancer efficacy. *Cancer Biol and Therapy* 7: 1952-58.

Wendel H, Silva R, Malina A, Mills J, Zhu H, Ueda T *et al* (2007). Dissecting eIF4E action in tumorigenesis. *Genes and Dev* 21: 3232-37.

Wullschieger S, Loewith R, Hall M (2006). TOR signaling in growth and metabolism. *Cell* 124: 471-84.

Xu Q, Simpson SE, Scialla TJ, Bagg A, Carroll M. (2003) Survival of Acute Myeloid Leukemia cells requires PI3 kinase activation. Blood, 102, 972-80.

Zhang P, Iwama A, Datta MW, Darlington GJ, Link DC, Tenen DG. (1997). *39th Annual Meeting of the American Society of Hematology, San Diego, California, USA, December, Vol. 90.*

2

Physiological and Pathological Aspects of Human NK Cells

Chiara Vitale[1], Renato Zambello[2], Mirna Balsamo[3], Maria Cristina Mingari[1,4] and Massimo Vitale[4]

[1]*DI.ME.S. Università di Genova, Genova*

[2]*Padova University School of Medicine, Department of Clinical and Experimental Medicine, Hematology and Clinical Immunology Branch – Padova*

[3]*Istituto G. Gaslini – Genova*

[4]*IRCCS A.O.U. S.Martino-IST Istituto Nazionale per la Ricerca sul Cancro, S.C. Immunologia - Genova*

Italy

1. Introduction

Natural Killer (NK) cells were first defined, more than 30 years ago, on the basis of their unique capability of killing spontaneously different targets including tumor and virus-infected cells. Thus, since their first discovery, NK cells came across as a potential attractive tool for the implementation of immuno-therapeutic strategies for different diseases. Accordingly, besides the plethora of studies aimed at investigating their functional and phenotypic properties, considerable efforts have also been spent in the past several years to understand how these cells could be generated and how their functions could be regulated and/or manipulated. At the same time further attention has been paid on their alteration in vivo and their potential role in the occurrence of NK cell-based hematological malignancies.

2. NK cells: From a function to a multifaceted population

2.1 The discovery of NK cells

NK cells were originally identified on a functional basis. In the middle '70s, it was discovered that healthy individuals could display selective cytotoxic activity against tumor or virally infected cells and that this activity was hidden within the circulating lymphocyte population (West et al., 1977; Santoli et al., 1978). This implied the presence in the Peripheral Blood (PB) of a lymphocyte subset capable of killing different targets without previous sensitization. These cells, that for their functional properties were termed 'Natural Killer', were then characterized morphologically as Large Granular Lymphocytes (LGL) by virtue of their size and cytolytic granule content. Finally, in the late '80s, NK cells were more precisely defined with the $CD3^-CD56^+CD16^+$ surface immuno-phenotype. This also allowed the identification of the CD16/FcγRIII as the receptor responsible for the Antibody-Dependent Cell Cytotoxicity (ADCC) function shown by NK cells (Lanier et al., 1986; Trinchieri, 1989). In the same period, the circulating NK cell population, which represented approximately 10-15% of PB lymphocytes, was further split into CD56brightCD16dim/neg and CD56dimCD16bright cell subsets, expressing respectively low and high cytolytic properties. In the following 10 years great efforts were done to widen the list of NK cell markers and to define the surface receptors responsible for the regulation of NK cell cytotoxicity. Finally, in the last decade it was discovered that NK cells could exert different regulatory functions, and many studies were oriented to the definition of novel NK cell subsets involved in such unexpected functional features.

2.2 The regulation of NK cell function: Activating and inhibitory receptors

Once NK cells could be physically identified and isolated, the goal was to understand how these cells could work; and the first questions were: "How can a single NK cell kill different targets?" and "how do NK cells recognize and spare self normal cells?" The answer to these questions was indicated by Karre in his "missing self hypothesis". He postulated that NK cells could sense the absence (or reduction) of self MHC class I molecules (MHC-I) during cell-to-cell interaction: the missing recognition of self would allow NK cells to kill the targets, while recognition of self MHC-I would inhibit their cytolytic activity (Ljunggren & Karre, 1990). This would explain how NK cells could kill tumor or virus infected cells, which frequently undergo surface MHC-I down-regulation, and spare self non-pathogenic cells, equipped with appropriate levels MHC-I. The hypothesis was then confirmed, and the inhibitory MHC-I-specific receptors responsible for the recognition of Self were identified. In humans, major HLA-I-specific inhibitory receptors are represented by the C-type lectin CD94/NKG2A dimer that recognizes the non-classical HLA-E alleles, and the Killer Ig-like Receptors (KIR). The CD94/NKG2A encoding genes are located in the NK Receptor complex on chromosome 12, while the KIR locus is located in the Leukocyte Receptor Complex in Chromosome 19. The KIRs constitute a family of strictly homologous proteins characterized by the presence of two or three extracytoplasmic Ig-like domains (KIR2D or KIR3D) and a long cytoplasmic tail (KIR2DL or KIR3DL) containing Immuno Tyrosine-based Inhibitory Motifs (ITIMs) for the inhibitory signal transduction. Each KIR recognizes a specific epitope common to a defined group of HLA-I alleles. In particular, KIR2DL1 recognizes the Lys80 containing C2 epitope, that is shared by a group of HLA-C alleles; KIR2DL2/L3 recognize the Asn80 containing C1 epitope, that is shared by the remaining alleles of the locus HLA-C; KIR3DL1 recognizes the Ile/Thr80 containing HLA-Bw4 epitope, that is common to certain HLA-A and HLA-B alleles, while KIR3DL2 recognizes certain HLA-A alleles (Biassoni et al., 2001; Parham, 2005). Interestingly, KIR3DL2 has also been recently shown to bind microbial nucleic acids at the cell surface and to shuttle them to TLR9 in the endosome, suggesting for certain KIR a novel (or rather an ancient) function as pathogen sensors (Sivori et al., 2010). The HLA-I-specific inhibitory receptors are clonally distributed within the NK cell population of each individual. Most NK cells express one or more receptors and at least one that recognize an autologous HLA-I allele. Recently, a KIR- NKG2A- NK cell subset has been described in different donors. These cells, however, appeared to be poorly functional. This suggested that the expression and the engagement of inhibitory receptors during maturation of NK cells could dictate the acquisition of their cytolytic potential (Licensing theory) (Anfossi et al., 2006). The KIR family also includes activating KIRs. These are homologous to their inhibitory counterparts, but display a short cytoplasmic tail (KIR2DS or KIR3DS), lack ITIMs and associate an ITAM-bearing molecule (DAP12) to transduce activating signals. Similarly, also for NKG2A, does exist a short-tailed activating counterpart, termed NKG2C. The meaning of these receptors is poorly known. It has been hypothesized that they may recognize HLA-I molecules loaded with viral or tumor peptides, or, with low affinity, normal HLA-I molecules. In this latter case, when target cells selectively down-regulate HLA alleles, recognized by inhibitory KIR, the engagement of activating KIR may result in NK cell activation. The simultaneous expression of activating and inhibitory KIRs may therefore represent a strategy whereby NK cells can recognize and kill pathologic cells uniquely by detecting changes in their HLA alleles repertoire. At present, however, binding to HLA-I molecules has been formally demonstrated only for KIR2DS1 and NKG2C.

NK cells are also equipped with a large array of non-HLA-specific triggering receptors and co-receptors, whose engagement by specific Ligands expressed on target cells induces NK cell cytotoxicity and cytokine release (Moretta A. et al., 2001; Vivier et al., 2011). The group of NK-triggering receptors is largely heterogeneous: it encompasses molecules either structurally unrelated or belonging to different molecular families. At variance with KIRs, triggering receptors are expressed by virtually all NK cells and, in most cases, by different lymphocyte subsets or monocytes. The activating receptor Ligands till now identified, appear to be over-expressed in one or more of the following cases: tumor transformation, viral infection, cell stress or activation. Consistently, most of the activating receptors have been shown to be variably involved in the recognition and killing of virus infected and/or tumor cells. Two members of CD2 family: 2B4 (CD244) and NTBA, which recognize CD48 and NTBA respectively, have been involved in the clearance of EBV-infected cells. NKp80 and NKG2D, two Killer cell Lectin Receptors (KLR) encoded in the NK gene Complex on human chromosome 12, recognize molecules that can be expressed on tumor and/or virus infected cells. NKp80 recognizes AICL (encoded in the same NK gene complex) that is expressed on activated monocytes, but it can be also expressed on malignant myeloid cells (Welte et al., 2006). NKG2D recognizes MHC-I-related stress-inducible molecules of the MIC and ULBP families, that can be up-regulated on virus infected or tumor cells. Three receptors, that are expressed on cytotoxic lymphocytes (both NK and T cells), DNAM-1 (CD226), TACTILE (CD96) and CRTAM, recognize members of the Nectin/Nectin-Like (NecL) family (Fuchs & Colonna, 2006). In particular DNAM-1, that is the most highly espressed on NK cells, recognizes Nectin2 (CD112) and NecL5 (CD155 - poliovirus receptor) (Bottino et al., 2003). Nectin/NecL molecules are involved in the formation of various types of cell-to-cell junctions, especially in epithelial cells, neurons or fibroblasts. Nectins 1 and 2, and NecL5 can also serve as viral entry receptors. These molecules, however, are frequently up-regulated in tumor cells of different histotypes. In addition, CMV infection can alter NecL5-Nectin3 intercellular interaction: in this case NecL5 would be exposed outside the cellular junction and allow DNAM-1 recognition.

While all the above-mentioned activating receptors are expressed by different leukocyte subsets, NKp30, NKp46 and NKp44 triggering receptors are restricted to NK cells. NKp44 and NKp46 are involved in the recognition of both viral antigens (as the influenza virus HA) (Mandelboim et al., 2001) and ligands expressed by tumor cells. NKp30 recognizes B7H6 and BAT-3 (Brandt et al., 2009; Pogge von Strandmann et al., 2007). B7H6 is a member of the B7 family (which includes ligands for stimulatory/inhibitory T cell co-receptors CD28/CTLA4). B7H6 is poorly expressed on normal cells, while it is up-regulated in different tumor cell lines. BAT-3 is a nuclear factor released in exosomes by tumor cells and Dendritic Cells (DC) in response to stress/activation stimuli. The tumor ligands for NKp46 and NKp44 remain still undefined. The NKp30, NKp46 and NKp44 receptors are structurally and genetically unrelated. NKp46 encoding gene is located within the Leukocyte Receptor Complex in Chromosome 19, while the NKp30 and NKp44 encoding genes are located in separated regions in chromosome 6. However, for their expression pattern, restricted to NK cells, and their impressive capability of triggering NK cell cytotoxicity against an extremely wide range of tumor cell lines, they were grouped and collectively termed Natural Cytotoxicity Receptors (NCRs).

Among the triggering receptors, NKp30, NKp46, NKp44, NKG2D and DNAM-1 are indispensable for the NK-mediated recognition and killing of tumor cells. Different studies have demonstrated how their blockade, impairment of function, or expression failure, heavily compromise the efficacy of NK cells in killing tumor cells in vitro, or in containing tumor growth in animal models (Bottino et al., 2004; Iguchi-Manaka et al., 2008; Guerra et al., 2008; Halfteck et al., 2009). Notably, NK cells can significantly improve their functional capabilities in response to various cytokines including type I IFN, IL-2, IL-15, IL-12 and IL-18. In this context, exposure to IL-2, IL-15 and IL-12 can indeed induce up-regulation of NCRs, NKG2D and DNAM-1. In particular major effect is exerted on NKp44 that is not expressed at all on resting NK cells (Biron et al., 1999; Moretta A. et al., 2001; Della Chiesa et al., 2006; Balsamo et al., 2009; Vivier et al., 2011).

Thus, NK cells by their inhibitory and activating receptors can sense the altered expression of both protective self HLA-I molecules and a large array of pathogenic markers, and on this basis can discriminate which cells have to be killed.

The fact that, at variance with activating receptors, the inhibitory HLA-specific receptors are clonally distributed, allows the generation of a repertoire of NK cell subsets capable of sensing alteration of even single HLA-alleles. Importantly, this phenomenon is the basis for the exploitation of alloreactive NK cell subsets in aplo-identical Hematopoietic Stem Cell Transplanation (HSCT) in hematological malignancies (see section 2.4).

2.3 Multiple NK cell subsets and functions

Besides their involvement in direct pathogen clearance, NK cells are also implied in the regulation of the immune responses. Indeed they can produce and respond to various cytokines, functionally interact with different immune cell types and participate at regulation of T cell functions, in particular at Th1/Th2 polarization (Cooper et al., 2001; Moretta A. et al., 2005; Scordamaglia et al., 2008).

Up today several NK cell types, with distinct phenotype, function and anatomical location have been described (Table 1).

The $CD56^{bright}CD16^{dim/neg}KIR^{-}NKG2A^{+}$ NK cells are characterized by low granule content and low cytolytic activity but produce large amounts of cytokines, in particular IFN-γ. These cells cover 5-10% of circulating NK cells but represent the large majority of NK cells in Lymph Nodes (L.N.). At these sites, upon interaction with maturing DC, $CD56^{bright}$ NK cells can proliferate and produce IFN-γ, thus favoring Th1 response (Fehniger et al., 2003; Ferlazzo & Munz 2004).

The classical $CD56^{dim}CD16^{bright}$ NK cells (approx. 90% of circulating NK cells) are highly cytotoxic, and also produce cytokines, in particular IFN-γ and TNF-α and, to a lesser extent, chemokines, such as MIP-1β. These cells may migrate to peripheral tissues driven by chemokines and type I IFNs. Indeed, CD56^{dim}CD16^{bright} NK cells express receptors (CXCR1 ChemR23 and CX_3CR1) specific for chemokines (CXCL8, Chemerin and CX_3CL1 respectively) that are usually produced during inflammatory events by Macrophages, Neutrophils, DC and Endothelial cells (Moretta A. et al., 2005; Della Chiesa et al., 2006b; Parolini et al., 2007). In addition they also express GPR56, a molecule that would function as receptor for Extra Cellular Matrix components (Della Chiesa et al., 2010). In inflamed tissues, different viral or bacterial products (i.e. PAMPs - Pathogen Associated Molecular Patterns) may either directly activate NK cells (which express TLR6 and TLR9 PAMP receptors) or induce DC, plasmacytoid DC (pDC), M1 type Macrophages, to produce cytokines capable of activating NK cells. At these sites, CD56^{dim}CD16^{bright} NK cells can physically interact with immature DC (iDC) and, by the engagement of NKp30 and DNAM-1, they can release TNF-α and HMGB1 and promote DC maturation. Once activated, NK cells, by using the same receptors (NKp30 and DNAM-1), can also kill iDCs (and spare mature DC - mDC). As compared to mDC, iDC express lower HLA-I levels, and are not "protected" from activated NK cells. This phenomenon may represent either a mechanism to eliminate those DC that have not properly undergone maturation or a signal to terminate the response and avoid chronic inflammation (Zitvogel et al., 2002; Moretta A. et al., 2005).

Recently, a novel CD56^{+}NKp44^{+} NK cell type was described in MALT (tonsils and Peyer patches), and was called NK22, by virtue of its ability to produce IL-22 in response to IL-23 (Colonna, 2009). IL-22 is a IL-10 family cytokine with anti-bacterial effects, as it maintains epithelial-cell barrier function in the gut thus contrasting bacterial dissemination. The meaning of NK22 cells, as well as their ontogenesis, are not fully understood, nevertheless these cells may play an important role in constraining inflammation and in defense against bacterial infection in the mucosa.

A unique NK cell subset expressing the phenotype CD56^{bright}CD16$^{dim/neg}$KIR^{+}NKG2A^{+}, populates decidua in the first trimester of pregnancy (Moffet-King, 2002; Hanna et al., 2006). These cells display peculiar functional features: they express the NCRs but are poorly cytolytic; rather, the engagement of NKp30 and NKp44 would induce them to produce a defined pattern of chemokines and pro-angiogenic factors (see Table 1). These factors would favor trophoblast migration and decidua vascularization, ensuring an appropriate placenta and fetus development. Decidual NK (dNK) cells may also have a role in the induction of tolerance at the maternal/fetal interface. dNK cells, by producing IFN-γ, would induce expression of IDO in decidual myelomonocytic cells. In turn IDO, together with TGF-β, would favor induction and proliferation of Tregs. Interestingly, unlike PB NK cells (see section 2.4), dNK cells are resistant to the inhibition of the IDO-induced Trp-catabolite, L-kynurenine. This resistance implies that dNK cells can maintain production of IFN-γ and sustain the tolerogenic pathway over time (Vacca et al., 2010).

It has been recently proposed that the CD56^{bright}CD16$^{dim/neg}$KIR^{-}NKG2A^{++} cells could undergo further differentiation through different stages (Bjorkstrom et al., 2010; Lopez-Verges et al., 2010). The relatively immature and poorly cytotoxic CD56^{bright}CD16$^{dim/neg}$KIR^{-}NKG2A^{++} cells, would progressively increase the expression of cytolytic granules, CD16, KIRs and CD57, down-regulate NKG2A, and modify the kinetics of IFN-γ release. In line with this hypothesis, four phenotypically distinct NK cell populations, possibly representing sequential stages of this differentiation process, have been identified within circulating pool:

$CD56^{bright}CD16^{dim/neg}CD57^{-}KIR^{-}NKG2A^{++}perforin^{+/-}$, $CD56^{dim}CD16^{dim}CD57^{-}KIR^{-}NKG2A^{++}perforin^{+}$, $CD56^{dim}CD16^{bright}CD57^{+/-}KIR^{+}NKG2A^{+}perforin^{++}$, $CD56^{dim}CD16^{bright}CD57^{+}KIR^{+}NKG2A^{-}perforin^{+++}$.

Interestingly, along these putative differentiation steps NK cells would also progressively lose CCR7 and CD62L expression and acquire the fraktalkine receptor CX_3CR1, thus skewing their initial homing capabilities to L.N., towards inflamed Peripheral Tissues (Juelke et al., 2010; Hamann et al., 2011). This latter point should not be disregarded, especially in view of the future perspective of selecting appropriate NK cell subsets for cancer immunotherapy.

NK cell subpopulation (phenotype)	Anatomical/ tissue localization	Functional features
$CD3^{-}CD56^{bright}CD16^{dim/neg}$ $KIR^{-}NKG2A^{++}$ $CCR7^{++}CD62L^{++}$ $CD57^{-}$	Lymph Nodes 5-10% PB NK cells	Differentiation towards KIR+ cells Cytokines production (IFN-γ TNF-α) mDC-induced prolif. and IFN-γ prod. (promote Th1 polarization)
$CD3^{-}CD56^{dim}CD16^{bright}$ KIR^{+}/KIR^{-} $NKG2A^{+}/NKG2A^{-}$ $CCR7^{-}CD62L^{+/-}$ $ChemR23^{+}CX3CR3^{+}$ $GPR56^{+}$	90% PB NK cells inflamed periph. tissues?	Cytotoxicity Cytokines production (IFN-γ TNF-α) Induction of DC maturation
$CD56^{-}CD161^{+}$	5-10% PB NK cells	Produce type2 cytokines (IL-5 IL-13) Low cytotox. Expanded in HIV patients
$CD3^{-}CD56^{bright}CD16^{dim}$ KIR^{+}	Decidua (1st. trimester pregnancy)	Low cytotox. $IFN\text{-}\gamma^{+}$ $IL\text{-}8^{++}$ $IP\text{-}10^{+}$ $VEGF^{+}$ Regulatory interactions with Trophoblasts (Placenta development) Decidua vascularization Induction of Tregs
$CD3^{-}CD56^{+}NKp44^{+}$	MALT	$IL\text{-}22^{+}$ / mucosal immunity
$CD3^{-}CD56^{+}CD16^{+/-}$ KIR^{+}	Liver	Cytotoxicity

Table 1. Surface phenotype, anatomical localization and function of different NK cell subsets

2.4 Role of NK cells in the control of tumors

The impressive advances obtained in the last 15-20 years in the knowledge of the mechanism of action of NK cells and of their regulation, have been fuelled by the evident therapeutic potential that these cells have shown since their first discovery. However, although the efficacy of NK cells in containing tumors in vivo has been demonstrated in different animal models (Kim et al., 2000; Smyth et al., 2000; Guerra et al., 2008; Halftech et al., 2009), the way to develop effective NK-based immunotherapy has been elusive for many years and only very recently it yielded promising results.

After the initial attempts by Rosenberg's group (Rosenberg et al., 1985), several trials had been done to set protocols for the adoptive transfer of ex-vivo activated autologous NK cell populations or for the use of different cytokines to elicit NK cell responses in vivo (Sutlu & Alici, 2009). The advantages of these approaches, however, appeared minimal: both because of the technical limits in expanding ex vivo large bulk populations (as repeated infusions were necessary to overcome the short life-span of transferred mature NK cells), and because of the putative adverse effects induced by IL-2 in vivo (such as the possible expansion of $CD25^+$ Tregs or the induction the AICD) (Ghiringhelli et al., 2005; Rodella et al., 2001). In addition, another possible limitation could be that tumor cells could retain sufficient HLA-I expression to protect themselves from autologous NK cell attack. A turning point in the definition of efficient NK-based immunotherapeutic strategies against cancer, was represented by the study by Velardi and co-workers, primarily aimed at the evaluation of the clinical outcome of aplo-identical HSCT in Acute Myeloid Leukemia (AML) (Ruggeri et al., 2002). In this study the authors suggested that, in the presence of HLA/KIR mismatch (i.e. recipient and donor expressing different HLA-I alleles that are recognized by different KIRs), NK cells that developed from donor's progenitors could play an active role in reducing both the risk of leukemia relapse and even the Graft versus Host Disease (GvHD). This implied that heterologous NK cells could develop in the conditioned host, and kill Leukemic blasts more efficiently than autologous NK cells could do. Further studies by different groups have led to the current hypothesis that in the host, heterologous NK cell population expressing KIRs specific for donor's and not for recipient's HLA-I alleles can develop and be educated (licensed) by the donor's bone marrow cells, thus acquiring efficient killing capabilities towards host (allogeneic) malignant cells or activated leukocytes (Pende et al., 2009; Cooley et al., 2010; Haas et al., 2011; L. Moretta et al., 2011). The functional capabilities of allogeneic NK cells would also explain the reduction of GvHD observed in patients undergoing HLA/KIR mismatched HSCT, as, besides the elimination of heterologous Leukemic blasts (Graft-versus-Leukemia - GvL - effect), donor's NK cells would also be involved in the killing of those host's DC capable of priming donor's T cells. Interestingly, this alloreactive NK cell population may persist (and exert the its beneficial effect) for years (Pende et al., 2009; Haas et al., 2011) without causing apparent detrimental clinical signs ascribable to NK cell activity.

The above studies open new perspectives for the exploitation of NK cells in immunotherapy. In this context, different trials have been designed for the treatment of hematological malignancies, and in some cases also for solid tumors (Miller et al., 2005; Terme et al., 2008; Sutlu & Alici, 2009). Several problems, however, still remain to be solved. For example the fact that immature, not fully competent, NK cells may predominate (and persist) in circulation during (and after) the recipient immunological reconstitution (Nguyen et al., 2005) with negative effects on the anti-tumor activity and surveillance against viruses. Another problem regards a general negative effect that malignancies may exert on NK cell functions. In this context, different studies have reported a down-regulation of activating receptors in circulating NK cells from tumor patients (Sanchez et al., 2010; Le Maux-Chansac et al., 2005; Fregni et al., 2011). Moreover , in solid tumors, the tumor microenvironment may play an additional negative role by contrasting both the responses and the infiltration capabilities of the immune effector cells (Albertsson et al., 2003). In this context, different studies have indicated that in some tumors, infiltrating NK cells may be rare or poorly functional (Albertsson et al., 2003; Carrega et al., 2009; Platonova et al., 2011). At the tumor site several stromal components, induced by aberrant tumor-driven inflammation, can contribute to NK cell down-regulation (Mantovani et al., 2008). Tregs, by the release of TGF-β, may suppress NK cell functions (Zimmer et al., 2008). The induction of M2 macrophages may reduce the macrophage-mediated NK cell activation (as this effect is prominently sustained by M1 macrophages) (Bellora et al., 2010). Also the Tumor Associated Fibroblasts (TAF) may contrast NK cells in their anti-tumor activity. Indeed, fibroblasts derived from melanoma lesions were found to inhibit, by mean of cell-to-cell contact and PGE_2 release, the IL-2-driven up-regulation of NKp44, DNAM-1 and NKp30 on NK cells (Balsamo et al., 2009). Finally, even the tumor cells can induce down-modulation of activating NK receptors. Several tumor cell lines constitutively express IDO, an enzyme involved in the Trp catabolism. The IDO-induced Trp catabolite Kynurenine has been shown to down-regulate NKp46 and NKG2D (Della Chiesa et al., 2006). In addition, tumor cells can also induce down-regulation of NKG2D or DNAM-1 on NK cells by the release of soluble NKG2D-Ligands (Doubrovina et al., 2003) or by the prolonged engagement of DNAM-1 in cell-to-cell contact (Carlsten et al., 2009)

3. Human Natural Killer cell development

3.1 In vitro NK cell development

3.1.1 Acquisition of NK cell receptors and function

Most of information available on human NK cell development came from in vitro studies of NK cell differentiation from $CD34^+$ Hematopoietic Stem Cells (HSC) or $CD34^{+/-}CD45RA^+$ early lymphoid precursors. These cells can be isolated from different sources such as fetal liver, Bone Marrow (BM), Thymus, PB and Umbilical Cord Blood (UCB) and stimulated with IL-2 or IL-15, in the presence or in the absence of feeder cells, to obtain NK cell differentiation (Freud & Caligiuri , 2006). In the 90s' it was shown that it was possible to obtain $CD3^-CD56^+$ $CD94/NKG2A^+$ cytolytic NK cells from either $CD34^-CD45RA^+CD7^+CD1a^-$ early thymic precursors (Mingari et al., a1991,b1997; Lanier et al., 1992; Sanchez et al., 1994) or $CD34^+$HSC isolated from BM or UCB (Miller et al., 1994; Lotzova et al., 1993).

Currently, optimal culturing conditions require the simultaneous presence of different cytokines: Stem Cell Factor (SCF), FMS-Like Tyrosine Kynase Ligand (Flt3-L), IL-7, IL-15 and IL-21.

During in vitro differentiation the development of NK cells proceeds through a step-by-step process (figure 1) (Freud& Caligiuri, 2006). Freshly isolated HSC precursors already express CD117 and Flt3, which are the SCF and Flt3-L receptors, respectively, and play an important role for their proliferation and survival before any cell lineage commitment takes place . The first cell markers that would suggest a NK-lymphoid commitment are the IL-2/IL-15 receptors CD122, CD132 and the IL-7 α-chain receptor (CD127). These receptors play an important role in transducing proliferation and differentiation signals upon interaction with the appropriate cytokines (IL-15 and IL-7 respectively). However, in humans, these markers are rarely detectable on ex-vivo isolated $CD34^+CD45RA^+$ precursors, while they can be detected on small fractions of precursor after first days of culture (Freud& Caligiuri, 2006).

The first surface cell marker that clearly identify NK cell precursors is CD161 (Bennet et al., 1996). It can be detected on small percentages of $CD3^{-}CD56^{-}CD117^{+}$cells, which already express CD244 co-receptor: the acquisition of NKp44 activating receptor and CD56 represents the following differentiation step. Next, the expression of the NKp46, NKG2D and DNAM-1 activating receptors and of CD94/NKG2A inhibitory receptor occurs. The acquisition of CD16 and KIRs can be hardly observed in vitro (Mingari et al., 1997; Miller et al., 2001; Sivori et al., 2002). These receptors are typical of functionally differentiated circulating NK cells: their acquisition by small percentages of cell precursors undergoing differentiation, appears after long term cultures in the presence of IL-21, a pro-inflammatory cytokine (Sivori et al., 2003). On the other hand, the early expression of NKp44 may be related to the fact that recombinant IL-15, present in the culture, rapidly activates NKp44 gene transcription. Hence, NKp44 transcription could be differently regulated from that of the other activating receptors.

This sequential process of cell marker acquisition identifies NK cell precursor intermediates with different functional properties (Freud & Caligiuri, 2006; Grzywacz et al., 2006). Early NK cell precursors $CD117^{+}CD161^{+}CD244^{+}CD56^{+/-}$ $NKp44^{+/-}$ are not cytolytic but can secrete cytokines such as GM-CSF and IL-13. These cells lack the expression of all the other activating receptors and inhibitory receptors. The next stage of in vitro NK cell differentiation correlates with the definitive acquisition of CD56 and of NKp44 ($CD117^{+}CD161^{+}$ $CD244^{+}CD56^{+}NKp44^{+}$): these precursors can be defined as immature NK cells (iNK). Immature NK cells secrete large amounts of CXCL8 and low amounts of IL-22 while they do not produce IFN-γ (Freud & Caligiuri, 2006; Vitale et al., 2008; Tang et al., 2011). The production of CXCL8 could have a role in the modulation of hematopoietic cell lineage commitment. In particular, CXCL8 inhibits myelopoiesis (Youn et al., 2000) and, thus, might favour NK cell differentiation. On the other hand, iNK cells are not cytotoxic. Indeed they have not acquired yet cytolytic granules in their cytoplasm, important NK activating receptors (i.e. NKp46), and the adhesion molecule LFA-1, that strongly contribute to the activation of cytolytic machinery (Bryceson et al., 2006).

The acquisition of a weak cytolytic activity correlates with the expression of NKp46 activating receptor and LFA-1; however, at this stage of development, the NKp46-mediated cytotoxicity against susceptible cell targets may be inhibited by the CD244 co-receptor, that acts as inhibitory receptor on these iNK cells. CD244 works as an activating co-receptor on mature NK cells thanks to the recruitment of an intra-cytoplasmic adaptor molecule SAP. However, on $CD117^{+/-}CD161^{+}$ $CD244^{+}CD56^{+}NKp46^{+/-}CD94/NKG2A^{-}LFA\text{-}1^{+/-}$ iNK cells SAP it is not synthetized yet, leading to inhibitory rather than activating function of CD244 (Moretta et al., 2001; Sivori et al., a2002, b2003; Vitale et al., 2008).

The full acquisition of cell functions typical of mature NK cells, such as IFN-γ secretion and cytolytic activity, correlates with the surface bright expression of NKp46, the expression of NKG2D and DNAM-1 activating receptors, CD94/NKG2A inhibitory receptor and of LFA-1 molecule. At this stage, SAP starts to be synthesized, and CD244 acquires a co-stimulatory activity. These cells are defined as $CD56^{bright}$ NK cells since they are very similar to $CD56^{bright}$ $CD94/NKG2A^{+}CD16^{-}KIR^{-}$ NK cells present in the PB. Notably, differentiation is a continuous process and cells may not be synchronized in their maturation status: hence, a certain heterogeneity of the different cell subsets may be observed.

Altogether these experimental evidences indicate that NK cell development is tightly regulated and that evolution had particularly tuned the acquisition of cytolytic activity. NK cells, to become cytotoxic, must express at least the NKp46 activating receptor and the LFA-1 adhesion molecule. Simultaneously, they have to loose the inhibitory activity of CD244 co-receptor. The ability to control NK cytotoxicity by inhibitory CD244 could be a "safe" mechanism, important in the interactions between NK cell precursors and other hematopoietic cells. CD244 ligand is the CD48 molecule, which is expressed by different types of leucocytes and hematopoietic precursors (Cannons et al., 2011). On the other hand, iNK cells secrete a peculiar pattern of cytokines, such as IL-22 and CXCL8, involved in inflammatory process, defence against bacteria, neo-angiogenesis and modulation of haematopoiesis. Hence, iNK cells might exert important crosstalk with other cells present in microenvironment where their differentiation takes place.

3.2 Factors that modulate NK cell differentiation

Hematopoietic cell lineage commitment depends on a wide variety of factors. Genetic components dictate the initial commitment but the milieu that surrounds lineage precursors may have a key role in the fate of these cells. The balance between specific transcription factors and the appropriate cytokines and hormones can change the commitment of intermediate lymphoid precursors, inducing their switch towards alternative lineages (Laiosa et al., 2006; Doulatov et al., 2010). In this context, in vitro analysis have shown that NK cells can share intermediate precursors not only among lymphoid cells but also with dendritic cells and myeloid cells (Miller et al., 1999; Marquez et al., 1998; Perez et al., 2003; Vitale et al., 2008; Grzywacz et al., 2011).

3.2.1 Cytokines

Cytokines are important factors that modulate NK cell differentiation. SCF and Flt3-L have a role in the first days of in vitro development because they induce HSC to enter into the cell cycle, and sustain precursor proliferation and survival (Yu et al., 1998). Then, IL-7 supports the lymphoid lineage commitment, since this cytokine is involved in T cell homeostasis and lymphoid differentiation (Ma A. et al., 2006). However, it is IL-15 that plays a key role in NK cell differentiation, through the interaction with IL-2/IL-15 common β and γ chains receptors (CD122 and CD132, respectively). Indeed, IL-15 has been shown to be critical in the terminal differentiation of $CD117^{+/-}CD161^{+}CD56^{+}$ iNK towards mature NK cells (Mrozek et al., 1995; Freud & Caligiuri, 2006). In murine models, NK cell deficiencies are more pronounced in mice lacking IL-15 or its receptors, than in mice lacking IL-2 or IL-7 related products (Di Santo et al., 1990; Giliani et al., 2005; Kennedy et al., 2000). In vitro assays revealed that high dose soluble IL-15 binds to its receptors and promote NK cell differentiation but, in vivo, IL-15 is primarily detectable complexed to its IL-15 Receptor α (IL15-Rα) present on accessory (stromal) cells (Dubois et al., 2002). IL-15/IL15-Rα complex would then present the cytokine *in trans* to $CD122^{+}CD132^{+}$ cells, meaning that also stromal cells could exert an important role in the terminal differentiation of iNK cells (Miller et al., 1994; Briard et al., 2002; Vacca et al., 2011). Finally, IL-21 have been shown to increase the proportions of $CD56^{+}KIR^{+}$ cells undergoing in vitro differentiation (Sivori et al., 2003).

3.2.2 Transcription factors

In vitro and in vivo studies using mice with loss-of-function mutation helped to clarify the role of many transcription factors (TFs) involved in NK cell commitment, proliferation and maturation. Some of them, like the E proteins, orchestrate a lymphoid-biased cellular context versus myeloid compartment (de Pooter et al., 2010) but must be down-regulated to allow NK cell differentiation (Boos et al., 2007). Other TFs are important both in the NK cell and T cell commitment, such as Notch-1 or Id2 (Benne et al., 2009; Boos et al., 2007). Id2 is an helix loop helix TF, able to modulate the activation the E protein E2A, and have been shown to exert a prominent role in NK cell commitment. Recently, other two TF have been suggested to induce definitive early NK cell commitment: a High Mobility Group protein, called TOX, and a basic leucin zipper, E4PB4 (also known as NFIL3)(Aliahmad et al., 2010; Gascoyne et al., 2009; Kamizono et al., 2009). It has been shown that IL-15 activates E4PB4 that, in turn, would activate Id2 transcription, leading to a definitive NK cell commitment and expansion of NK cell precursors. In humans, E4BP4 and Id2 expression can be observed either in ex-vivo-isolated early committed CD34$^{+/-}$CD122^{+}CD127^{+} NK cell precursors either in in vitro-derived CD117$^{+/-}$CD161^{+}CD56^{+}LFA-1^{-}NKG2A^{-} iNK cells (Hughes et al., 2010; Vacca at al., 2011). On the other hand, TOX would influence the activation of T-bet, a TF that correlates with the acquisition of cytolytic activity and the ability to produce IFN-γ by more differentiated CD161^{+}CD56^{+}LFA-1^{+} NKp46^{+} CD94/NKG2A^{+} NK cells (Yun et al., 2011).

Expression of others TFs appears to correlate with the different stages of NK cell differentiation. RORC correlates with the secretion of IL-22 by iNK cells (Tang et al., 2011) while the expression of EOMES (a T-box TF), similar to T-bet, correlates with IFN-γ production by more differentiated NK cells (Glimcher et al., 2004).

3.2.3 Corticosteroids

In the last years the studies on in vitro NK cell development offered new important clues on NK cell lineage commitment and on the factors that may modulate this process.

The attempt to improve models of in vitro NK cell differentiation, induced many groups to test additional factors, besides cytokines, that could favour in vitro NK cell differentiation: in particular, stromal cells and/or corticosteroids. These new protocols revealed an unexpected function for glucocorticoids, which were already known to exert a modulatory effect on T cell development (Jondal et al., 2004). Studies with Hydrocortisone (HC) showed that it was possible to obtain NK cells from the in vitro culture of CD33^{+}CD14$^{+/-}$ myeloid progenitors isolated from UCB (Perez et al., 2003). These results suggested that, in cord blood, it was possible to switch the differentiation of monocyte precursors towards NK cells. We obtained similar results with Methylprednisolone (MePDN). This corticosteroid is commonly used as first line of treatment for acute GvHD after allogeneic HSCT. Our hypothesis was that MePDN could inhibit not only mature NK cell proliferation and functions but also the in vitro NK cell differentiation. Surprisingly, our results showed that pharmacological concentrations of MePDN accelerated NK cell differentiation and were able to induce myeloid precursors to switch their differentiation towards CD161^{+}CD56^{+}NKp44^{+} iNK cells (Vitale et al., 2008). More recently, Grwaycz et al., with an elegant in vitro experiment, provided evidence that HC, in combination with a stromal cell line, induce differentiation of CD33^{+}CD13^{+}CD115$^{+/-}$ myelomonocytic precursors into cytolytic CD56^{+}NKp46^{+}CD94/NKG2A^{+}KIR$^{+/-}$CD16$^{+/-}$ NK cells (Grwaycz et al., 2011).

These results offer important clues to better clarify some major issues that have been discussed in the last years.

The first one is related to the hematopoietic cell lineage commitment. Current models of haematopoiesis suggest that HSC may commit early to the erythroid/platelet lineages or to leukocyte lineages. However, once committed to the leukocyte lineage, hematopoietic precursors would retain a high plasticity. Thus, the choice to terminally differentiate towards myeloid or lymphoid lineages would then depend on the role of lineage-specific transcription factors and on a permissive milieu (Doulatov et al., 2010). This would be of particular interest for NK cells, which are the only lymphocytes assigned to natural immunity compartment and that appear to be the connection ring with acquired immunity.

The second issue regards the role of NK cells after HSCT and their use in immunotherapy to obtain GvL reaction. The possibility that myeloid precursors, in the presence of corticosteroids, could generate more rapidly functional NK cells offers important clues also in the clinical settings (Vitale et al., 2008; Grwaycz et al., 2011). It is conceivable that NK

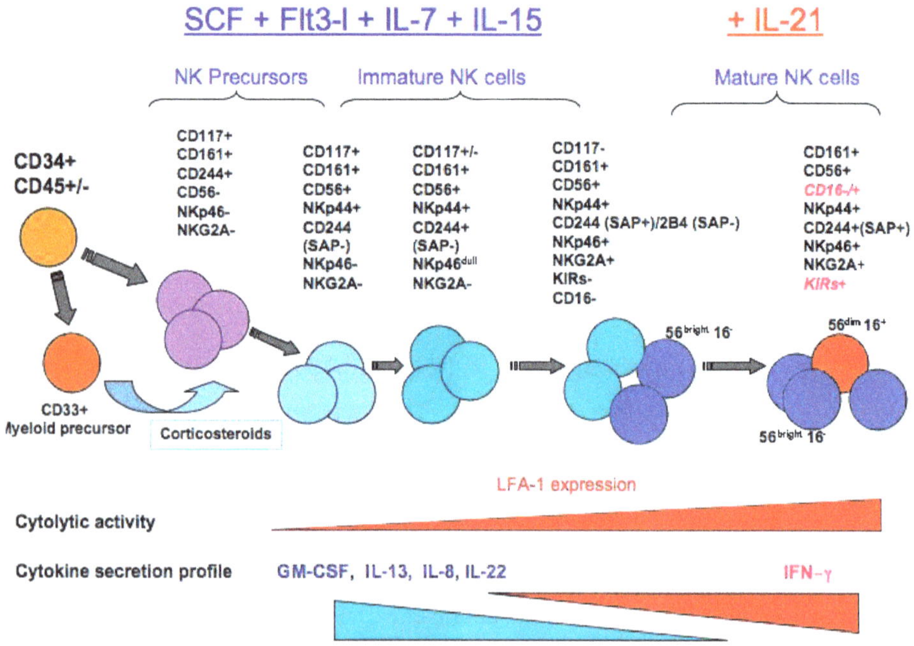

Fig. 1. Acquisition kinetic of receptors and functions by NK cells undergoing in vitro cell development.
Three main precursor subsets may be identified along different time intervals of culture: NK cell precursors, immature NK cells and more differentiated CD56^{bright} NK cells. The appearance of CD56^{dim} CD16^{+}KIR^{+} NK cells (red cell) is a late and rare event and is more achievable in the presence of IL-21. Stages of differentiation are endowed with a peculiar surface phenotype and functions. In particular the acquisition of cytolytic activity correlates with the expression of LFA-1, activating receptors and the production of IFN-γ, while high secretion of IL-8 correlates with the immature NK cell stage.

cells, present in high percentages in peripheral blood of patients at the earliest time intervals after HCST, may derive, at least in part, from myeloid precursors. Importantly, this maturation could not occur wholly in BM but also in PB and other sites. This is the third important issue that have been matter of debate of the last years: the site of in vivo human NK cell development and maturation.

3.3 In vivo NK cell development and maturation

NK cells were generally believed to differentiate into the BM from $CD34^{+}$ hematopoietic stem cells (Freud & Caligiuri, 2006). However, NK cell developmental intermediates were detectable in vivo neither in the BM nor in thymus. The possibility to observe in vivo any different NK cell developmental stages detectable in vitro, came from analysis of lymphocyte recovery in patients undergoing allogeneic HSCT. Analysis of PB of these patients revealed that, in some of them, the first waves of lymphocytes recovering at early time after transplant (2-3 weeks) are mostly NK cells. These lymphocytes are characterized by the $CD56^{bright}$ $CD16^{-}$ $CD94/NKG2A^{+}KIR^{-}$ phenotype and a dull expression of NCRs, while $CD56^{dim}CD16^{+}CD94/NKG2A^{+}KIR^{+}$ NK cells can be detected later, (4-8 weeks after transplant). (Vitale et al., 2000; Shilling et al., 2003; Vitale et al., 2004).

3.3.1 Sites of in vivo NK cell development: Stages of NK cell differentiation

The finding that in vitro models of NK cell differentiation led to the generation of $CD56^{bright}$ $CD16^{-}$ NK cells, supported the hypothesis that, in vivo, this subset could be a precursor reservoir, able to promptly differentiate towards more cytotoxic $CD56^{dim}CD16^{+}$ upon specific stimuli. However, experimental evidences that support this hypothesis have been acquired only recently. Freud and co-workers discovered that $CD45RA^{+}CD117^{-}$ and $CD34^{+}CD45^{+}CD117^{+}CD161^{+/-}$ cells were enriched in Secondary Lymphoid Tissue (SLT), particularly in lymphnodes and tonsils. Importantly, these precursors were able to generate selectively NK cells upon culture in the presence of appropriate cytokines. They defined these cells as pro-NK and pre-NK cells respectively. Further analysis revealed that in SLT, it was possible to detect and isolate four different subsets of NK cell precursors representing different stages of NK cell differentiation (Freud et al., a2005, b2006).

Stage 1: $CD34^{+}CD45RA^{+}CD117^{-}CD161^{-}$ pro-NK cells; stage 2: $CD34^{+}CD45RA^{+}CD117^{+}CD161^{+/-}$ pre-NK cells; stage 3: $CD34^{-}CD117^{+}CD161^{+}CD56^{+/-}$ $NKp46^{-}CD94/NKG2A^{-}KIR^{-}CD16^{-}$ immature NK cells; stage 4: $CD117^{+/-}$ $CD161^{+}CD56^{+}NKp46^{+}CD94/NKG2A^{+}KIR^{+/-}CD16^{-}$, defined as $CD56^{bright}$ NK cells. Further analysis suggested that also the expression of CD122 and CD127 could help to identify stage 1/2 of pre-NK cell precursors. These discoveries confirmed for the first time that in vitro models of NK cell differentiation may have in vivo similar counterpart. Indeed, the above stages 2, 3 and 4 remind the differentiation steps observed in vitro (Freud & Caligiuri et al., 2006; Caligiuri, 2008). This discovery suggests that hematopoietic precursors could migrate from BM to SLT and generate NK cells in organs far from the BM. It is possible that at least a fraction of $CD56^{bright}$ NK cells present in SLT could differentiate from these precursors upon interaction with DC and other cells capable of presenting membrane-bound IL-15.

As mentioned above a particular subset of NK cells has been found to be enriched in tonsils and gut-mucosa associated tissue: these cells are $CD56^{+/-}NKp46^{+/-}NKp44^{+}NKG2A^{-}$ and produce IL-22. Their development appears to be independent from IL-15. However, whether these cells may represent a new subset of NK cells (called NK22 cells) or simply immature NK cells with peculiar in vivo functions is still a matter of debate (Colonna, 2009).

In conclusion, BM microenvironment may provide a fundamental support for the early stages of NK cell differentiation but peripheral tissues, in particular SLT, could provide a unique cell-to-cell interactions and cytokines to induce the terminal NK cell differentiation.

Surface markers	STAGE 1: Pro-NK	STAGE 2: Pre-NK	STAGE 3: iNK	STAGE 4: CD56 ^{bright}	STAGE 5: CD56 ^{dim} CD16 $^{+}$
CD34	+	+	-	-	-
CD45RA	+/-	+/-	(+)/-	+/(-)	+/(-)
CD117	-	+	+	+/-	-
CD122	-	-	-	+/-	+
CD127	dull	dull	+	+/-	-
CD161	-	+/-	+	+	+
CD244	+	+	+	+	+
CD56	-	(+)/-	+/-	+	+
NKp44	-	-	+/(-)	(+)/-	(+)/-
NKp46	-	-	-	+	+
NKG2A	-	-	-	+	+/-
KIR	-	-	-	(+)/-	+/-
CD16	-	-	-	-	-

Table 2. Expression of surface markers by NK cell precursor intermediates isolated in SLT, according to model proposed by Freud and co. Legend: +/- variable expression; (+)/- majority of cells negative; +/(-) majority of cells positive; dull= weak expression

3.3.2 Other sites of in vivo NK cell development

The next step was to verify the possibility that NK-committed cell precursors could be isolated in other peripheral tissues, where peculiar NK cell subsets were enriched. Indeed NK-committed precursors were found in gut, endometrium and placenta (Chinen at al., 2007; Male et al., 2010; Vacca et al., 2011). In all these districts there is a high concentration of $CD56^{bright}$ NK cells characterized by immune-regulatory activity. In particular, NK cells present in human decidua (dNK) during the first trimester of pregnancy display a peculiar phenotype ($CD56^{bright}CD16^{-}NKG2A^{+}KIR^{-/+}$) and exert peculiar functions. For long time dNK cells were supposed to derive from PB NK cells undergone phenotypic and functional modifications upon interaction with decidual microenvironment. Recently, different experimental evidences suggested that dNK cells could derive from NK precursors already present in endometrium or in decidua, able to promptly differentiate upon stimuli given by the onset of pregnancy (Male et al., 2010; Vacca et al., 2011). In particular, it has been shown that NK cell lineage-committed $CD34^{+}CD127^{+}CD122^{+}$ cells expressing E4BP4 and Id2 TFs are present in human decidua ($dCD34^{+}$) during the first trimester of pregnancy. They can undergo in vitro differentiation into functional $CD56^{bright}CD16^{-}$ NK cells in the presence of suitable cytokines. More importantly, they could also differentiate without exogenous cytokines when co-cultured with decidual stromal cells (dSC), able to express endogenous membrane-bound IL-15. These results suggest that interaction between $CD34^+$ cell and decidual stromal cells would be sufficient to promote in situ NK cell differentiation.

3.3.3 The stage five of human NK cell differentiation: $CD56^{dim}$ $CD16^+CD94/NKG2A^{+/-}$ KIR^+ NK cells

As already discussed, several evidences suggest that $CD56^{dim}$ NK cells may derive from $CD56^{bright}$ NK cells. After HSCT the first wave of NK cells is represented by $CD56^{bright}CD16^-CD94/NKG2A^+KIR^-$ cells while $CD56^{dim}CD16^+CD94/NKG2A^{+/-}KIR^+$ cells appear later. Importantly, $CD56^{bright}$ display longer telomeres than $CD56^{dim}$ NK cells. Moreover, different phenotypically defined NK cell subsets have been recently proposed as functional intermediates between the $CD56^{bright}$ and $CD56^{dim}$ cell types (see section 2.3) (Romagnani et al., 2007; Juelke et al., 2010).

However, in in vitro assay, it is almost impossible to observe significant expansions of KIR^+ NK cells from any type $CD34^+$ cell precursors. Similar problems must be related to our inability to fully recreate the in vivo milieu in in vitro assay. $CD56^{dim}$ may acquire their surface phenotype and functional properties upon peripheral tissues/blood microenvironment stimuli. However, signals that drive the differentiation of $CD56^{dim}$ NK cells, both during normal homeostasis and infections, remain still elusive. Recent studies provided evidence that $CD56^{dim}$ cells change their phenotypic properties and continue to differentiate throughout their lifespan. The loss of expression of NKG2A, the acquisition of KIRs and CD57 would allow the identification of sequential steps of cell maturation accompanied by a progressive decline of cell proliferation and of responsiveness to cytokine stimulation. In particular, CD16 and KIR would be acquired at late stages of peripheral blood NK cell maturation (Björkström et al., 2010; Lopez-Vergès et al., 2010). Since the acquisition of KIR repertoire in each single NK cell is a stochastic process, related to the KIR genotype and polymorphism, it is important to understand how NK cells may be educated to avoid auto-reactivity. They should acquire appropriate KIR able to prevent them from killing healthy self-cells. However, in PB of normal donors, it is possible to detect NK cells expressing KIR mismatched for self HLA-I ligands or not expressing any HLA-I inhibitory receptor at all. These cells could represent a danger as they would not recognize self HLA-I on self normal cells. As above mentioned, however, it has been recently proposed that during their development only those NK cells expressing inhibitory receptors specific for self HLA-I ligands would acquire full functional competence, while cells that fail to express such receptors (i.e. potentially autoreactive NK cells) would retain a state of hypo-responsiveness. It has to be noted, however, that the question on how such licensing/educational process could actually occur in vivo is still matter of debate (Parham, 2006; Vivier et al., 2011).

The interest for NK cells and their clinical application for the control of leukemic relapse after allogeneic HSCT is enormously increased in the last years: hence, it is mandatory trying to clarify the epigenetic factors that regulate KIR acquisition and functions, because their expression pattern on allogeneic donor NK cells play a crucial role in the eradication of recipient's leukemia (Moretta et al., 2011).

4. Classification of NK cell disorders

The World Health Organization (WHO) classification of tumors of hematopoietic and lymphoid tissues encompasses four distinct entities, two of which are provisional: 1) NK cell lymphoblastic leukemia/lymphoma (*provisional*) (Borowitz et al., 2008); 2) Chronic Lymphoproliferative Disorder of NK cells (*provisional*) (Villamor et al., 2008); 3) Aggressive NK cell leukemia (Chan et al., 2008a); and 4) Extranodal NK/T-cell lymphoma, nasal type (Chan et al., 2008b). In addition, on the basis of morphology, immuno-phenotype, functional NK cell activity, and expression of cytotoxic molecules, NK cell neoplasms can be divided into immature and mature categories (Jaffe, 1996).

In recent years rare cases of lymphoblastic lymphomas/leukemia arising from immature NK cells has been reported, although the lack of suitable markers for immature NK cells mentioned above makes it difficult to distinguish NK-cell lymphoblastic lymphoma (LBL) from precursor T-cell LBL. It is also worth mentioning that the plasticity of hematopoietic-cell lineage seems greater than previously thought, and relations between phenotypically dissimilar neoplastic disorders are being reassessed. In contrast, it is believed that chronic lymphoproliferative disorder of NK cells, aggressive NK cell leukemia and extranodal NK cell lymphoma, nasal type, originate from mature NK cells (Chan et al., 2008a and b). Relevant biological features of NK cell neoplasms are summarized in Table 3.

	NK cell lymphoblastic leukemia/ lymphoma	Extranodal NK/T-cell lymphoma, nasal type	Aggressive NK cell leukemia	Chronic Lymphoproliferative Disorder of NK cells
Age	Pediatric	Middle-aged adult	Young to Middle aged adult	Adults (6th decade)
Geographic distribution	Worldwide	Asia	Asia	Worldwide
Cell origin	Immature NK cell	Mature NK cell	Mature NK cell	Mature NK cell
Relevant phenotype	sCD3-CD4-CD13-CD33- CD16-CD7+ CD2+CD56+CD3e+	CD2+sCD3-cCD3e+CD56+CD16- CD57- Granzyme B+ Perforin+TIA1+	sCD3-cCD3e±CD56+CD16± CD57-, CD94+	CD3-CD8±CD16+CD56+CD57+ KIRs±CD94/NKG2A± Granzyme B+Perforin+
Relevant cytogenetic aberrations	Complex karyotype	Deletion 6q	Deletion 6q Complex Karyotype	Usually Normal Karyotype
EBV association	No	Yes	Yes	No
Clinical course	Aggressive	Aggressive	Very Aggressive	Indolent
Prognosis	Poor	Poor	Poor	Good

Table 3. Clinical and Biological features of NK cell neoplasms

4.1 Immature NK cell neoplasms

4.1.1 NK cell lymphoblastic leukemia/lymphoma, provisional

A considerable confusion has been generated in the literature concerning this type of disorder, mostly due to the definition of NK cell leukemia on the basis of expression of CD56 antigen. This is indeed the most important and sensitive NK marker; unfortunately, CD56 is not specific for NK cells and can be also expressed in AML and ALL and blastic plasmacytoid dendritic cell neoplasms (BPDCN). On the other hand it may not be expressed by immature NK cells. NK cell lymphoblastic leukemia/lymphoma can be considered in cases showing blastic morphology, expressing CD56, TdT, immature T associated markers such as CD7 and CD2, and cytoplasmic CD3ε, but lacking the expression of surface CD3, CD19, CD20, CD13, CD33, and MPO (Liang & Graam, 2008). These patients frequently presented with leukemia and lymphadenopathy without skin involvement and were negative for EBV. TCR and/or Ig genes were in germline configuration in all cases in which the tests were performed. Outcomes of these patients were absolutely unfavourable. The immature morphology with NK cell-associated phenotype and genotype suggests that these tumours represent the true precursor NK cell neoplasms.

Some well characterized cases of NK precursor tumours with lymphomatous presentation that expressed CD94 1A transcripts have been reported (Lin et al., 2005). CD94 1A, a distal promoter of the CD94 molecule, is activated only by IL-15 (Lopez-Botet et al., 1997). Lin et al., recently reported that CD94 1A is the predominant form found in immature NK cells and it is expressed in TCR^- lymphoblastic leukemia (NK lineage LBL) but not in TCR^+ LBL (T lineage LBL) (Lin et al., 2005). By studying 21 patients with LBL and, on the basis of the expression of CD94 1A transcripts and the lack of TCR, the above investigators identified 7 patients with LBL of immature NK cell origin (CD94 $1A^+$, TCR^-). It is noteworthy that those NK-LBLs occurred in young patients and had better outcomes as compared with patients who had T-LBL (CD94 $1A^-$, TCR^+); none of the tumours was positive for CD56 (Lin et al., 2005). Thus, the use of CD94 1A associated with TCR appears to be more suitable than CD56 for identifying an immature NK cell neoplasm.

A standard treatment protocol for immature NK cell neoplasms has not been established mainly because of the rarity of these cases. Current chemotherapy strategies for non-Hodgkin's lymphoma or acute lymphoblastic leukemia (ALL) were the most commonly used. However, the overall outcomes were dismal and HSCT represents the only effective therapy to achieve a complete remission (Lin et al., 2005).

4.2 Mature NK cell neoplasms

4.2.1 Extranodal NK/T cell lymphoma, nasal type

The WHO classification encompasses both nasal NK/T cell lymphoma and extra-nasal NK/T cell lymphoma in the same category (Chan et al., 2008a). They share the same histology, even though these lymphomas may have different clinical manifestations, treatment approaches, and prognoses (Oshimi, 2007). Although most cases are genuine NK cell neoplasms, the term "NK/T" rather than "NK" is used because this entity also includes cytotoxic T cell neoplasms (Sozumiya et al., 1994). Nasal and extra-nasal NK/T cell lymphoma are invariably associated with EBV and have a ethnic predisposition, being more prevalent in Asia, Mexico, and Central and South America (Chan et al., 2008b; Kwong, 2005) and rare in Western Countries, the Middle East and Africa.

Nasal NK/T cell lymphomas refer to tumours that occur in the nose and the upper aero digestive tract (Oshimi, 2007; Cheung et al., 1998). They are the most common type among primary lymphomas of the nasal cavity (Cheung et al., 1998). The site of disease is primarily in the midline and includes the nasal cavity in more than 80% of cases. The tumour is locally invasive and might infiltrate surrounding tissues and organs, such as oropharynx, palate, orbits, till the appearance of the characteristic mid-facial destructive lesions, the so called "lethal midline granuloma" (Cheung et al., 1998). Common symptoms include nasal discharge, nasal obstruction, purulent rhinorrhea, epitasis and local swelling of the nasal bridge. The tumours may be destructive, leading to the highly characteristic midline perforation.

Extra-nasal NK/T cell lymphomas represent the counterpart of nasal NK/T cell lymphomas and involve any other part of the body. Males are predominantly affected, and the median age of presentation is the fifth decade. Primary sites of involvement include the skin, gastrointestinal tract, salivary glands, spleen, and testis (Chan et al., 1997). Patients with extra-nasal NK/T cell lymphoma more likely exhibit an advanced stage of disease with significantly higher general involvement, high levels of lactate dehydrogenise and a significantly decrease of haemoglobin and platelet count as compared with patients who have nasal NK/T cell lymphoma (Chan et al., 1997). The histological features are similar, regardless of the involved sites. Mucosal sites often show ulceration. A diffuse infiltrate of lymphoid cells is found in association with tissue necrosis and coagulation, although in some cases infiltrating cells lack atypical morphology, resulting in misdiagnosis as chronic inflammation. An angiocentric and angiodestructive growth pattern with associated fibrinoid changes in the blood vessels is frequently observed. In most patients, the neoplastic cells are characterized by the $CD45^+$ surface (s)$CD3^-$ cytoplasm (c)$CD3\varepsilon^+$ $CD56^+$ phenotype and lack myeloid and B lymphoid markers. Proliferating cells are also positive for cytotoxic granules, granzyme B, perforin, TIA. Rarely cells express CD30 and CD7, while CD56 negative cases have also been reported. Association with EBV can be demonstrated in nearly all patients (Harabuchi et al., 1990). Using *in situ* hybridization technique, EBV-encoded RNA can be found in neoplastic cells and Southern Blot analysis can detect monoclonal proliferation of EBV. Analyses of the terminal repeat region of the EBV genome indicates that the virus is in a clonal episomal form. Other than providing an indirect proof of the clonal nature of the lymphoid proliferation, this finding suggests that the EBV might play an etiologic role in mature NK cell neoplasms (Minarovitz, 1994). A defect in immune surveillance for EBV infection is demonstrated by the high frequency of 30-base pair deletions of the LMP1 gene in EBV-infected Asians. In addition, amino acid changes in the sequence coding HLA-A2- restricted CTL epitopes of the LMP1 and LMP2 genes, and low frequency of HLA-A*0201 in NK/T cell lymphoma patients have been reported (Kanno et al., 2000; Harabuchi et al., 2009). Genetic alterations have been detected in the tumour suppression genes and several oncogenes enabling tumour cells to proliferate and resist apoptosis. Mutations of *p53* have been demonstrated, with variable frequencies (24 to 60%). Mutation of *c-kit* can also be frequently demonstrated, as far as *Fas* gene mutations (Hoshida et al., 2003; Shen et al., 2002). The most common cytogenetic aberration is deletion of 6q. A recent microarray study showed that several genes associated with vascular biology, EBV induced genes, and *PDGFRa* gene are over-expressed, pointing to the deregulation of the tumor suppressor HACE1 in the frequently deleted 6q21 region (Huang et al., 2010). Moreover, in NK/T cell lymphoma, gene signatures related to angiogenesis, genotoxic stress and proliferation, and signaling pathways (TGF-β, Notch and Wnt), were significantly enriched as compared to IL2-activated normal NK cells. Interestingly, NK/T lymphoma cells of NK lineage have a very similar molecular profile to that of NK/T-cell or peripheral T-cell lymphoma of γδ-T cell lineage (Iqbal et al., 2010).

The clinical outcome of patients with nasal NK cell lymphoma is variable. Most observational studies have consistently demonstrated that radiotherapy is superior to chemotherapy alone in patients with stage I/II disease (Sakata et al., 1997). Some patients with early-stage disease are cured by radiation therapy. It has been demonstrated that radiotherapy, either as initial treatment or as part of the chemotherapy regimen, is the single most important key to a successful outcome (Ribrag et al., 2001). However, some patients with early-stage disease have early local or systemic recurrences and die of disease. For patients with stage III/IV disease, chemotherapy is the treatment of choice (Kwong, 2005). In several published series, the median survival of patients with advanced-stage disease was approximately 12 months. Extra-nasal NK cell lymphomas are clinically aggressive, the response to therapy is poor, and most patients die within 6 months after diagnosis. The long-term remission rate with allogeneic HSCT is less than 10% (Cheung et al., 1998).

4.2.2 Aggressive NK cell leukemia

First described by Fernandez et al., (Fernandez et al., 1986), aggressive NK cell leukemia (ANKL) is a systemic disease, more common in Asians than in Caucasians (Chan et al., 2008a), which is characterized by the presence of neoplastic NK cells in the peripheral blood, bone marrow, liver and spleen and by a rapidly progressive clinical course with poor prognosis. There is an equal sex incidence in men and women. The disease typically affects young to middle-aged adults with a median age in the third decade. At presentation, patients usually are very compromised with systemic symptoms, liver dysfunction, and hepato-splenomegaly sometimes accompanied by systemic lymphoadenopathy. In contrast to extra-nodal NK cell lymphoma, skin lesions are uncommon. The clinical progression is devastating despite treatment, and most patients survive for only days to weeks. Disseminated intravascular coagulation and hemophagocytic syndrome are often seen during the course of disease (Oshimi, 2007). In tissue sections, the neoplastic infiltrate is diffuse and destructive with lymphoid cell population usually appearing monomorphous (Siu, Chan & Kwong, 2002). Morphologically, leukemic cells are slightly larger than normal LGLs (Oshimi, 2007). There is an ample amount of pale or slightly basophilic cytoplasm that contains fine or coarse azurophilic granules. These cells are $sCD3^{-}cCD3\varepsilon^{+}CD56^{+}CD16^{+}$ (75% of cases), $CD57^{-}$ $CD94^{+}$ with a germ line configuration of β and γ genes of TCR. The chemokine system plays a critical role in the tumor cell diffusion, leading to the fulminant clinical courses. Serum levels of soluble FasL, IL-8, MIP-1α, and MIP-1β are significantly elevated in ANKL patients and proliferating cells are highly positive for Fas, IL-8, RANTES, MIP-1α, and MIP-1β (Makishima et al., 2007). Although clonal EBV is found in tumour cells in most patients and EBV is considered to be the etiological agent (Oshimi, 2007), little is known about the mechanisms through which EBV infection triggers clonal proliferation of NK cells. A defective T cell and NK cell response to EBV infection may play a role in the development of this disorder. However up to 10% of cases have been shown to be EBV-negative (Suzuki et al., 2004).

Several chromosomal abnormalities have been reported. In particular, the finding of abnormalities involving del(6q) in aggressive NK cell leukemia and in extranodal NK/T lymphoma provides a biological link between these two diseases (Wong, Chan & Kwong, 1997). A recent array-based comparative genomic hybridization study on 27 NK cell lymphoma/leukemia cases, classified into two disease groups based on the World Health Organization Classification (10 ANKL cases and 17 extranodal NK/T lymphomas, nasal type), showed recurrent gain of 1q and loss of 7p15.1-p22.3 and 17p13.1 in ANKL (Nakashima et al., 2005). The same study also demonstrated clear genetic differences between aggressive NK cell leukemia and extranodal NK/T cell lymphoma, suggesting that these are two separate entities (Nakashima et al., 2005).

Aggressive NK cell leukemia is a catastrophic disease with an almost uniform mortality. A few patients have a clinical response with conventional chemotherapy (Kwong, 2005), although the response is typically transient and survival is measured in days to weeks. Allogeneic HSCT results in short-term remission in a few patients (Kwong, 2005). Taking together, big efforts for the recognition of new therapeutical targets and for development of new experimental protocols are urgently required to address the issue of ANKL therapy. As a matter of fact, recent data in a murine model have reported impressive response by targeting of survivin by nanoliposomal ceramide (Liu et al., 2010).

4.2.3 Chronic lymphoproliferative disorder of NK cells (provisional)

The chronic lymphoproliferative disorders of NK cells (CLPD-NK) are included among the novelties of the current WHO classification (Villamor et al., 2008). These rare and heterogeneous disorders are characterized by a chronic expansion of mature appearing NK cells (usually more than 2,000/μl) in peripheral blood for more than 6 months (Loughran, 1993; Semenzato et al., 1987; Tefferi et al., 1994; Semenzato et al., 1997; Oshimi, 1996), without a clearly identified cause (Figure 2). Patients are usually adults with a mean age of 60 years without gender and racial predisposition (Pandolfi et al., 1990). In recent years several studies have been published focusing on the pathogenetic mechanisms of this disease (Zambello & Semenzato, 2009; Loughran et al., 1997; Zambello et al., 2003; Hodge et al., 2009; Gattazzo et al., 2010; Epling-Burnette et al., 2008). NK cell activation in response to an unknown stimulus, likely of viral origin, is postulated to play a role in the initial steps of CLPD-NK by selecting NK clones (Zambello & Semenzato, 2009). No prototypical HTLV infection was demonstrated in these patients. However, the evidence that sera from a series of patients from Europe and USA reacted with the recombinant HTLV env protein p21E, suggests that exposure to a protein containing homology to BA21 may be important in the pathogenesis of this lymphoproliferative disorder (Loughran et al., 1997). In contrast with other mature NK cell neoplasms, EBV is not usually detected within affected lymphocytes (Zambello & Semenzato, 2009). It is believed that BM, which is frequently involved in CLPD-NK patients, represents the setting where the putative inciting antigen could reside. In this compartment, DCs may represent the target of infection (Zambello et al., 2005). Bone marrow biopsies demonstrated a topographic distribution of DCs and NK cells that indicates a close contact between the two cell types (Zambello et al., 2005). Patients' NK cells also showed a reduced capability of promoting Mo-DC maturation and of killing iDC (Balsamo et al., 2009). These findings could be explained, at least in part, by the low expression levels of NKp30 activating receptor, usually involved in the molecular interactions occurring between NK cells and DC. It is suggested that impairment of DC killing capabilities detected in patients' NK-GLs may allow an accumulation of DC that, at certain sites, may sustain the chronic proliferation of NK cells themselves. DCs are also likely to represent the source of IL-15 that is crucial in the mechanisms sustaining the maintenance of NK proliferation. IL-15 has been found to mediate its activity by interfering with Bcl-2 family members, and more specifically by modulating Bid expression (Hodge et al., 2009). Hodge et al., demonstrated that CLPD-NK cells express low levels of Bid, that are reversed by blockade of IL-15 signaling (Hodge et al., 2009). Bid is also increased following bortezomib (Velcade/PS341) treatment and this effect is coordinate with increased susceptibility to Fas- or TRAIL- independent apoptosis. In fact, bortezomib increased cell surface expression of DR4, a TRAIL death receptor decoy. The inability of death receptors to account for the apoptosis may be explained by the putative role of Bid in DNA damage and repair. It is possible that elevation of Bid expression in CLPD-NK cells promotes S phase cell cycle block and death (Hodge et al., 2009).

A genetic susceptibility for this disease has been suggested and has been related to the detection of type B *KIR gene* repertoire which is characterized by a high number of activating genes (Zambello & Semenzato, 2009). In fact, a restricted pattern of KIR expression has usually been reported in these patients. A typical feature is the preferential expression of the KIR activating receptor isoforms and this pattern correlates with a reduced expression of other activating receptors, such as NCRs (Zambello et al., 2003). Together with a bias towards activating KIR expression, a deep silencing of inhibitory KIR through increased gene methylation has been recently demonstrated by our group (Gattazzo et al., 2010). More specifically, we showed the complete lack of KIR3DL1 expression in most analyzed patients, being the receptor expressed in 13% of patients as compared to 90% of controls ($p<0.01$). Interestingly, the results of methylation patterns of *KIR3DL1* promoter showed a significantly higher methylation status (0.76 ± 0.12 SD) in the patients with respect to the healthy subjects (0.49 ± 0.10 SD, $p<0.01$). These data suggest that together with the increased expression of activating receptors, the lack of the inhibitory signal could also play a role in the pathogenesis of disease (Gattazzo et al., 2010). Recent data on the pathogenesis of CLPD-NK are summarized in Figure 2.

Biochemical studies on the mechanisms sustaining the growth of NK cells in these patients have demonstrated a role of RAS farnesil transferase (Epling-Burnette et al., 2008), with clinical implications (see below). Pathological NK cells express CD16 and usually low levels of CD56 and CD57. As expected, cells express TIA1, granzyme and perforins, which correlate with the cytotoxic potential of these cells. CD94 is expressed at high density on patients' NK cells, frequently associated with the inhibitory subunit NKG2A, although, in a relevant number of cases, the dimer CD94/NKG2C has been reported (Zambello & Semenzato, 2003). Patients' NK cells express functional β and γ chains of IL-2/IL-15 receptor, which are strictly related to the role of these cytokines in the pathogenesis of disease (Zambello & Semenzato, 2009).

Most patients are asymptomatic, and the disease has a chronic indolent clinical course, similar to that reported for patients with T-LGL leukemia (Loughran, 1993; Semenzato et al., 1987; Tefferi et al., 1994; Semenzato et al., 1997; Oshimi 1996). In some cases this disorder is associated with other conditions, including pure red cell aplasia, vasculitic syndromes, solid and hematologic tumors, splenectomy, neuropathy and autoimmune disorders (Loughran,

1993; Semenzato et al., 1987; Tefferi et al., 1994; Semenzato et al., 1997; Oshimi, 1996). Recently, in patients with chronic myelogenous leukaemia, the association has been reported between treatment with dasatinib and the development of CLPD-NK. It has been suggested that the development of CLPD-NK might contribute on the control of Ph positive leukemic cells proliferation (Kim et al., 2009). Systemic symptoms, such as cytopenia (mostly neutropenia and anemia), are rare. Lymphoadenopathy, hepatomegaly, splenomegaly and cutaneous lesions are uncommon. Occasionally, patients present a slow progressive increase of peripheral blood NK cells and organ involvement. Several cases with a spontaneous complete remission have been reported (Zambello & Semenzato, 2009). Cytologically, the circulating cells show typical granular lymphocyte morphology, with moderate amount of pale cytoplasm that contains $\geq$ 3 azurophilic granules. Bone marrow biopsy is characterized by interstitial infiltration of cells with small nuclei and pale cytoplasm, which are difficult to recognize without the help of immunohistochemical techniques. Cytogenetic is normal in most cases (Zambello & Semenzato, 2009) and the germ line configuration of TCR is demonstrated, as expected for normal NK cells. Since clonality of proliferating cells is difficult to detect in these patients, the analysis of restriction fragment length polymorphism (RLFP) has been used as an indirect marker to demonstrate the clonality in some but not all patients. In rare case, in which EBV can be demonstrated in plasmid form within NK cells, the clonality of cells might be easily examined by Southern Blot analysis using probes recognizing the EBV terminal repeats (Kawa-Ha et al., 1989). Patients with CLPD-NK usually have an indolent clinical course and respond to immunosuppressive therapy with low doses of methotrexate (usually 10 mg/m^2/week) or of cyclophosphamide (50 or 100 mg/day) or cyclosporin (3-5 mg/kg/day) with or without inclusion of low doses of steroids (Lamy & Loughran, 2011).

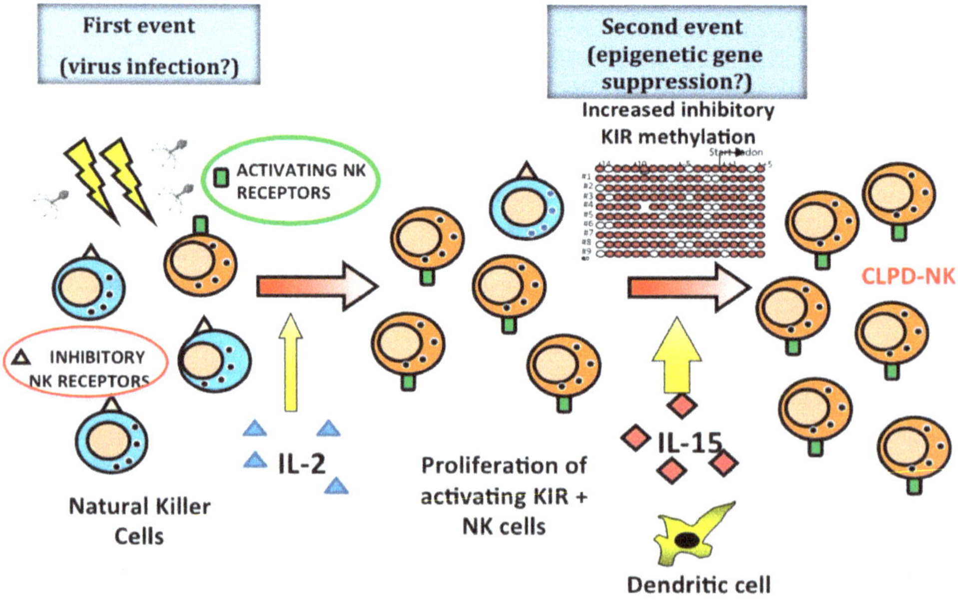

Fig. 2. Possible mechanisms of CLPD-NK pathogenesis.

5. Conclusions

NK cells are bone marrow-derived granular lymphocytes that have a key role in the recognition and in the killing of tumor- or virus-infected cells. The identification of a large array of surface NK receptors capable of transducing inhibitory or activating signals, let to explain how their effector functions could be regulated.

In recent years, it has also been shown that NK cells may play a role in the regulation of the immune response. This has been based on the finding that NK cells were able to functionally interact with different cells of the innate immune system including DCs, pDCs and macrophages. Besides the well known $CD56^{dim}CD16^{+}$ cytotoxic PB NK cells, different NK cell subsets located in specific tissue/organ compartments have been shown to exert various, alternative, regulatory functions. NK cells homing in SLT promote Th1 polarization. Conversely, decidual NK cells favour Treg expansion and play an important role in tissue remodelling and neo-angiogenesis process. In MALT, NK22 cells may support immune defence against bacteria invasion by their peculiar cytokine and chemokine secreting profile.

Whether the above described different NK cell subsets may derive from the same lineage or from different ones, is still a matter of debate. Studies on NK cell development may help to clarify the possible lineage relationship between the different NK cell subsets. In vitro models of NK cell development helped to define phenotypically and functionally different maturation stages that were, at least in part, confirmed by in vivo analysis. For example, the $CD56^{bright}CD16^{-}CD94/NKG2A^{+}KIR^{-}$ subset, that is largely represented at the end on in vitro development, represents the first wave of lymphocytes appearing in PB at early time intervals after HSCT. NK cells originate from $CD34^{+}$ hematopoietic precursors but several experimental evidences suggest that the NK cell development and terminal maturation does not occur wholly in the BM. Other secondary lymphoid organs, including L.N. and MALT, as well as decidua, may represent sites where NK cell development occurs. This suggest how defined subsets of NK cells may differentiate in peculiar tissues and point the attention on the role of the microenvironment in such a process. The full characterization of the genetic and epigenetic factors that may contribute to determine the type of NK cell that will develop is still in process and it will be important also to better define mechanisms leading to NK cell malignant transformation.

It is hopeful that investigation on NK cell neoplasm pathogenesis could lead to identify molecular targets and discovery of more efficient and less toxic treatments. The elucidation of pathways by which EBV transform NK cells might help to identify new molecular targets. Furthermore, the mechanisms of resistance to therapy, including alteration of apoptosis pathways should be deeply characterized. Thus, the definition the NK neoplasm pathophysiology and the identification of possible biological targets may help to improve therapeutical approaches.

6. References

Albertsson PA, Basse PH, Hokland M, Goldfarb RH, Nagelkerke JF, Nannmark U, Kuppen PJ. (2003) NK cells and the tumour microenvironment: implications for NK-cell function and anti-tumour activity. *Trends Immunol.* 24:603-609.

Aliahmad P, de la Torre B, Kaye J. (2010). Shared dependence on the DNA-binding factor TOX for the development of lymphoid tissue-inducer cell and NK cell lineages. *Nat Immunol* 11: 945-52

Anfossi N, André P, Guia S, Falk CS, Roetynck S, Stewart CA, Breso V, Frassati C, Reviron D, Middleton D, Romagné F, Ugolini S, Vivier E. (2006) Human NK cell education by inhibitory receptors for MHC class I. *Immunity*. 25:331-342.

Balsamo M, Scordamaglia F, Pietra G, Manzini C, Cantoni C, Boitano M, Queirolo P, Vermi W, Facchetti F, Moretta A, Moretta L, Mingari MC and Vitale M. (2009) Melanoma-associated fibroblasts modulate NK cell phenotype and antitumor cytotoxicity. *Proc Natl Acad Sci U S A*. 106:20847-20852

Balsamo M., Zambello R., Teramo A., Pedrazzi M., Sparatore B., Scordamaglia F., Pende D., Mingari M.C., Moretta L., Moretta A., Semenzato G. and Vitale M. (2009) Analysis of NK cell/DC interaction in NK-type Lymphoproliferative Disease of Granular Lymphocytes (LDGL): role of DNAM-1 and NKp30. *Exp. Hematol.* 37:1167-1175

Bellora F, Castriconi R, Dondero A, Reggiardo G, Moretta L, Mantovani A, Moretta A, Bottino C. (2010) The interaction of human natural killer cells with either unpolarized or polarized macrophages results in different functional outcomes. *Proc Natl Acad Sci U S A*. 107:21659-21664.

Benne C, Lelievre JD, Balbo M, Henry A, Sakano S, Levy Y. (2009). Notch increases T/NK potential of human hematopoietic progenitors and inhibits B cell differentiation at a pro-B stage. *Stem Cells* 27: 1676-85

Bennett IM, Zatsepina O, Zamai L, Azzoni L, Mikheeva T, Perussia B. (1996). Definition of a natural killer NKR-P1A+/CD56-/CD16- functionally immature human NK cell subset that differentiates in vitro in the presence of interleukin 12. *J Exp Med* 184: 1845-56

Biassoni R, Cantoni C, Pende D, Sivori S, Parolini S, Vitale M, Bottino C, Moretta A. (2001) Human natural killer cell receptors and co-receptors. *Immunol Rev.* 181:203-214.

Biron CA, Nguyen KB, Pien GC, Cousens LP and Salazar-Mather P. (1999) Natural Killer cells in antiviral defense: function and regulation by innate cytokines. *Annu Rev Immunol.* 17:189-220.

Bjorkstrom NK, Riese P, Heuts F, Andersson S, Fauriat C, Ivarsson MA, Bjorklund AT, Flodstrom-Tullberg M, Michaelsson J, Rottenberg ME, Guzman CA, Ljunggren HG, Malmberg KJ. (2010). Expression patterns of NKG2A, KIR, and CD57 define a process of CD56dim NK-cell differentiation uncoupled from NK-cell education. *Blood* 116: 3853-64

Boos MD, Yokota Y, Eberl G, Kee BL. (2007). Mature natural killer cell and lymphoid tissue-inducing cell development requires Id2-mediated suppression of E protein activity. *J Exp Med* 204: 1119-30

Borowitz M.J., Béné M.C., Harris N.L., Porwit A., Matutes E. Acute leukemias of ambigous lineage. *In*: Swerdlow S.H., Campo E., Harris N.L., Jaffe E.J., Pileri S.A., Stein H., Thiele J., Vardiman J. eds. (2008) WHO *Classification of Tumours of Haematopoietic and Lymphoid Tissues*. IARC Lyon: 155.

Bottino C, Castriconi R, Pende D, Rivera P, Nanni M, Carnemolla B, Cantoni C, Grassi J, Marcenaro S, Reymond N, Vitale M, Moretta L, Lopez M, Moretta A. (2003) Identification of PVR (CD155) and Nectin-2 (CD112) as cell surface ligands for the human DNAM-1 (CD226) activating molecule. *J Exp Med.* 198:557-567.

Bottino, C., L. Moretta, D. Pende, M. Vitale, and A. Moretta. (2004) Learning how to discriminate between friends and enemies, a lesson from Natural Killer cells. *Mol. Immunol.* 41: 569-575.

Brandt CS, Baratin M, Yi EC, Kennedy J, Gao Z, Fox B, Haldeman B, Ostrander CD, Kaifu T, Chabannon C, Moretta A, West R, Xu W, Vivier E, Levin SD. (2009) The B7 family member B7-H6 is a tumor cell ligand for the activating natural killer cell receptor NKp30 in humans. *J Exp Med.* 206:1495-1503.

Briard D, Brouty-Boye D, Azzarone B, Jasmin C. (2002). Fibroblasts from human spleen regulate NK cell differentiation from blood CD34(+) progenitors via cell surface IL-15. *J Immunol* 168: 4326-32

Bryceson YT, March ME, Ljunggren HG, Long EO. (2006). Activation, coactivation, and costimulation of resting human natural killer cells. *Immunol Rev* 214: 73-91

Caligiuri MA. (2008). Human natural killer cells. *Blood* 112: 461-9

Cannons JL, Tangye SG, Schwartzberg PL. (2011). SLAM family receptors and SAP adaptors in immunity. *Annu Rev Immunol* 29: 665-705

Carlsten M, Norell H, Bryceson YT, Poschke I, Schedvins K, Ljunggren HG, Kiessling R, Malmberg KJ. (2009) Primary human tumor cells expressing CD155 impair tumor targeting by down-regulating DNAM-1 on NK cells. *J Immunol.* 183:4921-4930.

Carrega P, Morandi B, Costa R, Frumanto G, Forte G, Altavilla G, Ratto G.B., Mingari M.C., Moretta L., Ferlazzo G.. (2008) Natural killer cells infiltrating human nonsmall-cell lung cancer are enriched in CD56 bright CD16(-) cells and display an impaired capability to kill tumor cells. *Cancer* 112:863-875.

Chan J.K., Sin V.C., Wong K.F., et al., (1997) Nonnasal lymphoma expressing the natural killer cell marker CD56: a clinicopathologic study of 49 cases of an uncommon aggressive neoplasm. *Blood* 89: 4501-4514.

Chan J.K.C., Jaffe E.S., Ralfkiaer E., Ko Y.K. Aggressive NK-leukemia. *In*: Swerdlow S.H., Campo E., Harris N.L., Jaffe E.J., Pileri S.A., Stein H., Thiele J., Vardiman J. eds. (2008a) *WHO Classification of Tumours of Haematopoietic and Lymphoid Tissues.* IARC Lyon 276-277.

Chan J.K.C., Quintanilla-Martinez N.L., Ferry J.A., Peh S.C. Extranodal NK/T-cell lymphoma, nasal type. *In*: Swerdlow S.H., Campo E., Harris N.L., Jaffe E.J., Pileri S.A., Stein H., Thiele J., Vardiman J. eds. (2008b) *WHO Classification of Tumours of Haematopoietic and Lymphoid Tissues.* IARC Lyon 285-288.

Cheung M.M., Chan J.K., Lau W.H., et al., (1998) Primary non-Hodgkin's lymphoma of the nose and nasopharynx: clinical features, tumor immunophenotype, and treatment outcome in 113 patients. *Journal of Clinical Oncology* 16: 70-77.

Chinen H, Matsuoka K, Sato T, Kamada N, Okamoto S, Hisamatsu T, Kobayashi T, Hasegawa H, Sugita A, Kinjo F, Fujita J, Hibi T. (2007). Lamina propria c-kit+ immune precursors reside in human adult intestine and differentiate into natural killer cells. *Gastroenterology* 133: 559-73

Colonna M. 2009. Interleukin-22-producing natural killer cells and lymphoid tissue inducer-like cells in mucosal immunity. *Immunity* 31: 15-23

Cooley S, Weisdorf DJ, Guethlein LA, Klein JP, Wang T, Le CT, Marsh SG, Geraghty D, Spellman S, Haagenson MD, Ladner M, Trachtenberg E, Parham P, Miller JS. (2010) Donor selection for natural killer cell receptor genes leads to superior survival after unrelated transplantation for acute myelogenous leukemia. *Blood.* 116:2411-2419.

Cooper MA, Fehniger TA and Caligiuri MA. (2001) The biology of human natural killer-cell subsets. *Trends Immunol.* 22:633-640.

de Pooter RF, Kee BL. (2010). E proteins and the regulation of early lymphocyte development. *Immunol Rev* 238: 93-109

Della Chiesa M, Carlomagno S, Frumento G, Balsamo M, Cantoni C, Conte R, Moretta L, Moretta A and Vitale M. (2006a) The tryptophan catabolite L-kynurenine inhibits the surface expression of NKp46- and NKG2D-activating receptors and regulates NK-cell function. *Blood.* 108:4118-4125.

Della Chiesa M, Romagnani C, Thiel A, Moretta L, Moretta A. (2006b) Multidirectional interactions are bridging human NK cells with plasmacytoid and monocyte-derived dendritic cells during innate immune responses. *Blood.* 108:3851-3858.

Della Chiesa M, Falco M, Parolini S, Bellora F, Petretto A, Romeo E, Balsamo M, Gambarotti M, Scordamaglia F, Tabellini G, Facchetti F, Vermi W, Bottino C, Moretta A and Vitale M. (2010) GPR56 as a novel marker identifying the $CD56^{dull}$ $CD16^{+}$ NK cell subset both in Blood Stream and Inflamed Peripheral Tissues. *Int. Immunol.* 22:91-100

DiSanto JP, Keever CA, Small TN, Nicols GL, O'Reilly RJ, Flomenberg N. (1990). Absence of interleukin 2 production in a severe combined immunodeficiency disease syndrome with T cells. *J Exp Med* 171: 1697-704

Doubrovina ES, Doubrovin MM, Vider E, Sisson RB, O'Reilly RJ, Dupont B, Vyas YM. (2003) Evasion from NK cell immunity by MHC class I chain-related molecules expressing colon adenocarcinoma. *J Immunol.*171:6891-6899.

Doulatov S, Notta F, Eppert K, Nguyen LT, Ohashi PS, Dick JE. (2010). Revised map of the human progenitor hierarchy shows the origin of macrophages and dendritic cells in early lymphoid development. *Nat Immunol* 11: 585-93

Dubois S, Mariner J, Waldmann TA, Tagaya Y. (2002). IL-15Ralpha recycles and presents IL-15 In trans to neighboring cells. *Immunity* 17: 537-47

Epling-Burnette P.K., Sokol L., Chen X., Bai F., Zhou J. et al., (2008) Clinical improvement by farnesyltransferase inhibition in NK large granular lymphocyte leukemia associated with imbalanced NK receptor signaling. *Blood* 112: 4694-4698.

Fehniger TA, Cooper MA, Nuovo GJ, Cella M, Facchetti F, Colonna M, Caligiuri MA. (2003) CD56bright natural killer cells are present in human lymph nodes and are activated by T cell-derived IL-2: a potential new link between adaptive and innate immunity. *Blood.* 101:3052-3057.

Ferlazzo G, Munz C. (2004) NK cell compartments and their activation by dendritic cells. *J. Immunol.* 172:1333-1339.

Fernandez L.A., Pope B., Lee C., Zayed E. (b1986) Aggressive natural killer cell leukemia in an adult with establishment of an NK line. *Blood* 67: 925-930.

Fregni G, Perier A, Pittari G, Jacobelli S, Sastre X, Gervois N, Allard M, Bercovici N, Avril MF, Caignard A. (2011) Unique functional status of natural killer cells in metastatic stage IV melanoma patients and its modulation by chemotherapy. *Clin Cancer Res.* 17:2628-2637.

Freud AG, Becknell B, Roychowdhury S, Mao HC, Ferketich AK, Nuovo GJ, Hughes TL, Marburger TB, Sung J, Baiocchi RA, Guimond M, Caligiuri MA. (2005). A human CD34(+) subset resides in lymph nodes and differentiates into $CD56^{bright}$ natural killer cells. *Immunity* 22: 295-304

Freud AG, Yokohama A, Becknell B, Lee MT, Mao HC, Ferketich AK, Caligiuri MA. (2006). Evidence for discrete stages of human natural killer cell differentiation in vivo. *J Exp Med* 203: 1033-43

Freud AG, Caligiuri MA. (2006). Human natural killer cell development. *Immunol Rev* 214: 56-72

Fuchs A. & Colonna M. (2006) The role of NK cell recognition of nectin and nectin-like proteins in tumor immunosurveillance. *Seminars in Cancer Biology.* 16:359-366.

Gascoyne DM, Long E, Veiga-Fernandes H, de Boer J, Williams O, Seddon B, Coles M, Kioussis D, Brady HJ. (2009). The basic leucine zipper transcription factor E4BP4 is essential for natural killer cell development. *Nat Immunol* 10: 1118-24

Gattazzo C., Teramo A., Miorin M., Scquizzato E., Cabrelle A., Balsamo M et al., (2010) Lack of expression of inhibitory KIR3DL1 receptor in patients with natural killer cell-type lymphoproliferative disease of granular lymphocytes. *Haematologica* 95:1722-1729.

Ghiringhelli F, Ménard C, Terme M, Flament C, Taieb J, Chaput N, Puig PE, Novault S, Escudier B, Vivier E, Lecesne A, Robert C, Blay JY, Bernard J, Caillat-Zucman S, Freitas A, Tursz T, Wagner-Ballon O, Capron C, Vainchencker W, Martin F, Zitvogel L. (2005) CD4+CD25+ regulatory T cells inhibit natural killer cell functions in a transforming growth factor-beta-dependent manner. *J Exp Med.* 202:1075-1085.

Giliani S, Mori L, de Saint Basile G, Le Deist F, Rodriguez-Perez C, Forino C, Mazzolari E, Dupuis S, Elhasid R, Kessel A, Galambrun C, Gil J, Fischer A, Etzioni A, Notarangelo LD. (2005). Interleukin-7 receptor alpha (IL-7Rα) deficiency: cellular and molecular bases. Analysis of clinical, immunological, and molecular features in 16 novel patients. *Immunol Rev* 203: 110-26

Glimcher LH, Townsend MJ, Sullivan BM, Lord GM. (2004). Recent developments in the transcriptional regulation of cytolytic effector cells. *Nat Rev Immunol* 4: 900-11

Grzywacz B, Kataria N, Sikora M, Oostendorp RA, Dzierzak EA, Blazar BR, Miller JS, Verneris MR. (2006). Coordinated acquisition of inhibitory and activating receptors and functional properties by developing human natural killer cells. *Blood* 108: 3824-33

Grzywacz B, Kataria N, Blazar BR, Miller JS, Verneris MR. (2011). Natural killer-cell differentiation by myeloid progenitors. *Blood* 117: 3548-58

Guerra N, Tan YX, Joncker NT, Choy A, Gallardo F, Xiong N, Knoblaugh S, Cado D, Greenberg NM, Raulet DH. (2008) NKG2D-deficient mice are defective in tumor surveillance in models of spontaneous malignancy. *Immunity.* 28:571-580.

Haas P, Loiseau P, Tamouza R, Cayuela JM, Moins-Teisserenc H, Busson M, Henry G, Falk CS, Charron D, Socié G, Toubert A, Dulphy N. (2011) NK-cell education is shaped by donor HLA genotype after unrelated allogeneic hematopoietic stem cell transplantation. *Blood.* 117:1021-1029.

Halfteck, G. G., M. Elboim, C. Gur, H. Achdout, H. Ghadially, and O. Mandelboim. (2009) Enhanced in vivo growth of lymphoma tumors in the absence of the NK-activating receptor NKp46/NCR1. *J. Immunol.* 182:2221-2230.

Hamann I, Unterwalder N, Cardona AE, Meisel C, Zipp F, Ransohoff RM, Infante-Duarte C. (2011) Analyses of phenotypic and functional characteristics of CX3CR1-expressing natural killer cells. *Immunology.* 133:62-73.

Hanna J, Goldman-Wohl D, Hamani Y, Avraham I, Greenfield C, Natanson-Yaron S, Prus D, Cohen-Daniel L, Arnon TI, Manaster I, Gazit R, Yutkin V, Benharroch D, Porgador

A, Keshet E, Yagel S and Mandelboim O. (2006) Decidual NK cells regulate key developmental processes at the human fetal-maternal interface. *Nat Med.* 12:1065-1074.

Harabuchi Y., Takahara M., Kishibe K., Moriai S., Nagato T., Ishii H. (2009) Nasal natural killer (NK)/T-cell lymphoma: clinical, histological, virological, and genetic features. *International Journal of Clinical Oncology* 14:181–190.

Harabuchi Y., Yamanaka N., Kataura N., Imai S., Kinoshita T., et al., (1990) Epstein-Barr virus in nasal T-cell lymphomas in patients with lethal midline granuloma. *Lancet* 335: 128-130.

Hodge D.L., Yang J., Buschman M.D., Schaughency P.M., Dang H. et al., (2009). Interleukin-15 enhances proteasomal degradation of Bid in normal lymphocytes: implications for large granular lymphocyte leukemias.*Cancer Res.* ;69:3986-94.

Hoshida Y., Hongyo T., Jia X., He Y., Hasui K., Dong Z., et al., (2003). Analysis of p53, K-ras, c-kit, and beta-catenin gene mutations insinonasal NK/T cell lymphoma in northeast district of China. *Cancer Sci.*94:297–301.

Huang Y., de Reynie`s A., de Leval L., Ghazi B., Martin-Garcia N., Travert M., et al., (2010) Gene expression profiling identifies emerging oncogenic pathways operating in extranodal NK/T-cell lymphoma,nasal type. *Blood* 115:1226–37.

Hughes T, Becknell B, Freud AG, McClory S, Briercheck E, Yu J, Mao C, Giovenzana C, Nuovo G, Wei L, Zhang X, Gavrilin MA, Wewers MD, Caligiuri MA. (2010). Interleukin-1beta selectively expands and sustains interleukin-22+ immature human natural killer cells in secondary lymphoid tissue. *Immunity* 32: 803-14

Iguchi-Manaka A, Kai H, Yamashita Y, Shibata K, Tahara-Hanaoka S, Honda S, Yasui T, Kikutani H, Shibuya K, Shibuya A. (2008) Accelerated tumor growth in mice deficient in DNAM-1 receptor. *J Exp Med.* 205:2959-2964.

Iqbal J., Weisenburger D.D., Chowdhury A., Tsai M.Y, Srivastava G., Greiner T.C., et al., (2010) The International Peripheral T-cell Lymphoma Project. Natural killer cell lymphoma shares strikingly similar molecular features with a group of non hepatosplenic γδ T-cell lymphoma and is highly sensitive to a novel aurora kinase a inhibitor in vitro. *Leukemia* 25: 348-358

Jaffe E.S. (1996) Classification of natural killer (NK) cell and NK-like T cell malignancies. *Blood* 87: 1207-1210.

Jondal M, Pazirandeh A, Okret S. (2004). Different roles for glucocorticoids in thymocyte homeostasis? *Trends Immunol* 25: 595-600

Juelke K, Killig M, Luetke-Eversloh M, Parente E, Gruen J, Morandi B, Ferlazzo G, Thiel A, Schmitt-Knosalla I, Romagnani C. (2010). CD62L expression identifies a unique subset of polyfunctional CD56dim NK cells. *Blood* 116: 1299-307

Kamizono S, Duncan GS, Seidel MG, Morimoto A, Hamada K, Grosveld G, Akashi K, Lind EF, Haight JP, Ohashi PS, Look AT, Mak TW. (2009). Nfil3/E4bp4 is required for the development and maturation of NK cells in vivo. *J Exp Med* 206: 2977-86

Kanno H, Kojya S, Li T, Ohsawa M, Nakatsuka S, Miyaguchi M, et al., (2000) Low frequency of HLA-A*0201 allele in patients with Epstein–Barr virus-positive nasal lymphomas with polymorphic reticulosis morphology. *Int J Cancer* ;87:195–9.

Kawa-Ha K., Ishihara S., Ninomiya T., Yumura-Yagi K., Hara J., et al., (1989) CD3-negative lymphoproliferative disease of granular lymphocytes containing Epstein-Barr viral DNA. *Journal of Clinical Investigation* 84: 51-55.

Kennedy MK, Glaccum M, Brown SN, Butz EA, Viney JL, Embers M, Matsuki N, Charrier K, Sedger L, Willis CR, Brasel K, Morrissey PJ, Stocking K, Schuh JC, Joyce S, Peschon JJ. (2000). Reversible defects in natural killer and memory CD8 T cell lineages in interleukin 15-deficient mice. *J Exp Med* 191: 771-80

Kim DH, Kamel-Reid S., Chang H., Sutherland R., et al., (2009) Natural Killer or natural killer/T cell lineage large granular lymphocytosis associated with dasatinib therapy for Philadelphia chromosome positive leukemia. *Haematologica* 94: 135-9.

Kim S, Iizuka K, Aguila HL, Weissman IL, Yokoyama WM. (2000) In vivo natural killer cell activities revealed by natural killer cell-deficient mice. *Proc Natl Acad Sci U S A.* 97:2731-2736.

Kwong YL, Chan AC, Liang R, et al., (1997) CD56+ NK lymphomas: clinicopathological features and prognosis. *Br J Haematol* 97: 821-829.

Kwong YL (2005) Natural killer-cell malignancies: diagnosis and treatment. *Leukemia* 19: 2186-2194

Laiosa CV, Stadtfeld M, Graf T. (2006). Determinants of lymphoid-myeloid lineage diversification. *Annu Rev Immunol* 24: 705-38

Lamy T., Loughran T.P. Jr. (2011) How we treat LGL leukemia. *Blood* 117:2764-74.

Lanier LL, Le AM, Civin CI, Loken MR, Phillips JH. (1986) The relationship of CD16 (Leu-11) and Leu-19 (NKH-1) antigen expression on human peripheral blood NK cells and cytotoxic T lymphocytes. *J Immunol.* 136:4480-4486.

Lanier LL, Spits H, Phillips JH. (1992). The developmental relationship between NK cells and T cells. *Immunol Today* 13: 392-5

Le Maux Chansac B, Moretta A, Vergnon I, Opolon P, Lécluse Y, Grunenwald D, Kubin M, Soria JC, Chouaib S, Mami-Chouaib F. (2005) NK cells infiltrating a MHC class I-deficient lung adenocarcinoma display impaired cytotoxic activity toward autologous tumor cells associated with altered NK cell-triggering receptors. *J Immunol.* 175:5790-5798.

Liang X., Graam G.K. (2008) Natural Killer cell neoplasms. *Cancer* 112:1425-1436.

Lin C.W., Liu T.Y., Chen S.U., et al., (2005) CD94 1A transcripts characterize lymphoblastic lymphoma/leukemia of immature natural killer cell origin with distinct clinical features. *Blood* 106: 3567-3574.

Liu X., Ryland L., Yang J., Liao A., Aliaga C., Watts R., Tan S.F., et al., (2010) Targeting of survivin by nanoliposomal ceramide induces complete remission in a rat model of NK-LGL leukemia. *Blood* 116:4192-201.

Ljunggren HG, Kärre K. (1990) In search of the 'missing self': MHC molecules and NK cell recognition. *Immunol Today*. 11(7):237-244.

Lopez-Botet M., Perez-Villar J.J., Carreterro M., et al., (1997) Structure and function of the CD94 C-type lectin receptor complex involved in recognition of HLA class I molecules. *Immmunology Reviews* 155: 165-174.

Lopez-Verges S, Milush JM, Pandey S, York VA, Arakawa-Hoyt J, Pircher H, Norris PJ, Nixon DF, Lanier LL. (2010). CD57 defines a functionally distinct population of mature NK cells in the human CD56dimCD16+ NK-cell subset. *Blood* 116: 3865-74

Lotzova E, Savary CA. (1993). Human natural killer cell development from bone marrow progenitors: analysis of phenotype, cytotoxicity and growth. *Nat Immun* 12: 209-17

Loughran T.P. Jr, Hadlock K.G., Yang Q., Perzova R., Zambello R. et al., (1997) Seroreactivity to an envelope protein of human T-cell leukemia/lymphoma virus in patients with

CD3- (natural killer) lymphoproliferative disease of granular lymphocytes. *Blood* 90:1977-1981.

Loughran T.P., Jr. (1993) Clonal diseases of large granular lymphocytes. *Blood* 82:1-14.

Ma A, Koka R, Burkett P. (2006). Diverse functions of IL-2, IL-15, and IL-7 in lymphoid homeostasis. *Annu Rev Immunol* 24: 657-79

Makishima H., Ito T., Momose K., Nakazawa H., Shimodaira S., Kamijo Y., et al., (2007) Chemokine system and tissue infiltration in aggressive NK-cell leukemia. *Leukemia Research* 31:1237–45.

Male V, Hughes T, McClory S, Colucci F, Caligiuri MA, Moffett A. (2010). Immature NK cells, capable of producing IL-22, are present in human uterine mucosa. *J Immunol* 185: 3913-8

Mandelboim O, Lieberman N, Lev M, Paul L, Arnon TI, Bushkin Y, Davis DM, Strominger JL, Yewdell JW, Porgador A. (2001) Recognition of haemagglutinins on virus-infected cells by NKp46 activates lysis by human NK cells. *Nature.* 409:1055-1060.

Mantovani A, Allavena P, Sica A, Balkwill F. (2008) Cancer-related inflammation. *Nature* 454:436-444.

Marquez C, Trigueros C, Franco JM, Ramiro AR, Carrasco YR, Lopez-Botet M, Toribio ML. (1998). Identification of a common developmental pathway for thymic natural killer cells and dendritic cells. *Blood* 91: 2760-71

Miller JS, Alley KA, McGlave P. (1994). Differentiation of natural killer (NK) cells from human primitive marrow progenitors in a stroma-based long-term culture system: identification of a CD34+7+ NK progenitor. *Blood* 83: 2594-601

Miller JS, McCullar V, Punzel M, Lemischka IR, Moore KA. (1999). Single adult human CD34(+)/Lin-/CD38(-) progenitors give rise to natural killer cells, B-lineage cells, dendritic cells, and myeloid cells. *Blood* 93: 96-106

Miller JS, McCullar V. (2001). Human natural killer cells with polyclonal lectin and immunoglobulinlike receptors develop from single hematopoietic stem cells with preferential expression of NKG2A and KIR2DL2/L3/S2. *Blood* 98: 705-13

Miller JS, Soignier Y, Panoskaltsis-Mortari A, McNearney SA, Yun GH, Fautsch SK, McKenna D, Le C, Defor TE, Burns LJ, Orchard PJ, Blazar BR, Wagner JE, Slungaard A, Weisdorf DJ, Okazaki IJ, McGlave PB. (2005) Successful adoptive transfer and in vivo expansion of human haploidentical NK cells in patients with cancer. *Blood.* 105:3051-3057.

Minarovits J., Hu L.F., Imai S., et al., (1994) Clonality, expression and methylation patterns of the EBV genomes in lethal midline granulomas classified as peripheral angiocentric T-cell lymphomas. *Journal Genetic Virology* 75: 77-84.

Mingari MC, Poggi A, Biassoni R, Bellomo R, Ciccone E, Pella N, Morelli L, Verdiani S, Moretta A, Moretta L. (1991). In vitro proliferation and cloning of CD3- CD16+ cells from human thymocyte precursors. *J Exp Med* 174: 21-6

Mingari MC, Vitale C, Cantoni C, Bellomo R, Ponte M, Schiavetti F, Bertone S, Moretta A, Moretta L. (1997). Interleukin-15-induced maturation of human natural killer cells from early thymic precursors: selective expression of CD94/NKG2-A as the only HLA class I-specific inhibitory receptor. *Eur J Immunol* 27: 1374-80

Moffett-King A. (2002). Natural killer cells and pregnancy. *Nat Rev Immunol* 2: 656-63

Moretta A, Bottino C, Vitale M, Pende D, Cantoni C, Mingari MC, Biassoni R, Moretta L. (2001). Activating receptors and coreceptors involved in human natural killer cell-mediated cytolysis. *Annu Rev Immunol* 19: 197-223

Moretta A., Marcenaro E., Sivori S., Della Chiesa M., Vitale M. and Moretta L. (2005) Early liaisons between cells of the innate immune system in inflamed peripheral tissues. *Trends Immunol.* 26:668-675.

Moretta L, Locatelli F, Pende D, Marcenaro E, Mingari MC, Moretta A. (2011) Killer Ig-like receptor-mediated control of natural killer cell alloreactivity in haploidentical hematopoietic stem cell transplantation. *Blood.* 117(3):764-771.

Mrozek E, Anderson P, Caligiuri MA. (1996). Role of interleukin-15 in the development of human CD56+ natural killer cells from CD34+ hematopoietic progenitor cells. *Blood* 87: 2632-40

Nakashima Y., Tagawa H., Suzuki R., Karman S., Karube K., et al., (2005) Genoma-wide array-based comparative genomic hybridization of natural killer cell lymphoma/leukemia: different genomic alteration pattern of aggressive NK-leukemia and extranodal NK/T cell lymphoma, nasal type. *Genes Chromosomes Cancer* 44: 247-255.

Nguyen S, Dhedin N, Vernant JP, Kuentz M, Al Jijakli A, Rouas-Freiss N, Carosella ED, Boudifa A, Debré P, Vieillard V. (2005) NK-cell reconstitution after haploidentical hematopoietic stem-cell transplantations: immaturity of NK cells and inhibitory effect of NKG2A override GvL effect. *Blood.* 105:4135-4142.

Oshimi K. (1996) Lymphoproliferative disorders of natural killer cells. *International Journal of Hematology* 63: 279-290.

Oshimi K. (2007) Progress in undestanding and managing natural killer cell-malignancies. *British Journal of Haematology* 139:532-544.

Pandolfi F., Loughran T.P.Jr, Starkebaum G., et al., (1990) Clinical course and prognosis of the lymphoproliferative disease of granular lymphocytes. A multicenter study. *Cancer* 65:341-348.

Parham P. (2005) MHC class I molecules and KIRs in human history, health and survival. *Nat Rev Immunol.* 5:201-214.

Parham P. (2006). Taking license with natural killer cell maturation and repertoire development. *Immunol Rev* 214: 155-60

Parolini S, Santoro A, Marcenaro E, Luini W, Massardi L, Facchetti F, Communi D, Parmentier M, Majorana A, Sironi M, Tabellini G, Moretta A, Sozzani S. (2007) The role of chemerin in the colocalization of NK and dendritic cell subsets into inflamed tissues. *Blood.* 109:3625-3632.

Pende D, Marcenaro S, Falco M, Martini S, Bernardo ME, Montagna D, Romeo E, Cognet C, Martinetti M, Maccario R, Mingari MC, Vivier E, Moretta L, Locatelli F, Moretta A. (2009) Anti-leukemia activity of alloreactive NK cells in KIR ligand-mismatched haploidentical HSCT for pediatric patients: evaluation of the functional role of activating KIR and redefinition of inhibitory KIR specificity. *Blood.* 113:3119-3129.

Perez SA, Sotiropoulou PA, Gkika DG, Mahaira LG, Niarchos DK, Gritzapis AD, Kavalakis YG, Antsaklis AI, Baxevanis CN, Papamichail M. (2003). A novel myeloid-like NK cell progenitor in human umbilical cord blood. *Blood* 101: 3444-50

Platonova S, Cherfils-Vicini J, Damotte D, Crozet L, Vieillard V, Validire P, André P, Dieu-Nosjean MC, Alifano M, Régnard JF, Fridman WH, Sautès-Fridman C, Cremer I. (2011) Profound coordinated alterations of intratumoral NK cell phenotype and function in lung carcinoma. *Cancer Res.* 71:5412-5422.

Pogge von Strandmann E, Simhadri VR, von Tresckow B, Sasse S, Reiners KS, Hansen HP, Rothe A, Böll B, Simhadri VL, Borchmann P, McKinnon PJ, Hallek M, Engert A.

(2007) Human leukocyte antigen-B-associated transcript 3 is released from tumor cells and engages the NKp30 receptor on natural killer cells. *Immunity.* 27:965-974.

Ribrag V., Ell Hajj M., Janot F., et al., (2001) Early locoregional high-dose radiotherapy is associated with long-term disease control in localized primary angiocentric lymphoma of the nose and nasopharynx *Leukemia* 15: 1123-1126.

Rodella L, Zamai L, Rezzani R, Artico M, Peri G, Falconi M, Facchini A, Pelusi G, Vitale M. (2001) Interleukin 2 and interleukin 15 differentially predispose natural killer cells to apoptosis mediated by endothelial and tumour cells. *Br J Haematol.* 115:442-450.

Romagnani C, Juelke K, Falco M, Morandi B, D'Agostino A, Costa R, Ratto G, Forte G, Carrega P, Lui G, Conte R, Strowig T, Moretta A, Munz C, Thiel A, Moretta L, Ferlazzo G. (2007). $CD56^{bright}CD16^{-}$ killer Ig-like receptor- NK cells display longer telomeres and acquire features of CD56dim NK cells upon activation. *J Immunol* 178: 4947-55

Rosenberg SA, Lotze MT, Muul LM, Leitman S, Chang AE, Ettinghausen SE, Matory YL, Skibber JM, Shiloni E, Vetto JT, Seipp C.A., R.N., Simpson C., and Reichert C.M. (1985) Observations on the systemic administration of autologous lymphokine-activated killer cells and recombinant interleukin-2 to patients with metastatic cancer. *N Engl J Med.* 313:1485-1492

Ruggeri L, Capanni M, Urbani E, Perruccio K, Shlomchik WD, Tosti A, Posati S, Rogaia D, Frassoni F, Aversa F, Martelli MF, Velardi A. (2002) Effectiveness of donor natural killer cell alloreactivity in mismatched hematopoietic transplants. *Science.* 295:2097-2100.

Sakata K., Hareyama M., Ohuchi A., et al., (1997) Treatment of lethal midline granuloma type nasal T-cell lymphoma. *Acta Oncologica* 36: 307-311.

Sanchez CJ, Le Treut T, Boehrer A, Knoblauch B, Imbert J, Olive D, Costello RT. (2011) Natural killer cells and malignant haemopathies: a model for the interaction of cancer with innate immunity. *Cancer Immunol Immunother.* 60:1-13.

Sanchez MJ, Muench MO, Roncarolo MG, Lanier LL, Phillips JH. (1994). Identification of a common T/natural killer cell progenitor in human fetal thymus. *J Exp Med* 180: 569-76

Santoli D., G. Trinchieri and F.S. Lief (1978) Cell-mediated cytotoxicity against virus-infected terget cells in humans. I. Characterization of the effector lymphocyte. *J. Immunol.* 121:526-531.

Scordamaglia F, Balsamo M, Scordamaglia A, Moretta A, Mingari MC, Canonica GW, Moretta L, and Vitale M. (2008) Perturbations of natural killer cell regulatory functions in respiratory allergic diseases. *J Allergy Clin Immunol.* 121: 479-485.

Semenzato G., Pandolfi F., Chisesi T., et al., (1987) The lymphoproliferative disease of granular lymphocytes. A heterogeneous disorder ranging from indolent to aggressive conditions. *Cancer* 60: 2971-2978.

Semenzato G., Zambello R., Starkebaum G., Oshimi K, Loughran T.P., Jr. (1997) The lymphoproliferative disease of granular lymphocytes: updated criteria for diagnosis. *Blood* 89: 256-260.

Shen L, Liang ACT, Lu L, Au WY, Kwong YL, Liang RHS, et al., (2002) Frequent deletion of Fas gene sequences encoding death and transmembrane domains in nasal natural killer/T-cell lymphoma. *Am J Pathol.* 161:2123–31.

Shilling HG, McQueen KL, Cheng NW, Shizuru JA, Negrin RS, Parham P. (2003). Reconstitution of NK cell receptor repertoire following HLA-matched hematopoietic cell transplantation. *Blood* 101: 3730-40

Siu L.L.P., Chan J.K.C., Kwong Y.L. (2002) Natural killer cell malignancies: clinicopathologic and molecular features. *Histol Histopathol* 17: 539-554.

Sivori S, Cantoni C, Parolini S, Marcenaro E, Conte R, Moretta L, Moretta A. (2003). IL-21 induces both rapid maturation of human CD34+ cell precursors towards NK cells and acquisition of surface killer Ig-like receptors. *Eur J Immunol* 33:3439-47

Sivori S, Falco M, Carlomagno S, Romeo E, Soldani C, Bensussan A, Viola A, Moretta L, Moretta A. (2010) A novel KIR-associated function: evidence that CpG DNA uptake and shuttling to early endosomes is mediated by KIR3DL2. *Blood.* 116:1637-1647.

Sivori S, Falco M, Marcenaro E, Parolini S, Biassoni R, Bottino C, Moretta L, Moretta A. (2002). Early expression of triggering receptors and regulatory role of 2B4 in human natural killer cell precursors undergoing in vitro differentiation. *Proc Natl Acad Sci U S A* 99: 4526-31

Smyth MJ, Thia KY, Street SE, Cretney E, Trapani JA, Taniguchi M, Kawano T, Pelikan SB, Crowe NY, Godfrey DI. (2000) Differential tumor surveillance by natural killer (NK) and NKT cells. *J Exp Med.* 191:661-668.

Sozumiya J., Takeshita M., Kimura N., Kikuchi M., Uchida T., et al., (1994) Expression of adult and fetal natural killer cell markers in sinunasal lymphomas. *Blood* 83: 2255-2260.

Sutlu T, Alici E. (2009) Natural killer cell-based immunotherapy in cancer: current insights and future prospects. *J Intern Med.* 266:154-181.

Suzuki R., Suzumiya J., Nakamura S., Aoki S., Notoya A., Ozaki S. (2004) NK-cell Tumor Study Group, et al., Aggressive natural killer-cell leukemia revisited: large granular lymphocyte leukemia of cytotoxic NK cells. *Leukemia* 18(4):763–70.

Tang Q, Ahn YO, Southern P, Blazar BR, Miller JS, Verneris MR. (2011). Development of IL-22-producing NK lineage cells from umbilical cord blood hematopoietic stem cells in the absence of secondary lymphoid tissue. *Blood* 117: 4052-5

Tefferi A., Li C.Y., Witzig T.E., Dhodapkar M.V., Okuno S.H., Phyliky R.L. (1994) Chronic natural killer cell lymphocytosis: a descriptive clinical study. *Blood* 84: 2721-2725.

Terme M, Ullrich E, Delahaye NF, Chaput N, Zitvogel L. (2008) Natural killer cell-directed therapies: moving from unexpected results to successful strategies. *Nat Immunol.* 9:486-494.

Trinchieri G. (1989) Biology of natural killer cells. *Adv Immunol.* 47:187-376

Vacca P, Cantoni C, Vitale M, Prato C, Canegallo F, Fenoglio D, Ragni N, Moretta L, Mingari MC. (2010) The crosstalk between decidual NK and CD14+ myelomonocytic cells results in induction of Tregs and immunosuppression. *Proc Natl Acad Sci U S A.* 107:11918-11923

Vacca P, Vitale C, Montaldo E, Conte R, Cantoni C, Fulcheri E, Darretta V, Moretta L, Mingari MC. (2011). CD34+ hematopoietic precursors are present in human decidua and differentiate into natural killer cells upon interaction with stromal cells. *Proc Natl Acad Sci U S A* 108: 2402-7

Villamor N., Morice W.G., Chan W.C., Foucar K. Chronic lymphoproliferative disorders of NK cells. In: Swerdlow S.H., Campo E., Harris N.L., Jaffe E.J., Pileri S.A., Stein H., Thiele J., Vardiman J. eds. (2008) *WHO Classification of Tumours of Haematopoietic and Lymphoid Tissues*. IARC Lyon 274-275.

Vitale C, Chiossone L, Morreale G, Lanino E, Cottalasso F, Moretti S, Dini G, Moretta L, Mingari MC. (2004). Analysis of the activating receptors and cytolytic function of human natural killer cells undergoing in vivo differentiation after allogeneic bone marrow transplantation. *Eur J Immunol* 34: 455-60

Vitale C, Cottalasso F, Montaldo E, Moretta L, Mingari MC. (2008). Methylprednisolone induces preferential and rapid differentiation of CD34+ cord blood precursors toward NK cells. *Int Immunol* 20: 565-75

Vitale C, Pitto A, Benvenuto F, Ponte M, Bellomo R, Frassoni F, Mingari MC, Bacigalupo A, Moretta L. (2000). Phenotypic and functional analysis of the HLA-class I-specific inhibitory receptors of natural killer cells isolated from peripheral blood of patients undergoing bone marrow transplantation from matched unrelated donors. *Hematol J* 1: 136-44

Vivier E, Raulet DH, Moretta A, Caligiuri MA, Zitvogel L, Lanier LL, Yokoyama WM, Ugolini S. (2011). Innate or adaptive immunity? The example of natural killer cells. *Science.* 331: 44-49

Vivier E, Tomasello E, Baratin M, Walzer T, Ugolini S. (2008) Functions of natural killer cells. *Nat Immunol.* 9:503-510.

Welte S, Kuttruff S, Waldhauer I, Steinle A. (2006) Mutual activation of natural killer cells and monocytes mediated by NKp80-AICL interaction. *Nat Immunol.* 7:1334-42.

West W. H., G.B. Cannon, H.D. Kay, G.D. Bonnard, and R.B. Herberman (1977) Natural Cytotoxic Reactivity of human lymphocytes against a myeloid cell line: characterization of effector cells. *J. Immunol.* 118: 355-361.

Wong K.F., Chan J.K., Kwong Y.L. (1997) Identification of del (6)(q21q25) as a recurring chromosomal abnormality in putative NK cell lymphoma/leukemia. *British Journal of Haematology* 98: 922-926.

Youn BS, Mantel C, Broxmeyer HE. (2000). Chemokines, chemokine receptors and hematopoiesis. *Immunol Rev* 177: 150-74

Yu H, Fehniger TA, Fuchshuber P, Thiel KS, Vivier E, Carson WE, Caligiuri MA. (1998). Flt3 ligand promotes the generation of a distinct CD34(+) human natural killer cell progenitor that responds to interleukin-15. *Blood* 92: 3647-57

Yun S, Lee SH, Yoon SR, Kim MS, Piao ZH, Myung PK, Kim TD, Jung H, Choi I. (2011). TOX regulates the differentiation of human natural killer cells from hematopoietic stem cells in vitro. *Immunol Lett* 136: 29-36

Zambello R., Berno T., Cannas G., Baesso I., Binotto G., Bonoldi E, Bevilacqua P, Miorin M, Facco M, Trentin L, Agostini C, and Semenzato G. (2005) Phenotypic and functional analyses of dendritic cells in patients with lymphoproliferative disease of granular lymphocytes (LDGL). *Blood* 102: 1797-1805.

Zambello R., Falco M., Della Chiesa M., Trentin L., Carollo D., Castriconi R, Cannas G, Carlomagno S, Cabrelle A, Lamy T, Agostini C, Moretta A, and Vitale M. (2003) Expression and function of KIR and natural cytotoxicity receptors in NK-type lymphoproliferative disease of granular lymphocytes. *Blood* 102:1797-1805

Zambello R., Semenzato G. (2003) Natural killer receptors in patients with lymphoproliferative diseases of granular lymphocytes. *Sem Hematol.* 40: 201-212.

Zambello R., Semenzato G. (2009) Large granular lymphocyte disorders: new etiopathogenetic clues as a rationale for innovative therapeutic approaches. *Haematologica* 94:1341-5.

Zimmer J, Andrès E, Hentges F. (2008) NK cells and Treg cells: a fascinating dance cheek to cheek. *Eur J Immunol.* 38:2942-2945.

Zitvogel L, Dendritic and Natural Killer Cells cooperate in the Control/Switch of innate immunity. (2002) *J. Exp. Med.* 195:9-14.

3

Molecular Mechanisms in Philadelphia Negative Myeloproliferative Neoplasia

Ciro Roberto Rinaldi[1], Ana Crisan[1] and Paola Rinaldi[2]
[1]*Department of Haematology – United Lincolnshire Hospital NHS Trust – Boston*
[2]*University Federico II and CEINGE Biotecnologie Avanzate – Naples*
[1]*UK*
[2]*Italy*

1. Introduction

The myeloproliferative neoplasia (MPNs) are a spectrum of clonal disorders of the hematopoietic system. The distinct clinical manifestations are dictated by the primary cell type affected, and thus chronic myeloid leukemia (CML) is a proliferation of mature granulocytes, polycythemia vera (PV) is an expansion or red blood cells, essential thrombocythemia (ET) results in an increase of platelets, etc.. The natural history of MPNs is generally chronic in nature, and patients come to medical attention either by coincidence (abnormal blood findings during routine exam) or by signs and symptoms related to the expansion of the hematopoetic system (e.g., an enlarged spleen). Common to most MPNs is a small but finite risk of disease evolution to an acute leukemia, where hematopoetic development is blocked at an early stage of differentiation, leading to the accumulation of poorly functioning myeloid blasts at an expensive of critical depletion of normal white blood cells and platelets, leading to morbidity and mortality from infections and bleeding complications. If they do not progress to an acute leukemia, the natural history of MPNs often results in fibrosis of the bone marrow, migration of hematopoesis to other organs (spleen and liver), and eventual complications of this secondary organ involvement, as well as from decreased normal blood counts from marrow fibrosis. A unifying theme in the pathogenesis of MPNs is the activation of tyrosine kinases. The "poster child" is CML, where the BCR-ABL translocation is found in all cases; the fusion BCR-ABL activates proliferative and antiapoptotic pathways; and most importantly, inhibition by tyrosine kinase inhibitors (TKIs) can markedly reverse the natural history of the disease. The molecular lesions responsible for PV, ET, and myelofibrosis (MF) were unknown until relatively recently. From 2005, a flurry of reports found that a point mutation in JAK2, resulting in a valine for phenylalanine substitution at codon 617 (JAK2V617F), occurred at a high prevalence in these disorders. The mutation was found in roughly half of MF and ET cases and nearly all PV cases. Constitutive activation of JAK2 activates STAT and MAPK proliferative signaling pathways, leading to transformation of hematopoetic progenitors. Curiously, not all hematopoetic stem cells in cases with the JAK2V617F harbor the mutation. Moreover, the data suggested a differential dosage effect in the different diseases. Whereas in most cases the JAK2V617F is heterozygous with a normal JAK2 allele, in many cases of

PV the mutation is homozygous through the process of acquired uniparental disomy. Curiously, in vitro cultures of PV cases will often show homozygous JAK2V617F erythroid colonies, whereas similar colonies from ET patients are heterozygous for the mutation. There has been a substantial body of work attempting to study the effects of the JAK2V617F in mouse models. Early reports focused on a bone marrow transplantation model, where mouse bone marrow cells harboring exogenous JAK2-V617F were transplanted into irradiated mice. These models produced a syndrome of what appeared mostly like PV, but most failed to completely recapitulate the spectrum of leukocytosis, thrombocytosis, and myelofibrosis found in human disease. Transgeneic models followed, which again produced a spectrum of MPN disorders, with a suggestion of phenotype relating to the JAK2V617F expression levels. Very recently, several groups have created knockin systems placing a conditionally inducible JAK2V617F allele under control of the endogenous JAK2 promoter. This allows for control of the JAK2V617F expression in only hematopoetic tissues, getting one closer to replicating the disease experience of the human patient. Marty et al. found that the heterozygous expression of JAK2V617F produced a PV-like syndrome, not like human where heterozygousity is more often associated with ET. However, Akada et al. demonstrated that both heterozygous and homozygous JAK2V617F caused a PV syndrome, with a demonstration of a dose effect, as indicated by the fact that homozygous expressors had a greater manifestation of elevated blood counts and spleen size, compared to those mice with lower levels of JAK2V617F. In addition, Li et al. have produced a very provocative study in which a human JAK2V617F knockin was created. This model produced a transplantable disease with some features of both ET and PV. Of interest is the finding that affected mice had reduced numbers of primitive hematopoetic cells that had evidence of impaired normal function (cell cycling, apoptosis, and DNA damage). Moreover, competitive marrow transplantation showed impaired hematopoetic stem cell function. Recently, Mullally and colleagues used a conditional JAK2V617F expression model to yield physiological levels of the mutated allele. The phenotype in the mice resembled much of the cellular biology and clinical features of human PV, and it was serially transplantable with great efficiency. Separation of the bone marrow into immature Lineage- SCA-1+ c-Kit+ (LSK) and more mature myeloid erythroid progenitor (MEP) and granulocytic monocytic progenitor (GMP) subpopulations demonstrated that the "MPN-initiating" JAK2V617F cell capable of transplantation resided in the LSK population, but not in the committed myeloid MEP or GMP progenitors. Surprisingly, several studies showed that mutant cells in the LSK compartment were quite similar to wildtype cells in regard to cell cycle status, STAT signaling, and gene expression (though JAK2V617F cells showed enrichment of the erthyroid, myeloid, and megakaryocytic differentiation pathways). Similar to the Li et al. paper, competitive transplantation experiments showed that mutant cells had at best a minor competitive edge compared to wild-type, and a small number of mutated cells nonetheless causes a PV phenotype. Lastly, the authors demonstrated that the MPN initiating cell was not killed by JAK2 inhibition. Mice treated with the inhibitor had a dramatic decrease in spleen size and a reduction of erthyroid precursors in the marrow, but LSK cells from treated mice were able to cause the PV phenotype in subsequently transplanted mice. These studies in total offer an increased understanding of the MPN that may usher in a new era of therapy, much like what occurred in the study of CML. Similar to CML, these studies suggest the initiating cell resides in the primitive compartment but is genetically and phenotypically quite similar to its normal complement. Like CML, mutated cells in the stem cell compartment appear resistant to kinase inhibition. However, as we move toward better therapies for MPN, these findings have implications in the feasibility of ''stem cell'' therapy, because there may not be a large therapeutic window to selectively kill MPN ''stem cells.'' In addition, a limitation of murine systems is that however eloquent, they are still only models of human disease. For example, human MPN may well have additional genetic lesions contributing to initiation and progression, and mouse models cannot easily recapitulate this complexity. In this regard it is interesting that several other mutations have recently been discovered in MPN (e.g., TET2, ASXL1, IDH1, and IDH2); TET2 mutations have been found in JAK2V617F-positive and -negative clones from the same patient, suggesting that TET2 mutations may be a relatively early event in MPN. Moreover, if tumor initiation and progression is influenced by interactions with a host's innate immunological system, then disease in the mouse model might be expected to be very different than in humans. Nonetheless, the work presented by Mullally and others are quite significant, and provide us with powerful tools to better understand disease and test new agents of therapy.However, it should be noted that some mutations might possess more than one mechanism of action, for example, *JAK2*V617F results in dysregulation of kinase signaling but might also have an epigenetic effect. Recently, Dawson et al.identified a novel nuclear role of JAK2 in the phosphorylation of Tyr 41 of histone H3 leading to chromatin displacement of HP1a. The authors suggested that the inability of HP1a to regulate chromatin could reduce the potential tumor suppressive functions of HP1a resulting in erratic mitotic recombination and transcription deregulation of several JAK2-regulated genes such as *LMO2*. These results were confirmed in hematopoietic cell lines and in the CD34+ cells collected from the peripheral blood of one PMF patient with JAK2V617F mutation. Our group defined the subcellular localization of JAK2 in total BM cells and in sorted cell populations collected from MPN (ET, PV, PMF) patients with the JAK2V617F mutation or from MPN patients with wild type (wt) JAK2. We find that in contrast to cells with normal JAK2 in which the protein is detected predominantly in the cytoplasm, JAK2 is mostly nuclear in V617F-positive CD34+ cells. However, this nuclear localization is no longer observed in V617F-positive differentiated cells. After expressing JAK2V617F in K562 cells, we observe a similar preferential accumulation of JAK2 in the nucleus in contrast to untrasfected- and wt JAK2-expressing cells in which the protein is found in the cytoplasm. The mutated-JAK2 nuclear translocation is mainly reverted by the addiction of the JAK2 inhibitor AG490.

1.1 Functional hallmarks of myeloid progenitors in myeloproliferative neoplasms

The BCR-ABL-negative myeloproliferative diseases, which include polycythemia vera (PV), essential thrombocythemia (ET) and primary myelofibrosis (PMF), were recently renamed myeloproliferative neoplasms (MPNs).[1] PV, ET and PMF are disorders of hematopoietic stem cells (HSCs) and early myeloid progenitors,[2, 3] where myeloid progenitors are hypersensitive and/or independent of cytokines for survival, proliferation and differentiation. For instance, the majority of PV patients harbor erythropoietin (Epo)-independent erythroid colonies.[4] Several intracellular anti-apoptotic pathways and molecules, such as STAT3, Akt or BclXL, are activated/induced constitutively in such MPN myeloid progenitors,[5, 6, 7] along with hypersensitivity to insulin-like growth factor 1 (IGF-1), granulocyte macrophage colony-stimulating factor, interleukin 3 (IL-3), granulocyte colony-stimulating factor (G-CSF) or thrombopoietin (Tpo).[8,9, 10, 11] Unlike many malignancies, where the INK4a locus is inactivated, erythroid progenitors from PV patients exhibit increased expression of the INK4a/ARF locus.[12]

1.2 Mutations involved in PV, ET and PMF

The acquired somatic *JAK2* V617F mutation is harbored by the majority of PV patients and by more than 50% of ET and PMF patients.[13, 14, 15, 16, 17]Subsequent identification of exon 12 mutants of *JAK2* in a minority of PV patients gave a molecular lesion to virtually all PV cases.[18] Sequencing of the gene coding for the Tpo receptor (TpoR/c-Mpl) identified mutations in the juxtamembrane tryptophan residue W515 (W515L and W515K) in a low percentage of PMF and ET patients, the majority of which are *JAK2* V617F-negative.[19, 20] The W515 residue of TpoR is required to maintain the receptor inactive in the absence of ligand.[21] All these mutations lead to constitutively active JAK–STAT pathway, especially JAK2, STAT5, STAT3, MAP kinase ERK1,2 and Akt.[13, 16, 21]Advancement over the past 3 years in the MPN research field has raised several major questions, such as: (i) What are the molecular bases for the significant differences in the *in vivo* phenotypes induced by *JAK2* V617F and TpoR W515L? (ii) How can a unique somatic mutation, *JAK2* V617F, be involved in the induction of three different diseases ET, PV or PMF? (iii) What mechanisms are responsible for the evolution of MPNs toward acute myeloid leukemia? (iv) What are the effects of *JAK2* V617F and of the other JAK2 and TpoR mutants at the level of HSC? and (v) What preceding and subsequent (to *JAK2* V617F) genetic events contribute to myeloproliferative diseases?Answers to these questions have begun to emerge. Gene dosage, as initially suggested by genotype/phenotype studies in patient cells,[22] by retroviral bone marrow reconstitution studies[23] and most recently probed in transgenic mice,[24]could be critically involved in inducing one or the other of the MPN phenotypes. It is fascinating that progenitors homozygous for the *JAK2* V617F mutation occur in almost all PV patients, but very rarely in ET patients.[25, 26] Although this can be seen as an argument in favor of the gene dosage hypothesis, other preceding or subsequent genetic changes might have an important function. Interestingly, host-modifying influences might have a major part in establishing the disease phenotype.[27] A screen for genetic variation within the genes coding for EpoR, TpoR, G-CSF receptor (G-CSFR) and JAK2 led to the discovery of three JAK2 single nucleotide polymorphisms that were significantly but reciprocally associated with PV and ET, but not with PMF. Three additional JAK2 single nucleotide polymorphisms were uniquely associated with PV. Such single nucleotide polymorphisms, although not in the coding region of the genes, might affect the levels of gene transcription, regulation by other factors or possibly expression of other genes.

1.3 Unknown effects of JAK2 V617F signaling in HSCs

JAK2 V617F mutation was detected at the HSC and the common myeloid/lymphoid progenitor levels, it skews the HSC differential potential toward the erythroid lineage and gives a selective proliferative advantage to myeloid lineages.[28, 29] The HSC compartment of PV and PMF patients was found to contain *JAK2* V617F-positive long-term, multipotent and self-renewing cells, with a much higher proportion of mutated HSCs in PMF than in PV.[30] It is not clear at this moment whether *JAK2* V617F profoundly affects the biology of HSCs[30] or whether it only gives a strong selection advantage past the HSC stage. A certain degree of heterogeneity exists between HSC subsets.[31] HSCs exist in niches, some near osteoblasts and others near endothelial cells. Exactly where and in which HSC subset the *JAK2* V617F mutation initially occurs might have a major impact on the subsequent disease phenotype.The *JAK2* V617F mutation was present in 30–40% of splanchnic venous thrombosis patients (Budd–Chiari syndrome and portal vein thrombosis).[32, 33,34, 35] A 'special' stem cell with hematopoietic/endothelial potential was suggested to be at the origin of splanchnic venous thrombosis, and it might harbor *JAK2*V617F.[36] A recent case report described a human allogeneic transplantation with*JAK2* V617F-positive cells from such a splanchnic venous thrombosis donor (with one episode of *JAK2* V617F-positive splanchnic venous thrombosis), but no MPN, to her HLA-matched sister with high-risk myelodysplastic syndrome (RAEB2).[37]The recipient exhibited a *JAK2* V617F burden similar to the donor immediately after transplant, but this burden decreased over time, and 7 years later, the recipient continues to be in remission and to exhibit low levels of *JAK2* V617F positivity.[37] These data suggest that, indeed, the *JAK2* V617F mutation can occur in an HSC, but at least in the transplantation setting, this HSC has no proliferative advantage. A considerable amount of data suggests that in addition to the presence of the*JAK2* V617F mutation, preceding or subsequent genetic events might be necessary for developing the MPN disease. First, in certain MPN patients, the clonality of expanded myeloid progenitors is found to be larger than the *JAK2* V617F clone, with the acquisition of *JAK2* V617F being a late genetic event.[38] Second, acute myeloid leukemia cases developed in*JAK2* V617F-positive patients can occur with leukemic blasts not harboring *JAK2*V617F.[39] Third, Epo-independent colonies might not always harbor the *JAK2*mutation in patients with the *JAK2* V617F mutation.[40] Such preceding or subsequent events could be associated differently with the three diseases, namely ET, PV and PMF.

1.4 The signaling space

Molecular cell biology textbooks list eight major signaling pathways that control gene expression that are linked to eight classes of cell surface receptors: cytokine receptors, receptor tyrosine kinases, receptors for transforming growth factor (TGF)-β, Wnt, Hedgehog, tumor necrosis factor (TNF)-α, Notch (Delta) and G-protein-coupled receptors.[41] Nuclear and corticoid receptor pathways, as well as integrin signaling, complete the picture of intracellular cell signaling. In several paperit has been well described that aberrant signaling occurs in MPNs through some of the listed pathways, such as cytokine receptors, receptor tyrosine kinases, TGF-β and TNF-α. It is not clear whether aberrant signaling in MPNs is simply due to the constitutive nature of signaling induced by mutated JAK2 or TpoR, or whether specific cross-talk events occur to other pathways that might confer specificity to JAK2 V617F versus JAK2 signaling. It is important to recognize from the outset that the experimental systems used by signal transduction research, such as phosphorylation studies, co-immunoprecipitation, gene expression and determination of protein localization, may not be able to identify subtle relative changes, such as kinetics and amplitude differences, between signals engaging generic pathways that are redundantly triggered by many stimuli. Such subtle quantitative differences might, however, be crucial for the disease phenotypes *in vivo*. That is the reason why genetics, *in vivo* models, results obtained with inhibitors and data derived from primary cells, must be taken into account to draw a picture describing aberrant signaling in MPNs.

1.5 Constitutive signaling and kinase activity of JAK2 V617F

The mammalian genome codes for four Janus kinases (JAKs), JAK1, JAK2, JAK3 and Tyk2. On the basis of homology, JAKs share seven JAK homology domains (JH), denoted as JH1–JH7. From the C to the N terminus, JH1 represents the kinase domain, JH2 the pseudokinase domain, JH3 and JH4 contain an SH2-like domain and linker regions, whereas JH5–JH7 contain a FERM (band 4.1, ezrin, radixin, moesin) domain[42, 43] (Figure 1).

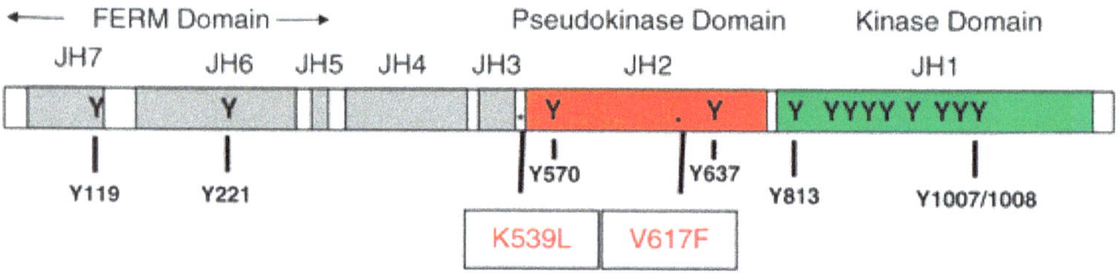

Fig. 1. Schematic illustration of Janus kinase (JAK)2 and the different JAK homology (JH) domains. The V617F mutation occurs in the pseudokinase domain rendering the kinase domain constitutively active. Exon 12 mutations, such as K539L, occur in the linker region between the JH3 and JH2 domains. Tyrosine residues that can be phosphorylated are depicted by their single letter. See text for details.

JAKs have been proposed to have a bipartite structure and the N terminus is required for binding to receptors, chaperoning and stabilizing them at the surface,[44, 45, 46, 47] whereas the kinase domain is absolutely crucial for signaling. The pseudokinase domain precedes the kinase domain, and because of sequence differences at key residues required for catalysis, it cannot transfer phosphate and thus is catalytically inactive.[42]Nevertheless, the pseudokinase domain is structurally required for the response of JAKs to cytokine receptor activation and for inhibiting the basal activity of the kinase domain.[48, 49] The V617F mutation occurs in the pseudokinase domain, leading to constitutive activation of the kinase domain (Figure 1). Although no X-ray crystal structure of full-length JAK2 exists, modeling has suggested that the pseudokinase domain of JAK2 maintains the kinase domain inactive in the basal state.[50] Thus, the V617F mutation is expected to relieve the inhibitory effect of JH2 on JH1 and to lead to basal kinase activity. The homologous V617F mutations in JAK1 and Tyk2 also lead to constitutive activation,[51] which strongly supports this model. Activating mutations in the pseudokinase domain of JAK1 at the homologous V658 position or at neighboring residues have been reported in 20% of patients with T-acute lymphoblastic leukemia.[52, 53] In transiently transfected JAK2-deficient cells, such as the γ-2A human fibrosarcoma cell line,[54] JAK2 V617F expression leads to constitutive activation of STAT5 and STAT3 signaling. In such transient transfection experiments, JAK2 V617F is constitutively tyrosine phosphorylated at the activation loop Y1007. Co-transfection of wild-type JAK2 reduces signaling by JAK2 V617F, presumably due to competition for an interaction partner, such as a cytokine receptor,[13] but does not prevent constitutive phosphorylation of JAK2 V617F.[16]To investigate the catalytic activity of JAK2 V617F mutation, kinase assays have been performed on GST fusion proteins. In COS7 overexpression conditions, when compared with wild-type JAK2, the JAK2 V617F mutated protein exhibits enhanced basal kinase activity on a reporter GST fusion protein containing the sequence of the activation loop of JAK2 containing tyrosine (Y) 1007.[17, 55] The kinase activity was clearly increased, but it appeared to be weak. In stably transfected Ba/F3 cells, JAK2 V617F also exhibits enhanced kinase activity on the same Y1007-containing GST fusion protein, but the levels of activation were also small (C Pecquet *et al.*, unpublished results). This is very different from BCR-ABL or other fusion proteins such as TEL-JAK2, where the kinase domain alone is oligomerized and activated by a fused exogenous oligomeric domain. In contrast, the kinase domain of JAK2 V617F is expected to maintain most of the negative regulatory intramolecular interactions that normally limit kinase domain activation.

1.6 JAK2 V617F and cytokine receptors

The FERM domain of JAKs is responsible for appending JAKs to cytokine receptors. Cytokine receptors contain in the cytosolic juxtamembrane region a proline-rich sequence, usually PxxPxP, denoted as Box 1, located 10–15 amino acid residues downstream of the TM domain, and further down 50–60 amino acid residues downstream of the TM domain, a sequence composed of hydrophobic and charged residues denoted as Box 2.[56]JAK2 binds to the region of EpoR that encompasses cytosolic residues of Box 1, Box 2 and also most of the residues between these boxes.[44, 56]Interaction between JAK2 and EpoR or TpoR is disrupted by a point mutation (Y114A) in the FERM domain.[47] Expression of the double-mutant JAK2 V617F Y114A in Ba/F3-EpoR cells did not lead to constitutive signaling through STAT5 or to autonomous growth,[57] suggesting that the V617F mutation does not suffice for activation in the absence of the assembly between the JAK2 V617F and a cytokine receptor. It can be noted that members of the JAK family are localized to membranes through recruitment by cytokine receptors, whereas mutations such as Y114A lead to cytosolic localization.[58] Furthermore, a mutation in the pseudokinase domain of JAK2 was identified (Y613 to glutamic acid, Y613E), which promotes constitutive activation only when JAK2 is in complex with the EpoR.[59] This result suggests that in the absence of an association with a cytokine receptor, JAK2 is locked into an inactive state and that receptor binding through the FERM domain is important for activation.[59]Another argument supporting the notion that binding to a cytokine receptor is important for the activity of the V617F mutant arises from the lack of activation of JH2–JH1 fusion proteins where the V617F mutation was introduced in the JH2 sequence.[60] The low basal activity of JH1 was shown to be suppressed by fusion with JH2.[49, 61] However, the presence of the FERM-SH2 domains is required for the activation effect exerted by the V617F mutation. JAK2 is crucial for signaling by EpoR[62] and TpoR,[63, 64] participates in signaling by G-CSFR[65, 66] (Figure 2) and also mediates signaling by the IL-3/IL-5/granulocyte macrophage colony-stimulating factor family of cytokines, as well as by several type-II cytokine receptors, such as interferon-γ receptor 2[67]. Given that MPNs mainly affect the erythroid, the megakaryocytic and the granulocyte lineages, as stated before, complexes between JAK2 V617F and EpoR, TpoR and G-CSFR may explain cytokine hypersensitivity and independence in these diseases (Figure 2).

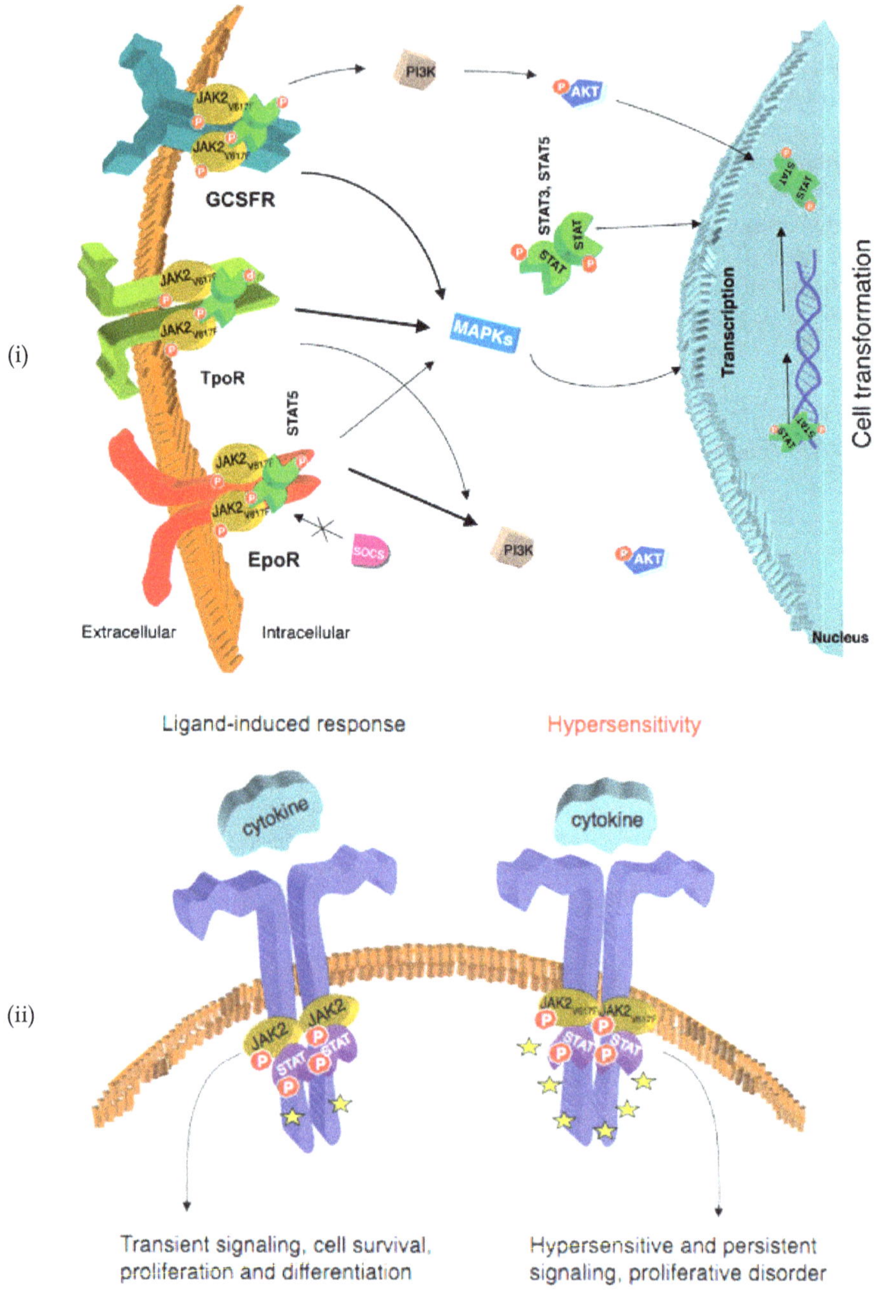

Fig. 2. Model of constitutive (ligand-independent) signaling induced by JAK2 V617F through erythropoietin receptor (EpoR), thrombopoietin receptor (TpoR) and granulocyte

colony-stimulating factor receptor (G-CSFR). (i) Janus kinase 2 (JAK2) is the main JAK used by EpoR and TpoR, but JAK1 is also used physiologically by G-CSFR. Primarily, EpoR and TpoR are expected to be bound by JAK2 V617F, whereas G-CSFR is expected to be in complex with JAK2 V617F at high JAK2 V617F levels, i.e., in homozygous *JAK2* V617F situations. Scaffolding of JAK2 V617F on the cytosolic tails of cytokine receptors leads to the enhanced activation of JAK2 V617F and downstream signaling through STATs, MAP kinase, PI-3-kinase (PI3K) and Akt. SOCS proteins are expected to engage both EpoR and activated wild-type JAK2, leading and down-modulation of JAK2 activity; the EpoR–JAK2 V617F complex appears to escape the down-modulation activity of SOCS3. (ii) Cytokine receptors that are in complex with JAK2 V617F are hypersensitive to their ligands for signaling. Cytokine binding to receptors coupled to wild-type JAK2 induce transient physiologic signals, leading to survival, proliferation and differentiation of myeloid progenitors. In contrast, receptors coupled to JAK2 V617F respond to lower levels of ligand, and are constitutively signaling after ligand withdrawal. It is not known whether dimeric receptor complexes, where one monomer is coupled to JAK2 V617F and the other to wild-type JAK2, are also hypersensitive to ligand or constitutively active.

1.7 EpoR and MPNs

EpoR functions as a preformed dimer on the cell surface, which upon cytokine binding undergoes a conformational change that triggers the activation of the receptor pre-bound JAK2.[68, 69] This involves a rotation of the receptor monomers within the dimer,[70] which is transmitted to JAK2 by switch residues, that is W258 in the juxtamembrane domain of EpoR.[69] Current data suggest that JAK2 V617F can scaffold on the cytosolic domain of EpoR and induce Epo-independent signaling, possibly by phosphorylating key cytosolic tyrosine residues on EpoR, which leads to strong STAT5 activation.[71]Early on after the identification of *JAK2* V617F, the need for a co-expressed type I dimeric cytokine receptor for constitutive signaling by JAK2 V617F provoked a controversy, which in the end led to a model of how dimeric receptors might actually promote JAK2 V617F activation. One study by Levine *et al.*[16] reported that JAK2 V617F readily induced autonomous growth in Ba/F3 cells engineered to express the EpoR (Ba/F3 EpoR cells), but not in parental Ba/F3 cells. In contrast, the study by James *et al.*[13] had shown that JAK2 V617F could induce autonomous growth in both Ba/F3 EpoR and parental Ba/F3 cells. This controversy (also described in Ihle and Gilliland[72]) was solved by carefully assaying the levels of JAK2 V617F transduction: at low levels, co-expression of a type I cytokine receptor was necessary for autonomous growth, whereas at higher levels JAK2 V617F alone induced autonomous growth, most likely by binding to an endogenous cytokine receptor, such as the IL-3-receptor β-subunit.[60] It is not clear whether other receptors—besides dimeric type I—could also promote signaling by low levels of transduced JAK2 V617F (Figure 2(ii)). Nevertheless, given that EpoR is a dimer in the absence of ligand, an insightful model was proposed by Harvey Lodish. In it, dimerization of JAK2 V617F by such a receptor is considered necessary for the activation of JAK2 V617F signaling, and the subtle V617F mutation promotes kinase activation when JAK2 is scaffolded on an inactive receptor dimer (Figure 2(i)).[71] Given that in MPNs the three lineages affected are controlled by the three type I dimeric cytokine receptors, EpoR, TpoR and G-CSFR, the model that JAK2 V617F mainly functions as a transforming kinase in association with these receptors is very plausible. EpoR signals mainly by JAK2-STAT5 and PI-3-kinase/Akt (Figure 2(i)) pathways. It is a weak activator of MAP kinase and of STAT3,[73] as it does not contain a consensus site for STAT3 binding, whereas several phosphorylated tyrosine residues (Y343, Y401, Y429 and Y431) can bind STAT5 and are required for maximal STAT5 activation.[74, 75] A consequence of STAT5 activation is induction of the anti-apoptotic BclXL protein expression,[76] which is constitutively expressed in PV erythroid progenitors.[7] The connection of EpoR with the PI-3-kinase pathway is accomplished by specific tyrosine residues, that is Y479, which appears to bind the regulatory subunit p85.[77, 78] PI-3-kinase and Akt activations are critically involved in erythroid differentiation,[79] possibly by the involvement of the transcription factor Forkhead family, FKHRL1.[80] Another mechanism appears to be the phosphorylation of S310 of GATA1.[81] Thus, scaffolding of an activated JAK2 to EpoR is predicted to activate the JAK2-STAT5 and PI-3-kinase/Akt pathways and stimulate proliferation and differentiation of erythroid progenitors.

1.8 EpoR and exon 12 JAK2 mutations

Patients with exon 12 *JAK2* mutations, such as JAK2 K539L, exhibit an erythrocytosis phenotype, without pathology changes to megakaryocytes typical for MPNs.[18] Unlike the uniqueness of the point mutation that generates JAK2 V617F, several deletions and insertions were noted in the case of exon 12 mutations.[18, 82] An attractive hypothesis is that exon 12 mutants of JAK2 favor interaction with EpoR over TpoR or G-CSFR, although a mechanistic basis for such a preference has yet to be found. Modeling of JAK2 suggests that the K539L falls in a loop in the linker region between the SH2 and the JH2 domain (Figure 1), which would be placed in space quite close to the loop represented by β4–β5 where V617 is located.

1.9 TpoR and MPNs

TpoR is coupled to and activates both JAK2 and Tyk2,[64, 83, 84] which appear to have comparable affinities for the receptor juxtamembrane domain and to promote cell surface traffic of the receptor to a similar extent.[47] However, JAK2 is much more effective than Tyk2 in transmitting the signals of the receptor.[47,64] TpoR activates JAK2, STAT5 and PI-3-kinase/Akt,[85] but in contrast to EpoR, it is a very strong activator of Shc, of the MAP kinase pathway and of STAT3 (Figure 2(i)).[83, 86, 87, 88, 89, 90] It is interesting that the first consequence of expressing the JAK2 V617F (at lower than physiologic levels in the transgenic model) mutation is to promote platelet formation.[24] Bipotential megakaryocyte-erythroid progenitors appear to be stimulated to engage on the platelet formation by STAT3 activation, whereas STAT5 activation favors erythroid differentiation programs.[91] STAT5 emerged as a critical factor for lineage commitment between erythroid and megakaryocytic cell fates. Depletion of STAT5 from CD34(+) cells in the presence of Tpo and stem cell factor favors megakaryocytic differentiation at the expense of erythroid differentiation.[91] Overexpression of an activated form of STAT5 impaired megakaryocyte development favoring erythroid differentiation at the expense of megakaryocyte differentiation.[91] Thus, at low levels of expression, JAK2 V617F might only activate STAT3, which might suffice for platelet formation. At higher expression levels, coupling to both TpoR and EpoR will lead to STAT5 activation, and this would favor the erythroid program. It is not clear at this point whether the PV phenotype is exclusively the result of EpoR activation or whether the pathologic activation of TpoR might also contribute to the PV phenotype. It is interesting to note that overexpression of TpoR in certain animal models led to an expansion of the erythroid compartment.[92]The SH2 and PH (pleckstrin homology domain) adapter protein Lnk was shown to not only bind to phosphorylated tyrosine residues of both TpoR and EpoR but also to exert a negative role on signaling by these receptors.[93, 94] It is not known whether the defects in this negative regulatory mechanism are operating in MPNs. Co-expression of JAK2 V617F and TpoR in Ba/F3 cells leads to down-modulation of TpoR, most likely due to internalization and down-modulation seen after excessive activation of cytokine receptors (J Staerk, C Pecquet, C Diaconu and SN Constantinescu, unpublished observations). This is consistent with early studies that have identified a maturation defect and down-modulation of cell surface TpoR in platelets and megakaryocytes from MPN patients.[95] More recently, an inverse correlation was reported between the burden of *JAK2* V617F and the levels of cell surface TpoR on platelets.[96] Although these results suggest that JAK2 V617F may contribute to the down-modulation of TpoR, several patients with MPNs in the absence of JAK2 V617F also exhibited down-modulated TpoR. Such down-modulation is not seen for EpoR. TpoR is a long-lived receptor at the cell surface[47] and recycles,[97] which is not the case for EpoR. Further experiments are necessary to follow up on the original observation of TpoR down-modulation in MPNs, which may be due to traffic alterations, excessive internalization and degradation or decreased protein synthesis. Several mutations in Mpl induce myeloid malignancies. A mutation in the transmembrane domain of Mpl, S505N, constitutively activates the receptor[98]and has been discovered in familial ET.[99] The S505N mutation in the transmembrane domain is expected to promote constitutive activation due to polar interactions between the asparagines that replace the natural serine. As stated earlier, mutations in Mpl at W515 induce severe MPNs with myeloprofibrosis.[19, 20] W515 mutations activate constitutive signaling by the receptor because W515 belongs to an amphipathic juxtamembrane helix (RWQFP in the human receptor), which is required for maintaining the un-liganded receptor in the inactive state. Another activating mutation was recently described for TpoR, where a threonine residue in the extracellular juxtamembrane region (located symmetrically from the W515 mutation on the N-terminal side of the transmembrane domain) is mutated to alanine (T487A) in a non-Down's syndrome childhood acute megakaryocytic leukemia.[100] In bone marrow transplantation assays, this Mpl T487A also induces a severe myeloproliferative disease, close to the phenotype induced by TpoR W515L.[100] Juxtamembrane mutations such as W515L/K or T487A may not only promote active dimeric conformations, but they could also induce receptor conformational changes by changing crossing angles between receptor monomers, whereas the S505N highly polar mutation in the transmembrane domain is predicted to stabilize an active dimeric conformation of the receptor. It will be interesting to test side by side in bone marrow transplantation experiments the effects of S505N, W515L and T487A mutations and to assess whether indeed the phenotype of the TpoR S505N mutation would be milder.

1.10 G-CSFR and MPNs

Bone marrow transplanted mice with HSCs expressing JAK2 V617F present not only an MPN phenotype, with low Epo, as predicted, but also with low G-CSF serum levels, suggesting that constitutive activation of G-CSFR occurs in these mice.[101]G-CSFR uses both JAK1 and JAK2 for signaling.[65, 66] JAK2 V617F may affect G-CSFR signaling with less efficiency than for EpoR and TpoR, as JAK1 may be the key JAK for G-CSFR. This is perhaps the reason why the granulocytic lineage is affected to a lower extent in MPNs, when compared with the erythroid and megakaryocytic lineages, especially at low levels of JAK2

V617F. Activation of the G-CSFR JAK2 V617F complexes may lead to enhanced numbers of granulocytes, constitutive activation of granulocytes (with release of enzymes) as well as interactions with platelets, which would contribute to thrombotic complications. It is not clear whether leukocytosis, which is seen in certain MPN patients and which appears to be associated with certain complications or evolution toward leukemia,[102] may be due to the pathologic activation of G-CSFR by JAK2 V617F. Granulocytes from patients with MPNs presented altered gene expression promoted by JAK2 V617F expression and confirmed a recapitulation of cytokine receptor signaling, resembling profiles of granulocytes activated by G-CSF.[103]Similar to TpoR, G-CSFR activates STAT3 and MAP kinase pathways, in addition to the JAK2-STAT5 and PI-3-kinase/Akt pathways. It can be noted that for this receptor, a very delicate balance has been identified between the activation of STAT3, required for differentiation and inducing a stop in cell growth (necessary for differentiation), and STAT5, which promotes proliferation.[102] Binding of SOCS3 through its SH2 domain to a phosphorylated tyrosine residue in the receptor's cytosolic end specifically downregulates STAT5 signaling. Deletion of the cytosolic region, which contains the binding site for SOCS3, leads to enhanced STAT5-to-STAT3 signaling ratio,[102] and this is associated with evolution toward acute myeloid leukemia of patients with severe congenital neutropenia. G-CSFR activation might synergize with other mechanisms and promote the mobilization of CD34(+) stem cells and progenitors from the bone marrow to the periphery. Interestingly, an increased number of circulating CD34(+) cells in MPN patients has been observed, and they exhibit granulocyte activation patterns similar to those induced by the administration of G-CSF.[104] The release of CD34(+) cells is generally due to a combination of increased levels of proteases[105] and especially due to the downregulation of the CXCR4 receptor on CD34(+) cells.[106] An altered SDF-1/CXCR4 axis was demonstrated in PMF patients with CD34(+) cells in the periphery.[107] These findings are supported by the rapid mobilization of CD34(+) cells with AMD3100, a CXCR4 antagonist.[108]

1.11 Tyrosine phosphorylation pattern of JAK2 V617F

JAK2 V617F is constitutively tyrosine phosphorylated. However, besides Y1007 in the activation loop, which is crucial for activation,[109] it is not known whether other phosphorylated tyrosines overlap with those phosphorylated in the wild-type JAK2. It can be noted that, JAK2 contains multiple tyrosine residues, of which at least 14 can be phosphorylated[110] (Figure 1). Some of these tyrosine residues exert positive (Y221) and other negative (Y119, Y570) effects on signaling by JAK2.[111, 112, 113] Y813 is a recruitment site for SH2-containing proteins,[114] such as SH2B, which can promote homodimerization of JAK2.[115] In theory, the constitutive activation of JAK2 V617F might promote a different pattern of phosphorylated tyrosines from that of wild-type JAK2.

1.12 STAT activation and MPNs

A hallmark of MPNs is constitutive or hypersensitive activation of the STAT family of transcription factors in myeloid precursors. As mentioned, the expressions of JAK2 V617F, TpoR mutants or exon 12 JAK2 mutants lead to constitutive STAT5 and STAT3 activation in various systems.[18, 116] As a function of the MPN disease type, one or the other of the STATs was suggested to be predominantly activated by JAK2 V617F. For example, in myelofibrosis, JAK2 V617F expression in neutrophils is associated with the activation of STAT3 but apparently not with that of STAT5.[117] In another study, in bone marrow biopsies and irrespective of JAK2 V617F, PV patients exhibited high STAT5 and STAT3 phosphorylation and ET patients exhibited high STAT3, but low STAT5 phosphorylation, whereas myelofibrosis patients exhibited low STAT5 and STAT3 phosphorylation.[118] Thus, constitutive activation of the STAT5/STAT3 signaling appears to be a major determinant of MPNs, irrespective of the particular JAK2 or receptor mutation. Furthermore, STAT3 activation by IL-6 has been shown in a murine model system to hold the potential to experimentally induce MPN. Mice homozygous for a knockin mutation in the IL-6 receptor gp130 (gp130(Y757F/Y757F)), which leads to gp130-dependent hyperactivation of STAT1 and STAT3 develop myeloproliferative diseases with splenomegaly, lymphadenopathy and thrombocytosis. gp130(Y757F/Y757F) is hyperactive owing to impaired recruitment of negative regulators such as SOCS3 and the SHP2 phosphatase.[119,120] The hematological phenotype disappeared when the knockin mice were crossed with heterozygous Stat3(+/-) mice.[121] Thus, the threshold of STAT3 signaling elicited by IL-6 family cytokines may have an important function in the myeloid lineage and may contribute to the development of MPN.

1.13 SOCS3 and JAK2 V617F

Suppressors of cytokine signaling (SOCS) proteins negatively regulate cytokine receptors and JAK-STAT signaling. There are eight members of the SOCS/CIS (cytokine-inducible SH2-domain-containing protein) family, namely SOCS1-SOCS7 and CIS. Each SOCS molecule contains a divergent N-terminal domain, a central SH2 domain, and a C-terminal 40 amino acid domain known as the SOCS box.[122] CIS/SOCS proteins are supposed to function as E3 ubiquitin ligases and target proteins bound to the SOCS N terminus, such as active JAKs, as well as themselves for proteasome-mediated degradation.[122] SOCS1 and SOCS3 can also inhibit the catalytic activity of JAK proteins directly, as they contain a kinase inhibitory region (KIR) that targets the activation loop of JAK proteins. SOCS proteins bind receptors and then target the activation loop of JAKs for inhibition by KIR and SH2 interactions.[122]SOCS3 is known to strongly down-modulate EpoR signaling.[123] JAK2 V617F appears not to be downregulated by SOCS3, possibly due to continuous phosphorylation of SOCS3, which can impair its E3 ligase activity.[124] Constitutive tyrosine phosphorylation of SOCS3 was also reported in peripheral blood mononuclear cells derived from patients homozygous for the JAK2 V617F mutant.[124] Taken together, a model was proposed in which JAK2 V617F may escape physiologic SOCS regulation by hyperphosphorylating SOCS3. It would be important to also determine whether exon 12 mutants of JAK2 are able to overcome down-modulation by SOCS3.Furthermore, one of the two tyrosine residues in the C terminus of SOCS3 that become phosphorylated upon ligand-activated cytokine receptors interacts with the Ras inhibitor p120 RasGAP.[125] This leads, in the case of IL-2 signaling, to sustained ERK activation, whereas the JAK-STAT pathway is down-modulated.[125]Whether part of the sustained ERK activation detected in cells transformed by JAK2 V617F may involve complexes of degradation-resistant SOCS3 and p120 RasGAP is yet to be determined.

1.14 Other JAK2 mutations activate JAK2

Substitution of pseudokinase domain residue V617 by large non-polar amino acids causes activation of JAK2.[126] Saturation mutagenesis at position 617 of JAK2 showed that, in addition to V617F, four other JAK2 mutants, V617W, V617M, V617I and V617L, were able to induce cytokine independence and constitutive downstream signaling. However, only V617W induced a level of constitutive activation comparable with V617F, and like V617F it was able to stabilize tyrosine-phosphorylated SOCS3.[126] Also, the V617W mutant induced a myeloproliferative disease in bone-marrow-reconstituted mice, mainly characterized by erythrocytosis and megakaryocytic proliferation. Although JAK2 V617W would predictably be pathogenic in humans, the substitution of the Val codon, GTC, by TTG, the codon for Trp, would require three base pair changes, which makes it unlikely to occur. Therefore, codon usage and resistance to SOCS3-induced down-modulation are two mechanisms that might explain the uniqueness of JAK2 V617F in MPNs.

2. Animal models of MPNs

2.1 JAK2 mutants

Mouse bone marrow reconstitution experiments with HSCs retrovirally transduced with JAK2 V617F resulted in strain-dependent myeloproliferative disease phenotypes. In these models, JAK2 V617F is expressed at ~10-fold higher than endogenous levels. In C57Bl6 mice, JAK2 V617F induces erythrocytosis, and in some animals myelofibrosis, although most reconstituted mice remain alive several months, and in some the erythrocytosis regresses; in Balb/c mice, the phenotype is more severe with erythrocytosis being followed by myelofibrosis.[13, 23, 127] Only very rarely, at low transduction levels, was a thrombocytosis phenotype observed, which, together with initial studies on primary patient cells,[22] led to the suggestion that gene dosage may be important for a particular phenotype to develop.[23] This hypothesis has been supported by studies in transgenic mice in which the expression of the JAK2 V617F was carefully regulated.[24] When JAK2 V617F levels were lower than endogenous JAK2 levels, an ET phenotype was obtained. When levels of JAK2 V617F were similar to those of endogenous wild-type JAK2, a PV-like phenotype was developed. Interestingly, upon development of the PV phenotype, a selection for higher levels of JAK2 V617F occurs, up to 5- to 6-fold higher than the endogenous JAK2 levels, which is not the case for the ET phenotype.[24] This indicates positive selection for JAK2 V617F expression in PV progenitors, a phenomenon that can be detected in stably transfected Ba/F3 cells.[51] In addition overexpression of several non-mutated JAK proteins, including JAK2, was shown to promote hematopoietic transformation to cytokine independence.[128]The phenotype induced by exon 12 mutants of JAK2 is more restricted to erythrocytosis, without the abnormal megakaryocyte clusters seen in the classical MPNs.[18] These *in vivo* data indicate that a difference must exist between signaling by JAK2 V617F and exon 12 JAK2 mutants.

2.2 Mpl (TpoR) mutants

The phenotype induced by TpoR W515L is different than that induced by JAK2 mutants, in that it is much more severe, with initial myeloproliferation, marked thrombocytosis, splenomegaly and myelofibrosis, and is established within 20–30 days after reconstitution.[19] At least one other mutation at W515 was identified in patients with PMF and ET, that is W515K.[20] W515 is located in an amphipathic motif (RWQFP) at the junction between the transmembrane and cytosolic domains. This motif is required to maintain the un-liganded TpoR in an inactive state. Given that a W515A mutation is also active,[21] it is not surprising that such different residues (Leu and Lys) are found in active TpoR mutants. We predict that other W515 mutations will be found in patients, as the loss of a Trp (W) residue is responsible for activation. The striking difference in severity and histopathology between the phenotypes induced by JAK2 V617F and Mpl 515 mutants is hard to understand when standard phosphorylation studies are performed on cell lines, such as Ba/F3 cells, where the same redundant pathways are activated by both JAK2 V617F and Mpl 515 mutants. Interestingly, deletion of the amphipathic motif (Δ5TpoR) that contains W515 or the mutation of either the lysine K514 (R514 in the human receptor) or the W515 in this motif to alanine leads to constitutive JAK2 and STAT activation and colony formation in primary cells and hypersensitivity to Tpo.[21] In hematopoietic cells transformed by Δ5TpoR (amphipathic motif deleted) or TpoR W515A, we noted enhanced STAT5 and MAP kinase activation in the absence of Tpo, and high levels of activation of STAT5, STAT3 and MAP kinase pathways on Tpo treatment.[21] Such TpoR mutants do not down-modulate cell surface levels of TpoR,[21] unlike TpoR in complex with JAK2 V617F, which is down-modulated (J Staerk *et al.*, unpublished observations). It is therefore tempting to speculate that prolonged activation of MAP kinase and STAT3 might be a distinct feature of TpoR W515 mutants, whereas JAK2 V617F, which couples not only to TpoR but also to other cytokine receptors expressed in myeloid progenitors, would generate a weaker or different signal. Taken together, these data suggest that some level of signaling specificity must exist, which would make the excessive activation of TpoR through JAK2 V617F qualitatively different from that induced by W515 mutations. Understanding this difference at the signaling level will be of utmost importance.

2.3 JAK2 inhibitors

Since 2005, mutations that directly or indirectly led to deregulated activation of non-receptor tyrosine kinase (TK) Janus activated kinase 2 (JAK2) have been implicated in the pathogenesis of MPN. These mutations activate the JAK2-signal transducer and activator of transcription (STAT) intracellular signaling pathways, which lead to increased cellular proliferation and resistance to apoptosis. These discoveries spurred the development of molecularly targeted agents (JAK2 inhibitors) as therapy for MPNs.

In clinical development, JAK2 inhibitors exhibit differential inhibitory activity against the JAK family members, and some exhibit effects on other receptor kinases and therefore are not selective forJAK2 TK. For example, INCB018424 inhibits JAK1, whereas CEP-701 and TG101348 inhibit FLT3. JAK2 inhibitors are small molecules that act by competing with adenosine triphosphate for the adenosine triphosphate-binding catalytic site in the TK domain. The V617F mutation locates outside the TK domain of JAK2. Therefore, the current JAK2 inhibitors target both wild-type and mutated JAK2 indiscriminately. This could explain why these drugs are active in patients with both wild-type and mutated JAK2. However, targeting the wild-type JAK2 is expected to lead to myelosuppression as a result of the exquisite signalling through JAK2 of thrombopoietin and erythropoietin receptors in normal hematopoiesis. This probably explains the reported therapy-related anaemia and thrombocytopenia observed with JAK2 inhibitors in clinical trials.

Previous research demonstrated that JAK2-deficiency is embryonically fatal in mice due to a lack of erythropoiesis. As a consequence, no in vivo JAK2 knock out animal model exists, which makes the biological characterization of JAK2 more difficult. siRNA knock down models may be useful for this purpose, but for the time being, they cannot be considered as therapeutic agents. JAK2 antagonists, however, could be used efficiently for analyzing the possible therapeutic benefit of JAK2 inhibition in hematologic malignancies and myeloproliferative disorders.

On the other hand, only a small number of JAK2 inhibitors have been reported in the literature so far. AG490 possesses significant JAK2 inhibition, for that reason it has been used extensively as a research tool. AG490 blocks leukemic cell growth significantly both in vitro and in vivo.[16] On the other hand, this compound lacks sufficient target specificity, therefore the interpretation of results obtained with AG490 may not be limited to JAK2 inhibition. Several other non-specific JAK2 inhibitors have already been reported in the literature (LFM-A13,21 INCB20,22 WP106623 and SD-100824). Since off-target effects may cause serious immune-modulative or proliferative side effects, specific JAK2 inhibition is highly desirable.

One molecule, TG101209, was able to inhibit proliferation of both JAK2 V617F- and TpoR W515L/K-expressing hematopoietic cells.[130] It may be recalled that TpoR W515-mutated proteins are expected to constitutively activate the wild-type JAK2.

TG101348, a nano-molar JAK2 inhibitor, was highly specific for JAK2 as evidenced by a 300-fold selectivity over JAK3. TG101348, was effective in a murine model of MPN induced by JAK2 V617F131 and inhibited the engraftment of JAK2 V617F-positive HSCs and myeloid progenitors in a bioluminescent xenogeneic transplantation assay.[132] Importantly, the inhibitor decreased GATA1 expression and phosphorylation of GATA1 at S310 and, as expected, STAT5 activation. These signaling events might be associated with erythroid-skewing of JAK2 V617F-positive progenitor differentiation, as phosphorylation at GATA1 S310 was shown to be important for erythroid differentiation.[81] GATA1 is absolutely required for erythroid and megakaryocyte formation.[133, 134] Although both EpoR and GATA1 are crucial for erythroid differentiation, this phosphorylation event, which depends on PI-3-kinase and Akt,81 appears to be the only one described where a direct EpoR downstream signal affects GATA1.

An experimental JAK2 inhibitor has been shown to be well tolerated and to produce a significant reduction in disease burden and durable clinical benefit in patients with myelofibrosis reports a study. [161] Currently there are no FDA approved treatments for myelofibrosis. Common treatments of the malignancy, which is associated with anaemia and splenomegaly, are palliative and do not alter the natural course of the disease. Median survival ranges from less than two years to greater than 15 years. Patients with myelofibrosis frequently harbour JAK-STAT activating mutations that are sensitive to TG101348, a selective small-molecule JAK2 inhibitor. It is estimated that JAK2 mutations occur in approximately 50 % of patients. Last September researchers reported positive results from a trial testing the experimental agent INCBO18424, (which inhibits JAK1 as well as JAK2) in patients with advanced myelofibrosis. In the current phase 1 study, Ayalew Tefferi and colleagues from the Mayo Clinic enrolled 59 patients, including 28 who took part in the dose-escalating phase. A substantial portion of patients experienced improvements in primary symptoms including splenomegaly, leukocytosis, thrombocytosis, and constitutional symptoms. There was also evidence for significant reductions in genomic disease burden, indicating the potential for disease-modifying activity. Although the drug was generally well tolerated, it caused anaemia in some patients, especially at higher doses.

A follow-up study is planned to see whether adjusting the dose will allow patients to achieve the benefits without the anaemia. In an accompanying editorial Srdan Verstovsek from the University of Texas MD Anderson Cancer Center wrote, "The development of JAK2 inhibitors has ushered in a new era of targeted therapies for Philadelphia-negative MPNs. These drugs do not eradicate the malignant clone, but they provide significant clinical benefit. Given that the current clinical management of patients with MF is largely palliative and minimally effective, significant improvements in two of the three most important clinical manifestations of MF (splenomegaly and systemic symptoms) seen with JAK2 inhibitors is significant therapeutic progress." Long term results, he added, are required to determine the full potential of JAK2 inhibitors in myelofibrosis and to determine whether they will have an impact on survival.

3. Cross-talk: JAK2 V617F and other pathways

3.1 JAK2 V617F and other tyrosine kinases

Tyrosine kinase receptors have been suggested to contribute to the pathogenesis of PV. In patients with PV, circulating erythroid progenitor cells are hypersensitive to IGF-1 and this effect requires the IGF-1 receptor.[10, 135]Expression of JAK2 V617F in Ba/F3 cells renders the cells responsive to IGF-1 at doses where parental Ba/F3 cells are unresponsive.[51] After selection for autonomous growth, these Ba/F3 JAK2 V617F cells acquire the ability to respond to IGF-1 by further tyrosine phosphorylation of the mutant JAK2 and of STAT5 and STAT3. Which adaptor/signaling protein mediates this cross-talk is not clear, but it might be relevant for the hypersensitivity of PV erythroid progenitors to IGF-1.

Treatment with imatinib, an inhibitor of the Abl, c-KIT and PDGF receptor kinase, leads to minimal responses in PV, but nevertheless some rare patients achieve remission and a decrease in the *JAK2* V617F allele burden.[136] Imatinib exerts a dose-dependent growth inhibitory effect on factor dependent cell paterson (FDCP) cells expressing JAK2 V617F, most likely by interrupting the cross-talk between JAK2 V617F and c-KIT.[137] Thus, this study predicts that in PV patients where imatinib exerts benefic effects, pathologic signaling occurs through c-KIT.Src tyrosine kinases have also been suggested to contribute to signaling by EpoR.[138] However, Src kinases were dispensable for the polycythemia phenotype induced by JAK2 V617F, as shown by bone marrow reconstitution studies in mice deficient for Lyn, Fyn or Fgr kinases.[139]

3.2 JAK2 V617F and TNF-α

In BALB/c mice reconstituted with HSCs transduced for the expression of JAK2 V617F, the PV-like phenotype is associated with increased serum levels of TNF-α.[101] TNF-α might be required for suppressing normal hematopoiesis, and in this manner it might favor the mutated clone. Reconstitution experiments in TNF-α knockout mice supported the notion that TNF-α might be required for the establishment of the MPN phenotype and for clonal dominance (Bumm TGP, VanDyke J, Loriaux M, Gendron C, Wood LG, Druker BJ, Deininger MW. TNF-α plays a crucial role in the JAK2-V617F-induced myeloproliferative disorder. *Blood*2007; 110. American Society of Hematology 2007 Abstract 675). Further studies will be required to firmly establish whether TNF signaling may contribute to clonal dominance. Erythroblasts from JAK2 V617F-positive PV patients show increased death receptor resistance, which may give them a proliferative advantage over the non-mutated erythroblasts.[101, 140] This effect was mediated by incomplete caspase-mediated cleavage of the erythroid transcription factor GATA-1, which in normal erythroblasts is completely degraded on CD95 stimulation.

3.3 MPNs and TGF-β

An increase of TGF-β expression in circulating megakaryocytic cells and platelets was demonstrated in PMF.[141] Fibroblasts participating in myelofibrosis were shown to be polyclonal, as opposed to the hematopoietic progenitors, thus suggesting that myelofibrosis is a reactive process.[141]In myelofibrosis induced by excessive levels of Tpo,[142] severe spleen fibrosis was seen only in wild-type mice but not in homozygous TGF-β1 null (TGF-β1 (-/-)) mice.[143] Studies using peripheral CD34(+) cells cultured in medium with Tpo and stem cell factor concluded that PMF is a consequence of an increased ability of PMF CD34(+) progenitor cells to generate megakaryocytes and a decreased rate of megakaryocyte apoptosis, which lead to high levels of megakaryocyte-produced TGF-β.[144] In other models with hyperactive JAK-STAT signaling, such as knock-in with a mutant hyperactive gp130 receptor, the activation of the JAK-STAT pathway led to the expression of the inhibitory Smad7, which prevents the anti-proliferative effect of TGF-β.[145] A pathway linking Tpo, GATA-1 and TGF-βin the development of myelofibrosis was invoked, given that mice expressing low levels of the transcription factor GATA-1 also develop myelofibrosis.[146]

3.4 JAK2 V617F and chromatin

Studies in *Drosophila melanogaster* show that persistent activation of D-STAT by mutated D-JAK leads to chromatin effects and gene induction other than the normal targets of D-STAT, with counteracting heterochromatic gene silencing.[147]A genome-wide survey of genes required for JAK/STAT activity identified a WD40/bromodomain protein *Drosophila* homolog of BRWD3,[148] a gene that is disrupted in human B-cell leukemia patients. Whether any histone acetylase, deacetylase, methyl-transferase or other proteins containing bromo-, chromo- or chromoshadow domains are direct targets of JAK2 V617F is not clear. Recently, encouraging results were obtained with an HDAC (histone deacetylase) inhibitor, which seems to target only *JAK2* V617F-positive cells among primary myeloid progenitors from PV patients.[149] Thus, like other cancers,[150] MPNs might also show restriction of fate options through hypermethylation. This notion is supported by the different effects of sequential treatment with the DNA methyltransferase inhibitor, decitabine, followed by the histone deacetylase inhibitor, trichostatin A (TSA), on normal CD34(+) versus PMF CD34(+) cells. In the former, the treatment led to the expansion of cells, whereas in the latter the total number of CD34(+) cells and hematopoietic cells was reduced.[151]Furthermore, promoter de-methylation appears to be at least partially at the basis of the dysregulated expression of the polycythemia rubra vera-1 (PRV-1) protein,[152] which is a key marker of PV.[153] Finally, hypermethylation of the SOCS1 promoter was reported approximately in 15% of MPN patients irrespective of *JAK2* V617F positivity.[154] SOCS1 promoter methylation may contribute to growth factor hypersensitivity, as SOCS1 appears to maintain the ability to down-modulate JAK2 V617F signaling.[124] Recently, Dawson et al.[155]identified a novel nuclear role of JAK2 in the phosphorylation of Tyr 41 of histone H3 leading to chromatin displacement of HP1a. The authors suggested that the inability of HP1a to regulate chromatin could reduce the potential tumor suppressive functions of HP1a resulting in erratic mitotic recombination and transcription deregulation of several JAK2-regulated genes such as *LMO2*[155,156]. These results were confirmed in hematopoietic cell lines and in the CD34+ cells collected from the peripheral blood of one PMF patient with JAK2V617F mutation. In this work we define the subcellular localization of JAK2 in total BM cells and in sorted cell populations collected from MPN (ET, PV, PMF) patients with the JAK2V617F mutation or from MPN patients with wild type (wt) JAK2. We find that in contrast to cells with normal JAK2 in which the protein is detected predominantly in the cytoplasm, JAK2 is mostly nuclear in V617F-positive CD34+ cells. However, this nuclear localization is no longer observed in V617F-positive differentiated cells. After expressing JAK2V617F in K562 cells, we observe a similar preferential accumulation of JAK2 in the nucleus in contrast to untrasfected- and wt JAK2-expressing cells in which the protein is found in the cytoplasm. The mutated-JAK2 nuclear translocation is mainly reverted by the addiction of the JAK2 inhibitor AG490.

4. Methods

4.1 Cell cultures

K562 were grown in RPMI 1640 medium (Sigma-Aldrich), supplemented with 10% fetal bovine serum (FBS), 1% penicillin/streptomycin, and 1% glutamine. The cells were maintained at 37 C and 5% CO2. Transfection was performed by AMAXA electroporation in accordance with the manufacturer's instructions. Stable cell lines were obtained by puromycin selection (3μg/ml). Leptomycine B was added to a final concentration of 1 uM and the cells were harvested after 24 h of incubation. The differentiation of K562 cells was obtained by culturing the cells with 10 nMol PMA.

4.2 Plasmids

pMSCV-puro-JAK2 and pMSCV-puro-JAK2V617F were kindly provided by Dr. J. Cools.

4.3 Confocal immunofluorescence (CFI) microscopy

The BM fractions of CD34+, CD15+, CD41+, CD71+ cells and the K562 cells were washed once in PBS before cytocentrifugation onto polylysine-coated microscope slides. The cells were fixed for 5 min in methanol at room temperature and 5 min in acetone at -20 C. After stepwise incubation with a primary antibody and a secondary fluorescent antibody, the cells were stained with DAPI and mounted with glycerol. Confocal laser images were captured with a laser scanning microscope LSM 510 META microscope equipped with a 403 oil-immersion lens.

4.4 Patients

BM aspirates and PB samples were obtained from 15 patients newly diagnosed with MPN according to the WHO criteria. Ten of the patients (ET n=4, PV n=3, PMF n=3) had the V617F mutation. The remaining 5 patients (PMF n= 2, ET n=3) had a normal JAK2. Informed consent for the study was obtained from all patients in accordance with the Declaration of

Helsinki. The study was conducted according to the guidelines of the Italian ethics committee.

4.5 Cell sorting

Mononucleated cells were isolated by Ficoll centrifugation. After erythrocyte lyses, 10 million BM (or PB) cells were labelled by incubation with the antibodies CD15-APC, CD41-FITC, CD71-PerCP, CD34-Pe (BD Biosciences, San Jose, CA), analyzed, and sorted with a fluorescence-activated cell sorter FACSAria (BD Biosciences) using FACS Diva software (BD Biosciences) according to the manufacturer's recommendations.

4.6 ASO-PCR and RT-PCR

The JAK2V617F mutation was identified by ASO-PCR as previously described[13-15]. Briefly, total RNA was isolated with the TRIzol reagent (Invitrogen) and cDNA was synthesised with the First Strand cDNA Synthesis kit (MBI Fermentas). Syber Green RQ-PCR was performed as previously described[155]. Quantitative values were obtained from the threshold cycle number (Ct) by subtracting the average Ct of the target gene from that of GAPDH and expressed as $2^{-\Delta Ct}$.

4.7 Cell fractionation and immunoblotting

Cytoplasmic and nuclear fractions were prepared using nuclei isolation KIT by Sigma-Aldrich according to the manufacturer's instructions. Equal amounts of cytoplasmic or nuclear fractions or total cell extracts were separated by SDS–PAGE, transferred to nitrocellulose and probed with relevant antibodies.

4.8 JAK2 inhibitor and antibodies

AG490 was provided by Invivogen. To establish the best experimental condition, the cells were cultured for 3 hours with 2 different concentrations of the inhibitor (12.5 uM and 25 uM). The following antibodies were used at the stated dilutions: anti-JAK2 antibodies (D2E12 no. 3230; Cell Signaling Technology), p-JAK2 (tyr1007/tyr1008)-R and p-JAK2 (tyr1007/tyr1008) (Santa Cruz), anti-b-tubulin (T5201; Sigma-Aldrich), anti-laminin A (Sigma-Aldrich); western blot 1:1000. Alex Fluor-488-conjugated IgG (Invitrogen) immunofluorescence 1:250.

4.9 Apoptotic rate

K562 cells were stained with propidium iodide and annexin V before and after 3 h incubation with AG490. Cell cycle parameters were assessed by FACS analysis using FACSCanto II flow cytometer (Becton Dickinson, San Jose, CA, USA).

4.10 Statistical analysis

Student *t* test was used to evaluate individual differences between means. $P \leq 0.05$ was considered significant.

5. Results and discussion

5.1 V617FJAK2 goes into the nucleus of JAK2 mutated K562

To determine whether the V617F mutation affects the sub-cellular localization of JAK2, we used CIF microscopy to analyze K562 cells stably transfected with pMSCV-puroJAK2V617F or pMSCV-puroJAK2. The results (Figure 3A) confirm the nuclear and cytoplasmic localization of JAK2 in K562 as reported by Dawson et al[155]. However, we consistently observed a much stronger nuclear signal in the cells expressing JAK2V617F than in those carrying wt JAK2, suggesting that the mutation leads to a nuclear accumulation of JAK2V617F. By CIF, this accumulation can be seen as a diffused nuclear pattern (Figure 3A top, upper and middle panels) or as nuclear spots (Figure 3A top, lower panel). This altered sub-cellular distribution was not affected by the addition of the nuclear export inhibitor leptomycin B (data not shown) and was confirmed by Western blot analysis of K562 cells (Figure 3A, bottom panels).

5.2 Preferential nuclear JAK2 in V617FJAK2 positive CD34+ but not in differentiated erythroid, granulocytic or megakaryocytic cells

To determine whether there is a preferential nuclear translocation of JAK2V617F *in vivo*, we analyzed by CIF microscopy the BM cells of 10 JAK2V617F-positive MPN patients (ET n=4, PV n=3, PMF n=3, allele burden median: 56%, 70%, 72% respectively) and of 5 MPN patients with wt JAK2 (PMF n= 2, ET n=3). We did not observe a significant signal in the nucleus of cells with wt JAK2 (Figure 3B). In contrast, we found a strong nuclear signal in 3%-5% of total BM mononucleated cells in 10 of 10 JAK2V617F-positive patients, suggesting that, unlike the wt JAK2, JAK2V617F has a predominantly nuclear homing. To identify the phenotype of these cells, we used fluorescence activated cell sorting (FACS) to isolate CD34+, CD15+, CD41+ and CD71+ fractions from the BM of three JAK2V617F-positive MPN patients (1 ET, 1 PV, 1 early PMF). We found nuclear JAK2 only in the fraction containing the CD34+ positive cells (Figure 3C, left panels). It should be noted that in these patients the CD34+ cells correspond to approximately 3% to 5% of total BM mononucleated cells. The nuclear localization of JAK2V617F was confirmed by WB analysis (Figure 3C, right panels). However, no predominant nuclear signal was detected in differentiated granulocytic, megakaryocytic and erythroid cells obtained from the patients (n=15) (Figure 3D). Similar results were obtained with PB cells (data not shown). The relocation of the mutated JAK2 to the cytoplasm was confirmed in K562 cells after their differentiation with PMA (Figure 4A). However, the relocation was not complete as observed for the primary BM cells and nuclear JAK2 was still observed. We believe that this is due to the nature of K562 cells, which are BCR-ABL-positive CML cells, and to the difficulty to obtain their terminal differentiation in vitro.

5.3 The JAK2 inhibitor AG490 relocate JAK2 in cytoplasm

To determine whether an alteration of JAK2 activity could interfere with the nuclear localization of JAK2, we incubated K562 cells expressing JAK2V617F or JAK2 with the selective JAK2 inhibitor AG490[158-160]. After 3 h of incubation at the IC50 dose of 25 uM, CIF images showed a relocalization of JAK2V617F to the cytoplasm in the vast majority of K562 cells (Figure 4B). Analyses with annexin V and propidium iodide did not reveal any significant change in the apoptotic rate of V617F-positive and wt-K562 cells.

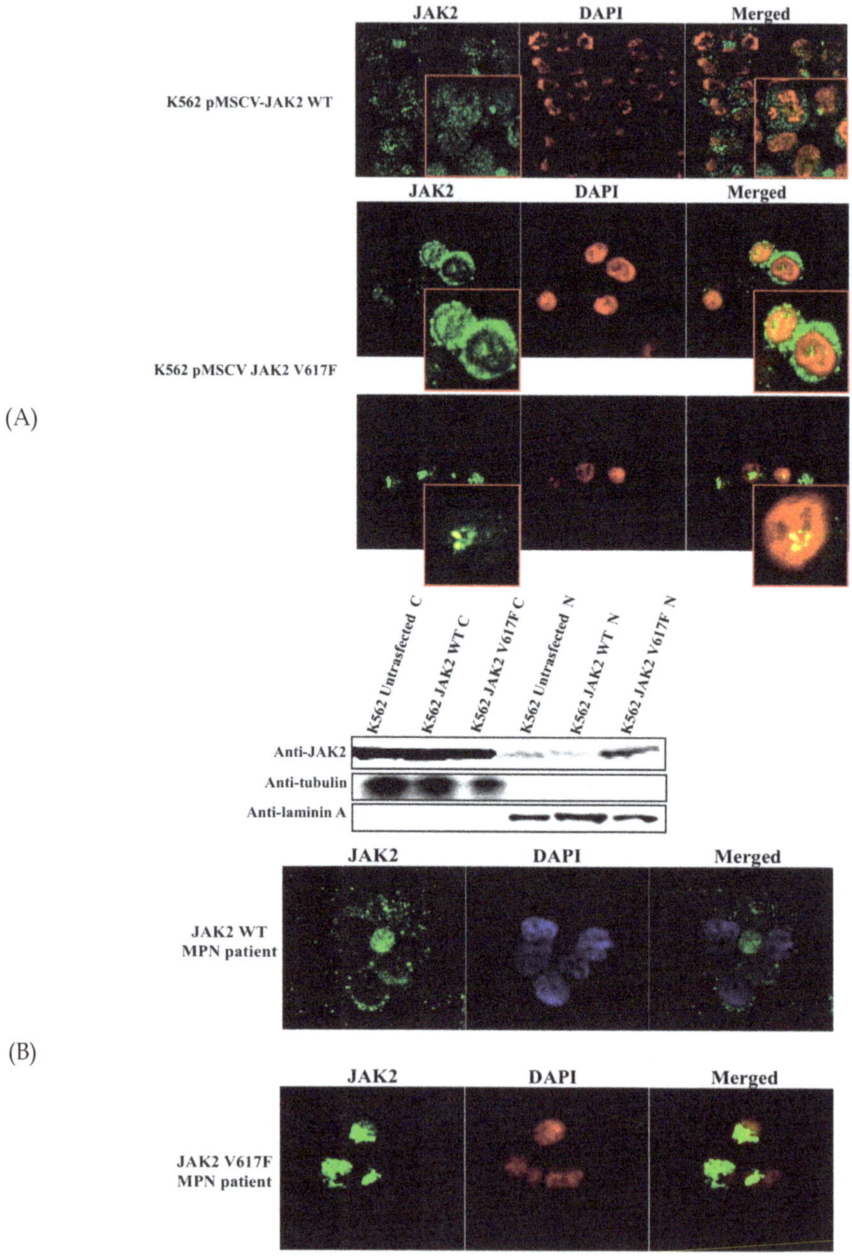

Fig. 3. V617F mutation favors nuclear translocation of JAK2 in K562 and early CD34+ progenitors isolated from BM of MPN patients. This translocation is not observed in differentiated cells.(A) CIF microscopy images of K562 cells stably transfected with pMSCV-JAK2 (upper panels) or pMSCV-JAK2V617F (middle and lower panels) and Western

blotting of cytoplasmic (C) and nuclear (N) fractions confirm that JAK2V617F is more abundant than JAK2 in K562 nuclei. (B)CIF images of BM cells from an MPN patient with wt JAK2 (upper panels) and an MPN patient with JAK2V617F (lower panels) confirm a nuclear increase of the mutated protein.

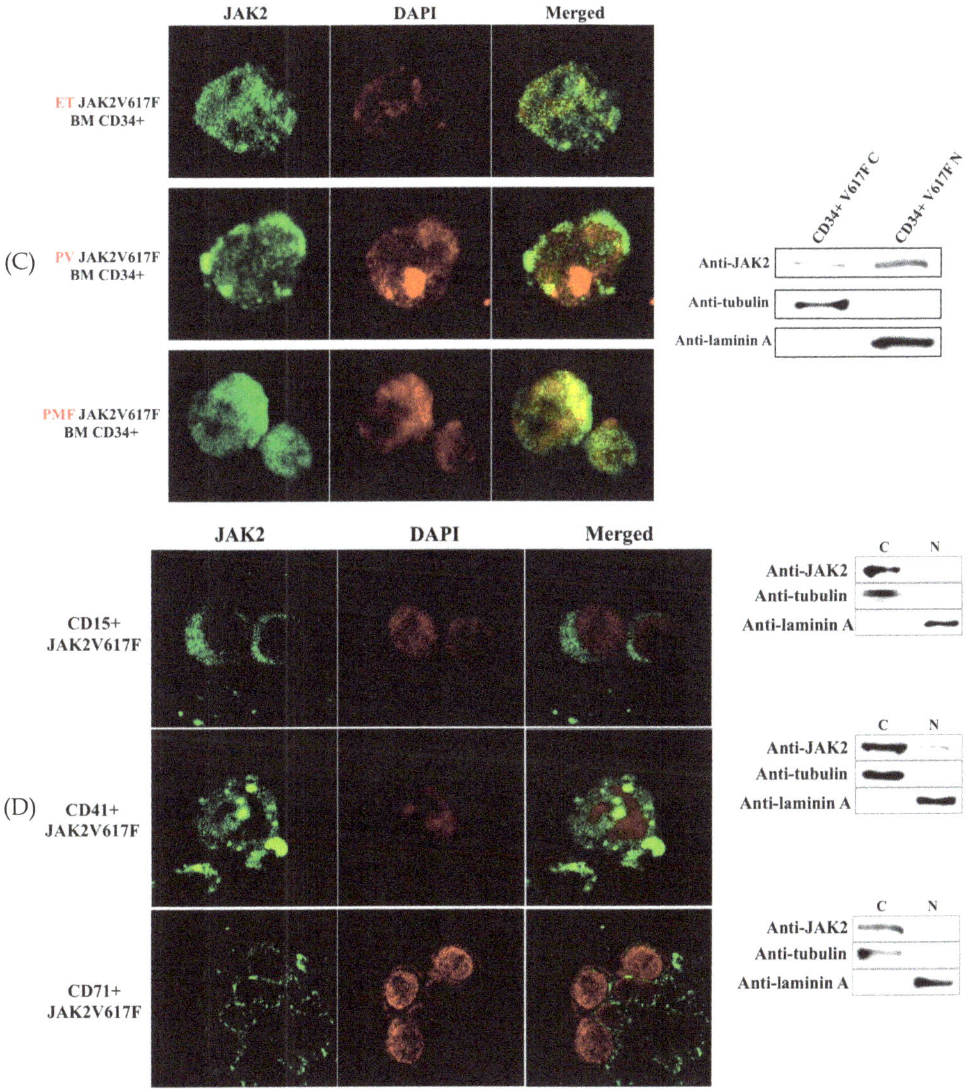

Fig. 3. V617F mutation favors nuclear translocation of JAK2 in K562 and early CD34+ progenitors isolated from BM of MPN patients. This translocation is not observed in differentiated cells.(C) Confocal IF demonstrates a predominantly nuclear accumulation of JAK2V617F in CD34+ cells isolated from BM of 1 ET, 1 PV and 1 earlyPMF (left panels) and Western blotting of cytoplasmic (C) and nuclear (N) extracts (right panel) confirm the data.

(D) Confocal IF images of CD15+, CD41+, CD71+ cells isolated from a JAK2V617F-positive MPN patient (PV, JAK2 allele burden 71%) and Western blotting of cytoplasmic (C) and nuclear (N) extracts (right panel). DAPI, 4,6-diamidino-2-phenylindole; Anti-JAK2, Cell Signaling monoclonal antibody; Anti-Tubulin and Anti-Laminin A, Sigma-Aldrich monoclonal antibodies.

5.4 V617F JAK2 up-regulates LMO2 and AG490 restores its level.

By QRT-PCR we show that the V617F mutation strongly up-regulates the expression of *LMO2* in K562 and in CD34+ cells (Figure 4C, left panels). The link between *LMO2* expression and JAK2 inhibition has been reported previously[156,157]. In our assay, the addition of AG490 progressively and completely restore*LMO2* levels in V617F expressing K562 (Figure 4C, right panels).

(A)

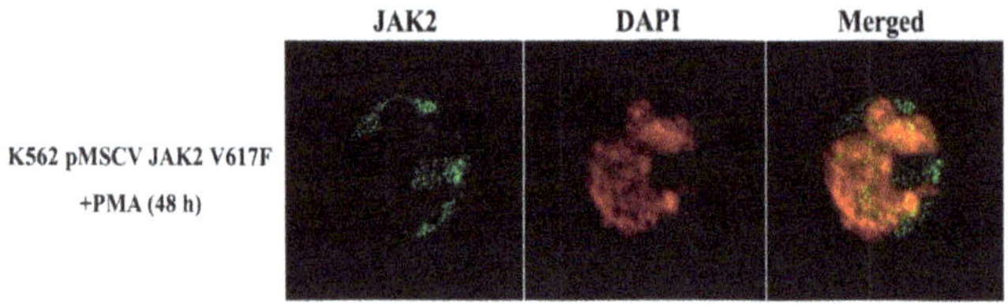

(B)

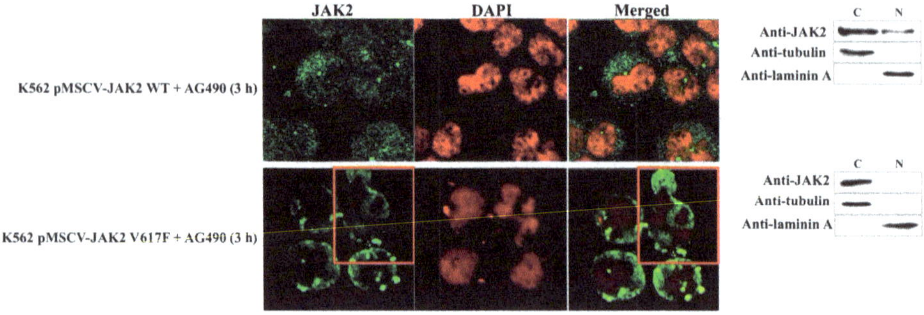

(C)

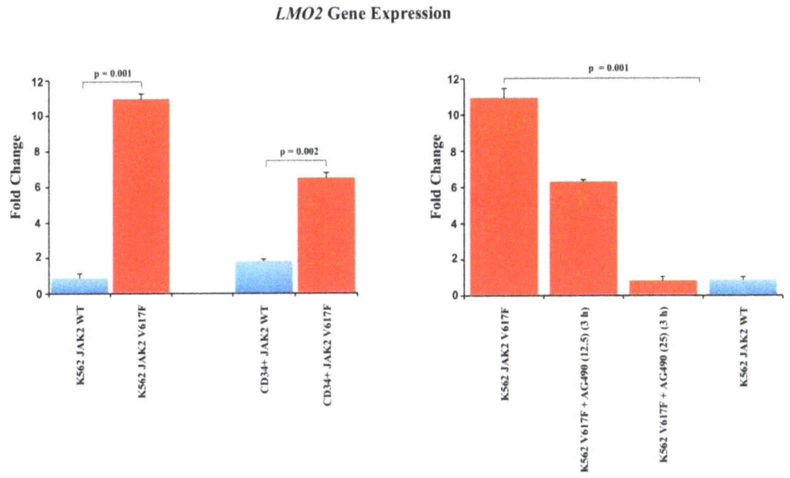

Fig. 4. V617F mutation causes up-regulation of *LMO2*. The JAK2 inhibitor AG490 replaces JAK2 into cytoplasm and restores LMO2 levels.(A) Confocal IF images show the redistribution of JAK2 and the replacement in the cytoplasm in V617F expressing K562 after PMA differentiation (B) Confocal IF images show the redistribution of JAK2 and the replacement in the cytoplasm in the vast majority of V617F expressing K562 (bottom panels) but not in wt cells (top panels) after AG490 incubation. (C) Quantitative RT-PCR revels that V617F mutation strongly up-regulates *LMO2* expression in K562 and in CD34+ cells (left panels). The addiction of AG490 progressively and completely restore*LMO2* levels in V617F expressing K562 (right panels). DAPI, 4,6-diamidino-2-phenylindole; Anti-JAK2, Cell Signaling monoclonal antibody.

6. Conclusions

Where do the major advances towards understanding the precise molecular bases of MPNs lead us? One striking observation is the key role played by various tyrosine kinases, constitutively activated either by balanced translocations or deletions generating fusion oncoproteins, or by activating point mutations. These mechanisms seem to be the molecular hallmark of MPNs, although there are probably alternative mechanisms directly involving cytokine receptors, adaptor proteins or transcription factors. All the molecular defects identified in MPNs to date confer proliferation and survival advantages on transformed cells, which retain the capacity to differentiate into mature cells. Differentiation may be disrupted by additional events, such as transcription factor deregulation, as frequently observed in acute myeloid leukaemia. *KIT* mutations and *FLT3* abnormalities are frequently found in cases of acute myeloid leukaemia. However, these molecular defects are now considered to be secondary events.

Strikingly, the diverse mutants and fusion proteins with constitutive tyrosine kinase activity each appear to stimulate a specific lineage. For example, PDGFR fusion proteins induce eosinophil differentiation, FGFR fusion proteins induce lymphoid malignancies, and

JAK2V617F mostly expands the erythroid compartment, whereas translocations involving the JAK2 kinase domain promote lymphoid proliferation as well. Thus, constitutive signalling via these different kinases is likely to result in effects on specific differentiation programs. Uncovering the molecular details of this specificity remains a major challenge, particularly as similar signalling molecules (*i.e.* STAT5, STAT3, RAS/MAPK, PI3K/AKT and others) are constitutively activated by all oncogenic fusion proteins.

Although the discovery of the JAK2V617F allele and the subsequent discovery of JAK2 exon 12 mutations and MPLW515L/K alleles have provided crucial insights into the genetic basis of PV, ET and PMF, many questions remain regarding the molecular pathogenesis of these MPNs. The activating mutations that cause JAK2 and MPL-negative MPN are not known, and the inherited and acquired alleles that can cooperate with JAK2V617F remain to be identified. In addition, the predominance of the JAK2V617F allele is surprising given that JAK2 exon 12 mutations, as well as activating JAK2 alleles identified in AML (JAK2T875N and JAK2ΔIREED), have similar in vitro and in vivo effects as JAK2V617F. The different JAK2 alleles might differentially interact with different cytokine receptor scaffolds, activate different signalling pathways, and/or be differentially affected by negative-feedback mechanisms; structural insight and additional in vitro and in vivo studies are needed to elucidate differences between JAK2V617F and the other activating JAK2 alleles. Another important question relates to the effects of JAK2V617F gene dosage on signalling and on phenotype. In vitro studies do not conclusively show whether the co-expression of wildtype JAK2 with JAK2V617F alters the signalling and/or transforming properties of the JAK2V617F kinase, and although retroviral models allow for an assessment of the in vivo effects of JAK2V617F expression, they do not provide the appropriate genetic context to investigate the importance of JAK2V617F gene dosage. Subsequent studies using more accurate genetic models will enable the delineation of the differential effects of JAK2V617F heterozygosity and homozygosity on signalling and on phenotype. Moreover, the role of the JAK2V617F allele in three distinct disorders of the myeloid lineage is not known, and the ability of different activated tyrosine kinases (for example, BCR-ABL and FIP1L1-PDGFRA) to cause distinct MPN remains to be delineated.

Dawson et al. identified a previously unrecognized nuclear role for JAK2 in the phosphorylation of the tyrosine 41 of the histone H3 with the exclusion of HP1a from chromatin and resulting in a disregulation of several JAK2-regulated genes such as LMO2 in haematopoietic cell lines and in one case on peripheral CD34+ cells from a JAK2V617F mutated PMF patient.

Our data corroborate recently published results of a nuclear localization of JAK2 in hematopoietic cells and they also extend these findings by showing that in all subtypes of MPN patients JAK2V617F accumulates in the nucleus of progenitor CD34+ cells while it remains mostly in the cytoplasm of their differentiated progeny. The chromatin alterations due to the preferential accumulation of JAK2V617F in the nucleus correlates with a significant increase in LMO2 expression in cell lines and in sorted CD34+ cells. The selective JAK2 inhibitor AG490 is able to revert nuclear JAK2 and normalize LMO2 levels in vitro, suggesting how the block in JAK2 nuclear translocation could be a new treatment strategy for JAK2 mutated patients. A question that remains to be answered is why mutated JAK2 is found only in the cytoplasm of the differentiated cells. MPN are clonal disorders arising in a pluripotent hematopoietic stem cell and it is well known that the constitutive activation of

JAK2 provides a sustained growth and survival advantage to the hematopoietic mutated stem cell clones. Signaling by the mutated kinase utilizes normal pathways, and normal or mutated JAK2 regulate EPO, TPO, and GCS-F response during differentiation, though they are probably not necessary to the differentiated cell. The signals that are required for the translocation of normal and mutated JAK2 to the nucleus are unknown. It is possible that the activation of the kinase by phosphorylation could be the first one of a number of modifications that control nuclear translocation, similarly to what happens to the STAT proteins. If this is true, then it is also possible that as the cell undergoes differentiaition these modifications are shut off, leaving mutated JAK2 predominantly in the cytoplasm.

7. Acknowledgements

The Authors thank Prof. Anthony R. Green (Cambridge Institute for Medical Research and Department of Haematology, University of Cambridge, Cambridge, United Kingdom) for his kind contribution and suggestions.

8. References

[1] Tefferi A, Gangat N, Wolanskyj AP, Schwager S, Pardanani A, Lasho TL *et al.* 20+ Year without leukemic or fibrotic transformation in essential thrombocythemia or polycythemia vera: predictors at diagnosis. *Eur J Haematol* 2008; 80: 386–390.

[2] Damashek W. Some speculations on the myeloproliferative syndromes.*Blood* 1951; 6: 372–375.

[3] Adamson JW. Analysis of haemopoiesis: the use of cell markers and *in vitro* culture techniques in studies of clonal haemopathies in man. *Clin Haematol* 1984; 13: 489–502.

[4] Prchal JF, Axelrad AA. Bone-marrow responses in polycythemia vera. *N Engl J Med* 1974; 290: 1382.

[5] Roder S, Steimle C, Meinhardt G, Pahl HL. STAT3 is constitutively active in some patients with polycythemia rubra vera. *Exp Hematol* 2001; 29: 694–702.

[6] Dai C, Chung IJ, Krantz SB. Increased erythropoiesis in polycythemia vera is associated with increased erythroid progenitor proliferation and increased phosphorylation of Akt/PKB. *Exp Hematol* 2005; 33: 152–158.

[7] Silva M, Richard C, Benito A, Sanz C, Olalla I, Fernandez-Luna JL. Expression of Bcl-x in erythroid precursors from patients with polycythemia vera. *N Engl J Med* 1998; 338: 564–571.

[8] Dai CH, Krantz SB, Dessypris EN, Means Jr RT, Horn ST, Gilbert HS. Polycythemia vera. II. Hypersensitivity of bone marrow erythroid, granulocyte-macrophage, and megakaryocyte progenitor cells to interleukin-3 and granulocyte gmacrophage colony-stimulating factor.*Blood* 1992; 80: 891–899.

[9] Dai CH, Krantz SB, Green WF, Gilbert HS. Polycythaemia vera. III. Burst-forming units-erythroid (BFU-E) response to stem cell factor and c-kit receptor expression. *Br J Haematol* 1994; 86: 12–21.

[10] Correa PN, Eskinazi D, Axelrad AA. Circulating erythroid progenitors in polycythemia vera are hypersensitive to insulin-like growth factor-1 *in vitro*: studies in an improved serum-free medium. *Blood* 1994; 83: 99–112.

[11] Axelrad AA, Eskinazi D, Correa PN, Amato D. Hypersensitivity of circulating progenitor cells to megakaryocyte growth and development factor (PEG-rHu MGDF) in essential thrombocythemia. *Blood* 2000; 96: 3310-3321.

[12] Dai C, Krantz SB. Increased expression of the INK4a/ARF locus in polycythemia vera. *Blood* 2001; 97: 3424-3432.

[13] James C, Ugo V, Le Couedic JP, Staerk J, Delhommeau F, Lacout C *et al.* A unique clonal JAK2 mutation leading to constitutive signalling causes polycythaemia vera. *Nature* 2005; 434: 1144-1148.

[14] Baxter EJ, Scott LM, Campbell PJ, East C, Fourouclas N, Swanton S *et al.* Acquired mutation of the tyrosine kinase JAK2 in human myeloproliferative disorders. *Lancet* 2005; 365: 1054-1061.

[15] Kralovics R, Passamonti F, Buser AS, Teo SS, Tiedt R, Passweg JR *et al.* A gain-of-function mutation of JAK2 in myeloproliferative disorders. *N Engl J Med* 2005; 352: 1779-1790.

[16] Levine RL, Wadleigh M, Cools J, Ebert BL, Wernig G, Huntly BJ *et al.* Activating mutation in the tyrosine kinase JAK2 in polycythemia vera, essential thrombocythemia, and myeloid metaplasia with myelofibrosis.*Cancer Cell* 2005; 7: 387-397.

[17] Zhao R, Xing S, Li Z, Fu X, Li Q, Krantz SB *et al.* Identification of an acquired JAK2 mutation in polycythemia vera. *J Biol Chem* 2005; 280: 22788-22792.

[18] Scott LM, Tong W, Levine RL, Scott MA, Beer PA, Stratton MR *et al.* JAK2 exon 12 mutations in polycythemia vera and idiopathic erythrocytosis. *N Engl J Med* 2007; 356: 459-468.

[19] Pikman Y, Lee BH, Mercher T, McDowell E, Ebert BL, Gozo M *et al.* MPLW515L is a novel somatic activating mutation in myelofibrosis with myeloid metaplasia. *PLoS Med* 2006; 3: e270.

[20] Pardanani AD, Levine RL, Lasho T, Pikman Y, Mesa RA, Wadleigh M *et al.* MPL515 mutations in myeloproliferative and other myeloid disorders: a study of 1182 patients. *Blood* 2006; 108: 3472-3476.

[21] Staerk J, Lacout C, Smith SO, Vainchenker W, Constantinescu SN. An amphipathic motif at the transmembrane-cytoplasmic junction prevents autonomous activation of the thrombopoietin receptor. *Blood* 2006; 107: 1864-1871.

[22] Campbell PJ, Scott LM, Buck G, Wheatley K, East CL, Marsden JT *et al.* Definition of subtypes of essential thrombocythaemia and relation to polycythaemia vera based on JAK2 V617F mutation status: a prospective study. *Lancet* 2005; 366: 1945-1953.

[23] Lacout C, Pisani DF, Tulliez M, Moreau Gachelin F, Vainchenker W, Villeval JL. JAK2V617F expression in murine hematopoietic cells leads to MPD mimicking human PV with secondary myelofibrosis. *Blood* 2006; 108: 1652-1660.

[24] Tiedt R, Hao-Shen H, Sobas MA, Looser R, Dirnhofer S, Schwaller J *et al.* Ratio of mutant JAK2-V617F to wild-type Jak2 determines the MPD phenotypes in transgenic mice. *Blood* 2008; 111: 3931-3940.

[25] Scott LM, Scott MA, Campbell PJ, Green AR. Progenitors homozygous for the V617F mutation occur in most patients with polycythemia vera, but not essential thrombocythemia. *Blood* 2006; 108: 2435-2437.

[26] Dupont S, Masse A, James C, Teyssandier I, Lecluse Y, Larbret F *et al.* The JAK2 617V>F mutation triggers erythropoietin hypersensitivity and terminal erythroid amplification in primary cells from patients with polycythemia vera. *Blood* 2007; 110: 1013-1021.
[27] Pardanani A, Fridley BL, Lasho TL, Gilliland DG, Tefferi A. Host genetic variation contributes to phenotypic diversity in myeloproliferative disorders. *Blood* 2008; 111: 2785-2789.
[28] Jamieson CH, Gotlib J, Durocher JA, Chao MP, Mariappan MR, Lay M *et al.* The JAK2 V617F mutation occurs in hematopoietic stem cells in polycythemia vera and predisposes toward erythroid differentiation. *Proc Natl Acad Sci USA* 2006; 103: 6224-6229.
[29] Delhommeau F, Dupont S, Tonetti C, Masse A, Godin I, Le Couedic JP *et al.* Evidence that the JAK2 G1849T (V617F) mutation occurs in a lymphomyeloid progenitor in polycythemia vera and idiopathic myelofibrosis. *Blood* 2007; 109: 71-77.
[30] James C, Mazurier F, Dupont S, Chaligne R, Lamrissi-Garcia I, Tulliez M *et al.* The hematopoietic stem cell compartment of JAK2V617F positive myeloproliferative disorders is a reflection of disease heterogeneity. *Blood*2008; e-pub ahead of print 8 July 2008; doi:10.1182/blood-2008-02-137877.
[31] Sieburg HB, Cho RH, Dykstra B, Uchida N, Eaves CJ, Muller-Sieburg CE. The hematopoietic stem compartment consists of a limited number of discrete stem cell subsets. *Blood* 2006; 107: 2311-2316.
[32] Pardanani A, Lasho TL, Schwager S, Finke C, Hussein K, Pruthi RK *et al.* JAK2V617F prevalence and allele burden in non-splanchnic venous thrombosis in the absence of overt myeloproliferative disorder. *Leukemia*2007; 21: 1828-1829.
[33] Pardanani A, Lasho TL, Hussein K, Schwager SM, Finke CM, Pruthi RK *et al.* JAK2V617F mutation screening as part of the hypercoagulable work-up in the absence of splanchnic venous thrombosis or overt myeloproliferative neoplasm: assessment of value in a series of 664 consecutive patients.*Mayo Clin Proc* 2008; 83: 457-459.
[34] Kiladjian JJ, Cervantes F, Leebeek FW, Marzac C, Cassinat B, Chevret S *et al.* The impact of JAK2 and MPL mutations on diagnosis and prognosis of splanchnic vein thrombosis. A report on 241 cases. *Blood* 2008; 111: 4922-4929.
[35] Patel RK, Lea NC, Heneghan MA, Westwood NB, Milojkovic D, Thanigaikumar M *et al.* Prevalence of the activating JAK2 tyrosine kinase mutation V617F in the Budd-Chiari syndrome. *Gastroenterology* 2006; 130: 2031-2038.
[36] Leibundgut EO, Horn MP, Brunold C, Pfanner-Meyer B, Marti D, Hirsiger H*et al.* Hematopoietic and endothelial progenitor cell trafficking in patients with myeloproliferative diseases. *Hematologica* 2006; 91: 1467-1474.
[37] Van Pelt K, Nollet F, Selleslag D, Knoops L, Constantinescu SN, Criel A *et al.* The JAK2V617F mutation can occur in a hematopoietic stem cell that exhibits no proliferative advantage: a case of human allogeneic transplantation. *Blood* 2008; 112: 921-922.
[38] Kralovics R, Teo SS, Li S, Theocharides A, Buser AS, Tichelli A *et al.* Acquisition of the V617F mutation of JAK2 is a late genetic event in a subset of patients with myeloproliferative disorders. *Blood* 2006; 108: 1377-1380.

[39] Theocharides A, Boissinot M, Girodon F, Garand R, Teo SS, Lippert E *et al.* Leukemic blasts in transformed JAK2-V617F-positive myeloproliferative disorders are frequently negative for the JAK2-V617F mutation. *Blood*2007; 110: 375–379.

[40] Nussenzveig RH, Swierczek SI, Jelinek J, Gaikwad A, Liu E, Verstovsek S *et al.* Polycythemia vera is not initiated by JAK2V617F mutation. *Exp Hematol*2007; 35: 32–38.

[41] Lodish HF, Berk A, Kaiser CA, Krieger M, Scott MP, Bretscher A *et al.Molecular Cell Biology, Chapter 16 Cell Signaling II: Signaling Pathways that Control Gene Activity*, 6th edn. WH Freeman and Company: New York, NY, 2007, pp 666–667.

[42] Wilks AF, Harpur AG, Kurban RR, Ralph SJ, Zurcher G, Ziemiecki A. Two novel protein-tyrosine kinases, each with a second phosphotransferase-related catalytic domain, define a new class of protein kinase. *Mol Cell Biol*1991; 11: 2057–2065.

[43] Girault JA, Labesse G, Mornon JP, Callebaut I. The N-termini of FAK and JAKs contain divergent band 4.1 domains. *Trends Biochem Sci* 1999; 24: 54–57.

[44] Huang LJ, Constantinescu SN, Lodish HF. The N-terminal domain of Janus kinase 2 is required for Golgi processing and cell surface expression of erythropoietin receptor. *Mol Cell* 2001; 8: 1327–1338.

[45] Radtke S, Hermanns HM, Haan C, Schmitz-Van De Leur H, Gascan H, Heinrich PC *et al.* Novel role for Janus kinase 1 in the regulation of oncostatin M receptor surface expression. *J Biol Chem* 2002; 10: 10.

[46] Ragimbeau J, Dondi E, Alcover A, Eid P, Uze G, Pellegrini S. The tyrosine kinase Tyk2 controls IFNAR1 cell surface expression. *EMBO J* 2003; 22: 537–547.

[47] Royer Y, Staerk J, Costuleanu M, Courtoy PJ, Constantinescu SN. Janus kinases affect thrombopoietin receptor cell surface localization and stability. *J Biol Chem* 2005; 280: 27251–27261.

[48] Yeh TC, Dondi E, Uze G, Pellegrini S. A dual role for the kinase-like domain of the tyrosine kinase Tyk2 in interferon-alpha signaling. *Proc Natl Acad Sci USA* 2000; 97: 8991–8996.

[49] Saharinen P, Silvennoinen O. The pseudokinase domain is required for suppression of basal activity of Jak2 and Jak3 tyrosine kinases and for cytokine-inducible activation of signal transduction. *J Biol Chem* 2002; 277: 47954–47963.

[50] Lindauer K, Loerting T, Liedl KR, Kroemer RT. Prediction of the structure of human Janus kinase 2 (JAK2) comprising the two carboxy-terminal domains reveals a mechanism for autoregulation. *Protein Eng* 2001; 14: 27–37.

[51] Staerk J, Kallin A, Demoulin J-B, Vainchenker W, Constantinescu SN. JAK1 and Tyk2 activation by the homologous polycythemia vera JAK2 V617F mutation: cross-talk with IGF1 receptor. *J Biol Chem* 2005; 280: 41893–41899.

[52] Jeong EG, Kim MS, Nam HK, Min CK, Lee S, Chung YJ *et al.* Somatic mutations of JAK1 and JAK3 in acute leukemias and solid cancers. *Clin Cancer Res* 2008; 14: 3716–3721.

[53] Flex E, Petrangeli V, Stella L, Chiaretti S, Hornakova T, Knoops L *et al.* Somatically acquired JAK1 mutations in adult acute lymphoblastic leukemia. *J Exp Med* 2008; 205: 751–758.

[54] Kohlhuber F, Rogers NC, Watling D, Feng J, Guschin D, Briscoe J *et al.* A JAK1/JAK2 chimera can sustain alpha and gamma interferon responses. *Mol Cell Biol* 1997; 17: 695–706.

[55] Li Z, Xu M, Xing S, Ho WT, Ishii T, Li Q *et al.* Erlotinib effectively inhibits JAK2V617F activity and polycythemia vera cell growth. *J Biol Chem* 2007;282: 3428-3432.

[56] Miura O, Cleveland JL, Ihle JN. Inactivation of erythropoietin receptor function by point mutations in a region having homology with other cytokine receptors. *Mol Cell Biol* 1993; 13: 1788-1795.

[57] Wernig G, Gonneville JR, Crowley BJ, Rodrigues MS, Reddy MM, Hudon HE*et al.* The Jak2V617F oncogene associated with myeloproliferative diseases requires a functional FERM domain for transformation and for expression of the Myc and Pim proto-oncogenes. *Blood* 2008; 111: 3751-3759.

[58] Behrmann I, Smyczek T, Heinrich PC, Schmitz-Van de Leur H, Komyod W, Giese B *et al.* Janus kinase (Jak) subcellular localization revisited: the exclusive membrane localization of endogenous Janus kinase 1 by cytokine receptor interaction uncovers the Jak.receptor complex to be equivalent to a receptor tyrosine kinase. *J Biol Chem* 2004; 279: 35486-35493.

[59] Funakoshi-Tago M, Pelletier S, Moritake H, Parganas E, Ihle JN. Jak2 FERM domain interaction with the erythropoietin receptor regulates Jak2 kinase activity. *Mol Cell Biol* 2008; 28: 1792-1801.

[60] Lu X, Huang LJ, Lodish HF. Dimerization by a cytokine receptor is necessary for constitutive activation of JAK2V617F. *J Biol Chem* 2008; 283: 5258-5266.

[61] Saharinen P, Takaluoma K, Silvennoinen O. Regulation of the Jak2 tyrosine kinase by its pseudokinase domain. *Mol Cell Biol* 2000; 20: 3387-3395.

[62] Witthuhn BA, Quelle FW, Silvennoinen O, Yi T, Tang B, Miura O *et al.* JAK2 associates with the erythropoietin receptor and is tyrosine phosphorylated and activated following stimulation with erythropoietin. *Cell* 1993; 74: 227-236.

[63] Tortolani PJ, Johnston JA, Bacon CM, McVicar DW, Shimosaka A, Linnekin D*et al.* Thrombopoietin induces tyrosine phosphorylation and activation of the Janus kinase, JAK2. *Blood* 1995; 85: 3444-3451.

[64] Drachman JG, Millett KM, Kaushansky K. Thrombopoietin signal transduction requires functional JAK2, not TYK2. *J Biol Chem* 1999; 274: 13480-13484.

[65] Shimoda K, Feng J, Murakami H, Nagata S, Watling D, Rogers NC *et al.* Jak1 plays an essential role for receptor phosphorylation and Stat activation in response to granulocyte colony-stimulating factor. *Blood* 1997;90: 597-604.

[66] Touw IP, van de Geijn GJ. Granulocyte colony-stimulating factor and its receptor in normal myeloid cell development, leukemia and related blood cell disorders. *Front Biosci* 2007; 12: 800-815.

[67] Watowich SS, Wu H, Socolovsky M, Klingmuller U, Constantinescu SN, Lodish HF. Cytokine receptor signal transduction and the control of hematopoietic cell development. *Annu Rev Cell Dev Biol* 1996; 12: 91-128.

[68] Constantinescu SN, Keren T, Socolovsky M, Nam H, Henis YI, Lodish HF. Ligand-independent oligomerization of cell-surface erythropoietin receptor is mediated by the transmembrane domain. *Proc Natl Acad Sci USA* 2001;98: 4379-4384.

[69] Constantinescu SN, Huang LJ, Nam H, Lodish HF. The erythropoietin receptor cytosolic juxtamembrane domain contains an essential, precisely oriented, hydrophobic motif. *Mol Cell* 2001; 7: 377-385.

[70] Seubert N, Royer Y, Staerk J, Kubatzky KF, Moucadel V, Krishnakumar S *et al.* Active and inactive orientations of the transmembrane and cytosolic domains of the erythropoietin receptor dimer. *Mol Cell* 2003; 12: 1239–1250.
[71] Lu X, Levine R, Tong W, Wernig G, Pikman Y, Zarnegar S *et al.* Expression of a homodimeric type I cytokine receptor is required for JAK2V617F-mediated transformation. *Proc Natl Acad Sci USA* 2005; 102: 18962–18967.
[72] Ihle JN, Gilliland DG. Jak2: normal function and role in hematopoietic disorders. *Curr Opin Genet Dev* 2007; 17: 8–14.
[73] Kirito K, Nakajima K, Watanabe T, Uchida M, Tanaka M, Ozawa K *et al.* Identification of the human erythropoietin receptor region required for Stat1 and Stat3 activation. *Blood* 2002; 99: 102–110.
[74] Gobert S, Chretien S, Gouilleux F, Muller O, Pallard C, Dusanter-Fourt I *et al.* Identification of tyrosine residues within the intracellular domain of the erythropoietin receptor crucial for STAT5 activation. *EMBO J* 1996; 15: 2434–2441.
[75] Klingmuller U, Bergelson S, Hsiao JG, Lodish HF. Multiple tyrosine residues in the cytosolic domain of the erythropoietin receptor promote activation of STAT5. *Proc Natl Acad Sci USA* 1996; 93: 8324–8328.
[76] Socolovsky M, Fallon AE, Wang S, Brugnara C, Lodish HF. Fetal anemia and apoptosis of red cell progenitors in Stat5a-/-5b-/- mice: a direct role for Stat5 in Bcl-X(L) induction. *Cell* 1999; 98: 181–191.
[77] Klingmuller U, Wu H, Hsiao JG, Toker A, Duckworth BC, Cantley LC *et al.* Identification of a novel pathway important for proliferation and differentiation of primary erythroid progenitors. *Proc Natl Acad Sci USA*1997; 94: 3016–3021.
[78] Damen JE, Cutler RL, Jiao H, Yi T, Krystal G. Phosphorylation of tyrosine 503 in the erythropoietin receptor (EpR) is essential for binding the P85 subunit of phosphatidylinositol (PI) 3-kinase and for EpR-associated PI 3-kinase activity. *J Biol Chem* 1995; 270: 23402–23408.
[79] Bao H, Jacobs-Helber SM, Lawson AE, Penta K, Wickrema A, Sawyer ST. Protein kinase B (c-Akt), phosphatidylinositol 3-kinase, and STAT5 are activated by erythropoietin (EPO) in HCD57 erythroid cells but are constitutively active in an EPO-independent, apoptosis-resistant subclone (HCD57-SREI cells). *Blood* 1999; 93: 3757–3773.
[80] Kashii Y, Uchida M, Kirito K, Tanaka M, Nishijima K, Toshima M *et al.* A member of Forkhead family transcription factor, FKHRL1, is one of the downstream molecules of phosphatidylinositol 3-kinase–Akt activation pathway in erythropoietin signal transduction. *Blood* 2000; 96: 941–949.
[81] Zhao W, Kitidis C, Fleming MD, Lodish HF, Ghaffari S. Erythropoietin stimulates phosphorylation and activation of GATA-1 via the PI3-kinase/AKT signaling pathway. *Blood* 2006; 107: 907–915.
[82] Butcher CM, Hahn U, To LB, Gecz J, Wilkins EJ, Scott HS *et al.* Two novel JAK2 exon 12 mutations in JAK2V617F-negative polycythaemia vera patients. *Leukemia* 2008; 22: 870–873.
[83] Miyakawa Y, Oda A, Druker BJ, Kato T, Miyazaki H, Handa M *et al.* Recombinant thrombopoietin induces rapid protein tyrosine phosphorylation of Janus kinase 2 and Shc in human blood platelets. *Blood* 1995; 86: 23–27.

[84] Sattler M, Durstin MA, Frank DA, Okuda K, Kaushansky K, Salgia R *et al.* The thrombopoietin receptor c-MPL activates JAK2 and TYK2 tyrosine kinases. *Exp Hematol* 1995; 23: 1040–1048.

[85] Miyakawa Y, Rojnuckarin P, Habib T, Kaushansky K. Thrombopoietin induces phosphoinositol 3-kinase activation through SHP2, Gab, and insulin receptor substrate proteins in BAF3 cells and primary murine megakaryocytes. *J Biol Chem* 2001; 276: 2494–2502.

[86] Drachman JG, Griffin JD, Kaushansky K. The c-Mpl ligand (thrombopoietin) stimulates tyrosine phosphorylation of Jak2, Shc, and c-Mpl. *J Biol Chem*1995; 270: 4979–4982.

[87] Miyakawa Y, Oda A, Druker BJ, Miyazaki H, Handa M, Ohashi H *et al.* Thrombopoietin induces tyrosine phosphorylation of Stat3 and Stat5 in human blood platelets. *Blood* 1996; 87: 439–446.

[88] Drachman JG, Kaushansky K. Dissecting the thrombopoietin receptor: functional elements of the Mpl cytoplasmic domain. *Proc Natl Acad Sci USA*1997; 94: 2350–2355.

[89] Rouyez MC, Boucheron C, Gisselbrecht S, Dusanter-Fourt I, Porteu F. Control of thrombopoietin-induced megakaryocytic differentiation by the mitogen-activated protein kinase pathway. *Mol Cell Biol* 1997; 17: 4991–5000.

[90] Filippi MD, Porteu F, Le Pesteur F, Schiavon V, Millot GA, Vainchenker W *et al.* Requirement for mitogen-activated protein kinase activation in the response of embryonic stem cell-derived hematopoietic cells to thrombopoietin *in vitro*. *Blood* 2002; 99: 1174–1182.

[91] Olthof SG, Fatrai S, Drayer AL, Tyl MR, Vellenga E, Schuringa JJ. Downregulation of STAT5 in CD34+ cells promotes megakaryocytic development while activation of STAT5 drives erythropoiesis. *Stem Cells*2008; 26: 1732–1742.

[92] Cocault L, Bouscary D, Le Bousse Kerdiles C, Clay D, Picard F, Gisselbrecht S *et al.* Ectopic expression of murine TPO receptor (c-mpl) in mice is pathogenic and induces erythroblastic proliferation. *Blood* 1996; 88: 1656–1665.

[93] Tong W, Lodish HF. Lnk inhibits Tpo-mpl signaling and Tpo-mediated megakaryocytopoiesis. *J Exp Med* 2004; 200: 569–580.

[94] Tong W, Zhang J, Lodish HF. Lnk inhibits erythropoiesis and Epo-dependent JAK2 activation and downstream signaling pathways. *Blood* 2005; 105: 4604–4612.

[95] Moliterno AR, Spivak JL. Posttranslational processing of the thrombopoietin receptor is impaired in polycythemia vera. *Blood* 1999; 94: 2555–2561.

[96] Moliterno AR, Williams DM, Rogers O, Spivak JL. Molecular mimicry in the chronic myeloproliferative disorders: reciprocity between quantitative JAK2 V617F and Mpl expression. *Blood* 2006; 108: 3913–3915.

[97] Dahlen DD, Broudy VC, Drachman JG. Internalization of the thrombopoietin receptor is regulated by 2 cytoplasmic motifs. *Blood* 2003; 102: 102–108.

[98] Onishi M, Mui AL, Morikawa Y, Cho L, Kinoshita S, Nolan GP *et al.* Identification of an oncogenic form of the thrombopoietin receptor MPL using retrovirus-mediated gene transfer. *Blood* 1996; 88: 1399–1406.

[99] Ding J, Komatsu H, Wakita A, Kato-Uranishi M, Ito M, Satoh A *et al.* Familial essential thrombocythemia associated with a dominant-positive activating mutation of the c-

MPL gene, which encodes for the receptor for thrombopoietin. *Blood* 2004; 103: 4198–4200.

[100] Malinge S, Ragu C, Della-Valle V, Pisani D, Constantinescu SN, Perez C *et al.* Activating mutations in human acute megakaryoblastic leukemia. *Blood*2008.

[101] Bumm TG, Elsea C, Corbin AS, Loriaux M, Sherbenou D, Wood L *et al.* Characterization of murine JAK2V617F-positive myeloproliferative disease.*Cancer Res* 2006; 66: 11156–11165.

[102] Gangat N, Strand J, Li CY, Wu W, Pardanani A, Tefferi A. Leucocytosis in polycythaemia vera predicts both inferior survival and leukaemic transformation. *Br J Haematol* 2007; 138: 354–358.

[103] Kralovics R, Teo SS, Buser AS, Brutsche M, Tiedt R, Tichelli A *et al.* Altered gene expression in myeloproliferative disorders correlates with activation of signaling by the V617F mutation of Jak2. *Blood* 2005; 106: 3374–3376.

[104] Passamonti F, Rumi E, Pietra D, Della Porta MG, Boveri E, Pascutto C *et al.* Relation between JAK2 (V617F) mutation status, granulocyte activation, and constitutive mobilization of CD34+ cells into peripheral blood in myeloproliferative disorders. *Blood* 2006; 107: 3676–3682.

[105] Xu M, Bruno E, Chao J, Huang S, Finazzi G, Fruchtman SM *et al.* Constitutive mobilization of CD34+ cells into the peripheral blood in idiopathic myelofibrosis may be due to the action of a number of proteases. *Blood* 2005; 105: 4508–4515.

[106] Rosti V, Massa M, Vannucchi AM, Bergamaschi G, Campanelli R, Pecci A *et al.* The expression of CXCR4 is down-regulated on the CD34+ cells of patients with myelofibrosis with myeloid metaplasia. *Blood Cells Mol Dis*2007; 38: 280–286.

[107] Migliaccio AR, Martelli F, Verrucci M, Migliaccio G, Vannucchi AM, Ni H *et al.* Altered SDF-1/CXCR4 axis in patients with primary myelofibrosis and in the Gata1 low mouse model of the disease. *Exp Hematol* 2008; 36: 158–171.

[108] Broxmeyer HE, Orschell CM, Clapp DW, Hangoc G, Cooper S, Plett PA *et al.* Rapid mobilization of murine and human hematopoietic stem and progenitor cells with AMD3100, a CXCR4 antagonist. *J Exp Med* 2005; 201: 1307–1318.

[109] Feng J, Witthuhn BA, Matsuda T, Kohlhuber F, Kerr IM, Ihle JN. Activation of Jak2 catalytic activity requires phosphorylation of Y1007 in the kinase activation loop. *Mol Cell Biol* 1997; 17: 2497–2501.

[110] Matsuda T, Feng J, Witthuhn BA, Sekine Y, Ihle JN. Determination of the transphosphorylation sites of Jak2 kinase. *Biochem Biophys Res Commun*2004; 325: 586–594.

[111] Argetsinger LS, Kouadio JL, Steen H, Stensballe A, Jensen ON, Carter-Su C. Autophosphorylation of JAK2 on tyrosines 221 and 570 regulates its activity. *Mol Cell Biol* 2004; 24: 4955–4967.

[112] Feener EP, Rosario F, Dunn SL, Stancheva Z, Myers Jr MG. Tyrosine phosphorylation of Jak2 in the JH2 domain inhibits cytokine signaling. *Mol Cell Biol* 2004; 24: 4968–4978.

[113] Funakoshi-Tago M, Pelletier S, Matsuda T, Parganas E, Ihle JN. Receptor specific downregulation of cytokine signaling by autophosphorylation in the FERM domain of Jak2. *EMBO J* 2006; 25: 4763–4772.

[114] Kurzer JH, Argetsinger LS, Zhou YJ, Kouadio JL, O'Shea JJ, Carter-Su C. Tyrosine 813 is a site of JAK2 autophosphorylation critical for activation of JAK2 by SH2-B beta. *Mol Cell Biol* 2004; 24: 4557–4570.

[115] Nishi M, Werner ED, Oh BC, Frantz JD, Dhe-Paganon S, Hansen L *et al.* Kinase activation through dimerization by human SH2-B. *Mol Cell Biol*2005; 25: 2607–2621.

[116] Vainchenker W, Constantinescu SN. A unique activating mutation in JAK2 is at the origin of polycythemia vera and allows a new classification of myeloproliferative diseases. *Hematology Am Soc Hematol Educ Program*2005; 2005: 195–200.

[117] Mesa RA, Tefferi A, Lasho TS, Loegering D, McClure RF, Powell HL *et al.* Janus kinase 2 (V617F) mutation status, signal transducer and activator of transcription-3 phosphorylation and impaired neutrophil apoptosis in myelofibrosis with myeloid metaplasia. *Leukemia* 2006; 20: 1800–1808.

[118] Teofili L, Martini M, Cenci T, Petrucci G, Torti L, Storti S *et al.* Different STAT-3 and STAT-5 phosphorylation discriminates among Ph-negative chronic myeloproliferative diseases and is independent of the V617F JAK-2 mutation. *Blood* 2007; 110: 354–359.

[119] Nicholson SE, De Souza D, Fabri LJ, Corbin J, Willson TA, Zhang JG *et al.* Suppressor of cytokine signaling-3 preferentially binds to the SHP-2-binding site on the shared cytokine receptor subunit gp130. *Proc Natl Acad Sci USA* 2000; 97: 6493–6498.

[120] Schmitz J, Weissenbach M, Haan S, Heinrich PC, Schaper F. SOCS3 exerts its inhibitory function on interleukin-6 signal transduction through the SHP2 recruitment site of gp130. *J Biol Chem* 2000; 275: 12848–12856.

[121] Jenkins BJ, Roberts AW, Najdovska M, Grail D, Ernst M. The threshold of gp130-dependent STAT3 signaling is critical for normal regulation of hematopoiesis. *Blood* 2005; 105: 3512–3520.

[122] Yoshimura A, Naka T, Kubo M. SOCS proteins, cytokine signalling and immune regulation. *Nat Rev Immunol* 2007; 7: 454–465.

[123] Hortner M, Nielsch U, Mayr LM, Heinrich PC, Haan S. A new high affinity binding site for suppressor of cytokine signaling-3 on the erythropoietin receptor. *Eur J Biochem* 2002; 269: 2516–2526.

[124] Hookham MB, Elliott J, Suessmuth Y, Staerk J, Ward AC, Vainchenker W *et al.* The myeloproliferative disorder-associated JAK2 V617F mutant escapes negative regulation by suppressor of cytokine signaling 3. *Blood* 2007;109: 4924–4929.

[125] Cacalano NA, Sanden D, Johnston JA. Tyrosine-phosphorylated SOCS-3 inhibits STAT activation but binds to p120 RasGAP and activates Ras. *Nat Cell Biol* 2001; 3: 460–465.

[126] Dusa A, Staerk J, Elliott J, Pecquet C, Poirel HA, Johnston JA *et al.* Substitution of pseudokinase domain residue V617 by large non-polar amino acids causes activation of JAK2. *J Biol Chem* 2008; 283: 12941–12948.

[127] Wernig G, Mercher T, Okabe R, Levine RL, Lee BH, Gilliland DG. Expression of Jak2V617F causes a polycythemia vera-like disease with associated myelofibrosis in a murine bone marrow transplant model. *Blood* 2006;107: 4274–4281.

[128] Knoops L, Hornakova T, Royer Y, Constantinescu SN, Renauld JC. JAK kinases overexpression promotes *in vitro* cell transformation. *Oncogene*2008; 27: 1511–1519.

[129] Ugo V, Marzac C, Teyssandier I, Larbret F, Lecluse Y, Debili N *et al.* Multiple signaling pathways are involved in erythropoietin-independent differentiation of erythroid progenitors in polycythemia vera. *Exp Hematol*2004; 32: 179–187.
[130] Pardanani A, Hood J, Lasho T, Levine RL, Martin MB, Noronha G *et al.* TG101209, a small molecule JAK2-selective kinase inhibitor potently inhibits myeloproliferative disorder-associated JAK2V617F and MPLW515L/K mutations. *Leukemia* 2007; 21: 1658–1668.
[131] Wernig G, Kharas MG, Okabe R, Moore SA, Leeman DS, Cullen DE *et al.* Efficacy of TG101348, a selective JAK2 inhibitor, in treatment of a murine model of JAK2V617F-induced polycythemia vera. *Cancer Cell* 2008; 13: 311–320.
[132] Geron I, Abrahamsson AE, Barroga CF, Kavalerchik E, Gotlib J, Hood JD *et al.* Selective inhibition of JAK2-driven erythroid differentiation of polycythemia vera progenitors. *Cancer Cell* 2008; 13: 321–330.
[133] Weiss MJ, Orkin SH. GATA transcription factors: key regulators of hematopoiesis. *Exp Hematol* 1995; 23: 99–107.
[134] Cantor AB, Orkin SH. Transcriptional regulation of erythropoiesis: an affair involving multiple partners. *Oncogene* 2002; 21: 3368–3376.
[135] Mirza AM, Correa PN, Axelrad AA. Increased basal and induced tyrosine phosphorylation of the insulin-like growth factor I receptor beta subunit in circulating mononuclear cells of patients with polycythemia vera. *Blood*1995; 86: 877–882.
[136] Jones AV, Silver RT, Waghorn K, Curtis C, Kreil S, Zoi K *et al.* Minimal molecular response in polycythemia vera patients treated with imatinib or interferon alpha. *Blood* 2006; 107: 3339-3341.
[137] Gaikwad A, Verstovsek S, Yoon D, Chang KT, Manshouri T, Nussenzveig R*et al.* Imatinib effect on growth and signal transduction in polycythemia vera. *Exp Hematol* 2007; 35: 931–938.
[138] Chin H, Arai A, Wakao H, Kamiyama R, Miyasaka N, Miura O. Lyn physically associates with the erythropoietin receptor and may play a role in activation of the Stat5 pathway. *Blood* 1998; 91: 3734–3745.
[139] Zaleskas VM, Krause DS, Lazarides K, Patel N, Hu Y, Li S *et al.* Molecular pathogenesis and therapy of polycythemia induced in mice by JAK2 V617F.*PLoS ONE* 2006; 1: e18.
[140] Zeuner A, Pedini F, Signore M, Ruscio G, Messina C, Tafuri A *et al.* Increased death receptor resistance and FLIPshort expression in polycythemia vera erythroid precursor cells. *Blood* 2006; 107: 3495–3502.
[141] Le Bousse-Kerdilès MC, Martyré MC. Involvement of the fibrogenic cytokines, TGF-beta and bFGF, in the pathogenesis of idiopathic myelofibrosis. *Pathol Biol (Paris)* 2001; 49: 153–157.
[142] Villeval JL, Cohen-Solal K, Tulliez M, Giraudier S, Guichard J, Burstein SA*et al.* High thrombopoietin production by hematopoietic cells induces a fatal myeloproliferative syndrome in mice. *Blood* 1997; 90: 4369–4383.
[143] Chagraoui H, Komura E, Tulliez M, Giraudier S, Vainchenker W, Wendling F. Prominent role of TGF-beta 1 in thrombopoietin-induced myelofibrosis in mice. *Blood* 2002; 100: 3495–3503.

[144] Ciurea SO, Merchant D, Mahmud N, Ishii T, Zhao Y, Hu W *et al.* Pivotal contributions of megakaryocytes to the biology of idiopathic myelofibrosis.*Blood* 2007; 110: 986–993.

[145] Jenkins BJ, Grail D, Nheu T, Najdovska M, Wang B, Waring P *et al.* Hyperactivation of Stat3 in gp130 mutant mice promotes gastric hyperproliferation and desensitizes TGF-beta signaling. *Nat Med* 2005; 11: 845–852.

[146] Vannucchi AM, Bianchi L, Paoletti F, Pancrazzi A, Torre E, Nishikawa M *et al.* A pathobiologic pathway linking thrombopoietin, GATA-1, and TGF-beta1 in the development of myelofibrosis. *Blood* 2005; 105: 3493–3501.

[147] Shi S, Calhoun HC, Xia F, Li J, Le L, Li WX. JAK signaling globally counteracts heterochromatic gene silencing. *Nat Genet* 2006; 38: 1071–1076.

[148] Muller P, Kuttenkeuler D, Gesellchen V, Zeidler MP, Boutros M. Identification of JAK/STAT signalling components by genome-wide RNA interference. *Nature* 2005; 436: 871–875.

[149] Guerini V, Barbui V, Spinelli O, Salvi A, Dellacasa C, Carobbio A *et al.* The histone deacetylase inhibitor ITF2357 selectively targets cells bearing mutated JAK2(V617F). *Leukemia* 2008; 22: 740–747.

[150] Schuebel KE, Chen W, Cope L, Glockner SC, Suzuki H, Yi JM *et al.* Comparing the DNA hypermethylome with gene mutations in human colorectal cancer. *PLoS Genet* 2007; 3: 1709–1723.

[151] Shi J, Zhao Y, Ishii T, Hu W, Sozer S, Zhang W *et al.* Effects of chromatin-modifying agents on CD34+ cells from patients with idiopathic myelofibrosis. *Cancer Res* 2007; 67: 6417–6424.

[152] Jelinek J, Li J, Mnjoyan Z, Issa JP, Prchal JT, Afshar-Kharghan V. Epigenetic control of PRV-1 expression on neutrophils. *Exp Hematol* 2007; 35: 1677–1683.

[153] Temerinac S, Klippel S, Strunck E, Roder S, Lubbert M, Lange W *et al.* Cloning of PRV-1, a novel member of the uPAR receptor superfamily, which is overexpressed in polycythemia rubra vera. *Blood* 2000; 95: 2569–2576.

[154] Jost E, do ON, Dahl E, Maintz CE, Jousten P, Habets L *et al.* Epigenetic alterations complement mutation of JAK2 tyrosine kinase in patients with BCR/ABL-negative myeloproliferative disorders. *Leukemia* 2007; 21: 505–510.

[155] Dawson MA, Bannister AJ, Gottgens B, et al. JAK2 phosphorylates histone H3Y41 and excludes HP1alpha from chromatin. Nature. 2009;461(7265):819-22.

[156] McCormack, M. P. & Rabbitts, T. H. Activation of the T-cell oncogene LMO2 after gene therapy for X-linked severe combined immunodeficiency. N Engl J Med. 2004;350:913–922.

[157] Yoshihiro Y, Warren AJ, Dobson C, Foster A, Pannel R, Rabbits TH. The T cell leukemia LIM protein Lmo2 is necessary for adult mouse hematopoiesis. Proc Natl Acad Sci USA. 1998; 95:3890–3895.

[158] Ma AC, Ward AC, Liang R, Leung AY. The role of jak2a in zebrafish hematopoiesis. Blood. 2007;110:1824–1830.

[159] Seo IA, Lee HK, Shin YK, Lee SH, et al. Janus Kinase 2 Inhibitor AG490 Inhibits the STAT3 Signaling Pathway by Suppressing Protein Translation of gp130. Korean J Physiol Pharmacol. 2009;13(2):131-138.

[160] Tsuchiya Y, Takahashi N, Yoshizaki T, et al. A Jak2 inhibitor, AG490, reverses lipin-1 suppression by TNF-alpha in 3T3-L1 adipocytes. Biochem Biophys Res Commun. 2009;382(2):348-352.

[161] A Pardanani, J Gotlib, C Jamieson, et al Safety and efficacy of TG101348, a selective JAK2 inhibitor, in myelofibrosis *Journal of Clinical Oncology* (2011)

4

Stratification of Patients with Follicular Lymphoma

Hasan A. Abd El-Ghaffar et al.*
Clinical Pathology Department, Faculty of Medicine, Mansoura University, Mansoura Oncology Center, Mansoura University, Mansoura Egypt

1. Introduction

Follicular lymphoma (FL) is an indolent lymphoid neoplasm that is derived from mutated germinal center B cells and exhibits a nodular or follicular histologic pattern. It is typically composed of a mixture of small, cleaved follicle center cells referred to as centrocytes and large noncleaved follicular center cells referred to as centroblasts. FL accounts for about 20 % of all lymphomas with the highest incidence in the USA and Western Europe. In Asia and in the developing countries the incidence is much lower [1].

2. The cell of origin of follicular lymphoma

The current theory that tumors are derived from mutated stem cells called cancer stem cells was suggested because stem cells and some cancer cells share self-renewal and differentiation capacities [2-4]. Although this hypothesis was postulated in early reports [5-7],definite proof of their existence came from recent studies in leukemia, where among the complete tumor cell population only a small subset of cells could initiate, regenerate and maintain the leukemia after transplantation into immunocompromised mice [8,9].Using similar functional approaches, a variety of cancer stem cells have been identified in an increasing number of epithelial tumors, including breast, prostate, pancreatic and head and neck carcinomas [10].Despite these outstanding discoveries in leukemias and solid tumors, the existence of lymphoma-originating cells with stem cell properties that may similarly generate lymphoma upon mutation remains a controversial and largely unexplored issue [11]. Recently, it has been proposed that commited lymphoid progenitors/precursor cells with an active V-D-J recombination program are the initiating cells of follicular lymphoma when targeted by immunoglobulin-gene translocations in the bone marrow. However, these pre-malignant lymphoma initiating cells cannot drive complete malignant transformation,

* Sameh Shamaa[2,4], Nadia Attwan[3], Tarek E. Selim[1], Nashwa K. Abosamra[1,4], Dalia Salem[1,4], Sherin M. Abd El-Aziz[1,4] and Layla M. Tharwat[1,4]
[1]*Clinical Pathology Department, Faculty of Medicine, Mansoura University, Mansoura, Egypt*
[2]*Internal Medicine Department, Faculty of Medicine, Mansoura University, Mansoura, Egypt*
[3]*Pathology Department, Faculty of Medicine, Mansoura University, Mansoura, Egypt*
[4]*Oncology Center, Mansoura University, Mansoura, Egypt*

requiring additional cooperating mutations in specific stem cell programs to be converted into the lymphoma originating cells able to generate and sustain lymphoma development [12].

3. Clinical aspects of follicular lymphoma

Signs and Symptom

Follicular lymphoma mainly affects older adults. The average age at diagnosis is about 55. Men and women are nearly equally affected. Follicular lymphoma is a slow-growing disease with minor warning signs that often go unnoticed for a long time before it is diagnosed. The disease is often advanced before a diagnosis is made. Most individuals are diagnosed in stage III or IV. However, even in advanced stages there is no immediate threat to life. The disease has a "waxing and waning" course, meaning that it flares up and regresses a number of times over years.

The first sign of the condition is often a painless swelling in the neck, armpit or groin that is caused by enlarged lymph nodes. However the majority of patients initially present with disseminated disease that follows a relatively indolent clinical course. Patients with follicular lymphoma typically present with superficial lymph nodes of small to medium size. All common superficial territories can be involved by the disease.

In some patients, the first symptoms are more insidious and related to the slow growth of lymph nodes in deep areas, usually in the infradiaphragmatic territories such as the retroperitoneum, the mesenteric, or the iliac areas. In those cases, patients may complain of atypical symptoms while the tumor bulk can be important, with single or confluent lymph nodes. Primary mediastinal involvement is uncommon, as well as isolated splenic enlargement[13]. Other symptoms may include loss of appetite and tiredness. The general status of the patient is usually preserved, Some people have night sweats, unexplained high temperatures and weight loss. These are known as B symptoms. Others have an altered performance status.

Primary involvement of extranodal areas is also very uncommon[14]. The bone marrow is involved in 50% to 60% of the cases. Follicular lymphoma can arise in the gastrointestinal (GI) tract, predominantly in the duodenum or the small intestine, [15,16]. where it can eventually represent the unique site of disease. Lymphoma infiltration may be unifocal or multifocal[13]. The new World Health Organization–European Organization for Research on Treatment of Cancer (WHO-EORTC) cutaneous lymphoma classification recognizes an entity called "primary cutaneous follicle center cell lymphoma" that includes what was previously known as "cutaneous follicular lymphoma variant" in the WHO classification. [17]. Other follicular lymphomas that may be considered as peculiar entities with a distinct behavior are those involving the testis [18] and the rare cases of follicular lymphoma encountered in children [19].

Follicular lymphoma is characterised by response to treatment with disease-free or asymptomatic disease intervals, alternating with recurrence/progression and may transform to aggressive lymphoma at a rate of around 3% per year [13]. This feature is usually—but not systematically—associated with a poor outcome [20].The clinical factors associated with the risk of transformation (as well as the biology underlying this phenomenon) are not fully characterized. Some reports indicated that early treatment and achievement of a complete response after the first-line therapy were associated with a lower risk of transformation in patients with follicular lymphoma [21].

4. Clinical prognostic factors

Several prognostic parameters for follicular lymphomas were identified in the last two decades, that led to the development of some prognostic indexes. The International Prognostic Index developed for aggressive lymphomas was also found to be able of predicting the outcome for patients with follicular lymphoma, but the proportion of patients in the higher-risk categories was usually limited. [13]

The first prognostic system specific to follicular lymphoma was developed by the Italian Lymphoma Intergroup (ILI) in the late 1990s [22]. Currently, the Follicular Lymphoma International Prognostic Index (FLIPI) [23] is deemed to be more applicable across a range of clinical settings . Both systems were developed prior to the introduction of monoclonal antibody therapy, which has profoundly changed the treatment and outcome of follicular lymphoma [24]. Hence, the FLIPI-2 was recently developed, in a prospective series of patients needing treatment, using parameters which were not previously amenable to retrospective analysis, and may represent a promising new tool for the identification of follicular lymphoma patients with different risk profiles in the era of immunochemotherapy [25].

The description of the Follicular Lymphoma International Prognostic Index (FLIPI) represents an important step in identifying patient subgroups with predictable outcome and comparing the results of clinical trials. Analyses of gene expression profiles or constitutive gene variations may also provide additional insights for prognostication in the near future. Furthermore, these data underline the complex interactions between the tumor cells and their microenvironment; recent attempts to translate these findings with immunohistochemical studies remain unable to robustly predict patient outcome. The therapeutic strategies in follicular lymphoma have been transformed by monoclonal antibodies, used alone or in combination with chemotherapy. Treatment options should be adapted to the clinical features at diagnosis and appear to be able to modify the overall survival of some subgroups of patients. Further efforts may focus on strategies that can alter the natural history of this disease [13].

5. Treatment

There is a general consensus that the natural history of advanced stages of low-grade or indolent lymphoma has not changed for the last 30 years. Patients with advanced stages of indolent non-Hodgkin's lymphoma have been treated for many years with various approaches, including deferred initial therapy (watch and wait), single-agent alkylating agents, radiation therapy, combination chemotherapy, and autologous stem-cell transplantation. Unfortunately, it has been impossible to demonstrate that the long-term prognosis for these patients has significantly changed with any these treatment options [26].

The decision to start first-line treatment depends not only on the stage but also on the symptoms of the disease [27].According to The Swiss Group for Clinical Cancer Research

(SAKK) trials at least one of the following signs is present in order to start treatment: B symptoms; symptomatic enlarged lymph nodes or spleen; steady, clinically significant progression of lymphadenopathy, splenomegaly or other follicular lymphoma lesions documented by a 50% increase in size over a period of at least 6 months; involvement of at least 3 nodal sites (>3 cm), bulky disease (>7 cm), haemoglobin <10g/dL, and platelets <100 x 10^9/L due to bone marrow infiltration or splenomegaly [28].

Inspite of encouraging early results [29],there is still no solid data to confirm that early treatment with rituximab significantly delays the need for new therapy,and whether this approach may alter the natural history of the disease and there is also conflicting results Whether early treatment of follicular lymphoma is associated with a decreased risk of transformation [27].

Horning [30],reported the results of sequential treatment studies conducted at Stanford University from 1960 to 1991. Median survival times have ranged from 7 to 10 years, and the OS for each group of studies was overlapping. Indolent lymphoma is generally considered incurable because no plateau in the survival curve has been demonstrable. However, the development of monoclonal antibodies (MoAbs) has revolutionized the treatment of patients with follicular lymphoma [26].

Many trials utilizing different protocols of combination chemotherapy plus rituximab,eg. CVP [31], CHOP [32,33] concluded that OS for patients with follicular lymphoma has improved over time and that the choice of initial therapy may matter. Sacchi et al [34],concluded that FFS and OS have significantly improved in advanced-stage follicular lymphoma patients treated on GISL(Gruppo Italiano Studio Linfomi) protocols during the last 18 years. These improvements are related to evolving front-line and salvage therapies, particularly the introduction of rituximab in combination with chemotherapy

For patients needing therapy, most patients are treated with chemotherapy plus rituximab, which has improved response rates, duration of response, and overall survival. Randomized studies have shown additional benefit for maintenance rituximab both following chemotherapy-rituximab and single agent rituximab [35]. Rituximab maintenance for up to 2 years has a favorable side effect profile and, based on a systematic meta-analysis, substantially prolongs PFS and OS in relapsed disease even after antibody-containing induction in patients who have not received antibody as first-line therapy [36].

Stem cell transplantation (SCT) including both autologous and allogeneic SCT or experimental agent therapy is considered for recurrent disease [35].

In the small proportion of patients with limited non-bulky stages I–II, radiotherapy (involved or extended field, 30–36 Gy) is the preferred treatment having a curative potential [37]. However, In selected cases a watchful waiting may be discussed to avoid the side effects of radiation [38]. Radioimmunotherapy or chlorambucil plus rituximab remains an alternative in patients with low risk profile or contraindications for a more intensive chemoimmunotherapy [39,40].

Therfore, the therapeutic strategies in follicular lymphoma have been transformed by monoclonal antibodies, used alone or in combination with chemotherapy. Treatment options should be adapted to the clinical features at diagnosis and appear to be able to modify the overall survival of some subgroups of patients. Further efforts may focus on strategies that can alter the natural history of this disease [13].

6. Cytomorphology of follicular lymphoma

Follicular NHLs are characterized by a follicular growth pattern , but a diffuse area may also be present. The follicles of follicular lymphoma were more closely packed together, more monotonous in size and shape, and frequently lacked an obvious mantle zone [41].

These follicles contained a comparatively monomorphic cellular phenotype, mostly of centrocytes (small cells with cleaved nuclei) and occasional centroblasts (large cells with multilobated nuclei and multiple nucleoli). Mitotic figures were fewer than in reactive follicular hyperplasia (RFH) and tingible body macrophages were sparse or absent. Polykaryocytes were not observed in RFH or follicular lymphoma and sclerosis was only focally present to a minimal degree [42].

The distinction of FL from RFH is essential, as the latter represents a benign condition [43].A number of morphological features are of value in making this distinction; in particular, a low density of follicles per unit area, The follicles are separated by wide interfollicular areas with prominent mantle zones. The variably sized follicles were composed of a polymorphic population of lymphocytes, dendritic cells, and tingible body macrophages that imparted a"starry sky" pattern. Mitotic figures were conspicuous. The presence of polarity within follicles and the lack of a monomorphic appearance within the follicles all favor RFH [42].

7. Immunophenotype

Being a mature B-cell lymphoma, FL express a large spectrum of B-cell markers, such as CD20, CD19, CD22, CD79a, and Pax5[1] [44].

FL cells express antigens of the germinal center including CD10 and Bcl-6. Most cases of FL express Bcl-2 protein which is highly correlated with the presence of the t(14;18) but may be expressed in cases with a clonal karyotype lacking the t(14;18) [45].

The follicles of RFH and follicular lymphoma stained positively for the B cell marker CD20 which highlight the difference in the width of the interfollicular region between the follicles. In RFH, T cells were predominantly located in the interfollicular zones but also lightly percolated throughout the center of the follicles, demonstrated by T cell marker CD3. CD5 stained T cells are in a nearly identical pattern. T cells stained positively for CD3 and CD5 in follicular lymphoma located within the interfollicular zones. The latter also displaying a more prominent spillover of CD20-positive cells than in RFH [42].

Follicles in both RFH and follicular lymphoma were positive for BCL-6. BCL-2 staining revealed that the follicular centers in RFH were negative and those in follicular lymphoma were positive. CD10 staining was positive for both RFH and follicular lymphoma but showed a greater interfollicular staining in follicular lymphoma [41].

Some cases of both RFH and follicular lymphoma manifested a vague follicular architecture that is difficult to detect. In these cases, CD23, a dendritic cell marker, outlined the follicles of RFH more clearly by disclosing a scaffolding or a cluster of interconnecting cells with elongated cytoplasmic processes. Follicular lymphoma manifested the same pattern of CD23 staining. Ki-67, a marker for cellular proliferation, showed dense positivity that was polarized (unevenly distributed or centered at one edge of the follicle) within RFH follicles. In contrast, follicular lymphoma demonstrated a more diffuse, evenly distributed staining pattern within the follicular centers. Polyclonality was evident in RFH, with in situ hybridization revealing roughly equal populations of both kappa and lambda light chains. In follicular lymphoma rare cells stained positive for kappa or lambda [42].

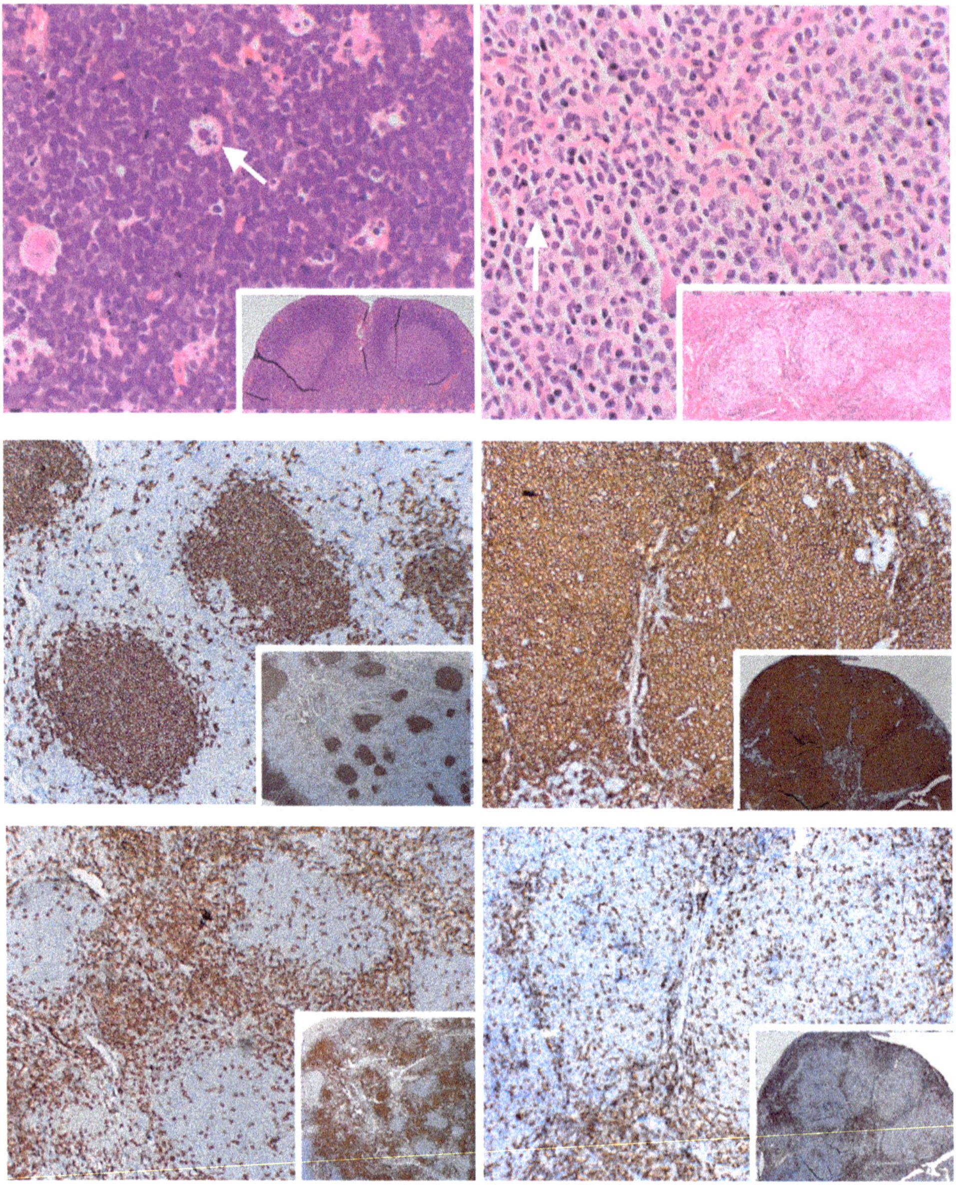

Fig. 1. Histopathological and immunohistochemical characterization of reactive lymphoid hyperplasia and follicular lymphoma.(Top left) Hematoxylin-eosin staining demonstrates follicles in reactive lymphoid hyperplasia (RLH) (inset). The follicles are composed of small

cells with mitotic figures and tingible body macrophages (arrow). (Top right) Hematoxylin-eosin-stainedsection of follicular lymphoma shows mostly small centrocytes with cleaved nuclei and an occasional centroblast (arrow) with a large nucleus and peripheral nucleoli. Inset shows the closer, less well-defined arrangement of several follicles. (Middle left) CD20 stains B cells within the follicles of RLH. The inset indicates the substantial width of the interfollicular zones. (Middle right) CD20 also stains the B cells in the follicles of follicular lymphoma; the close arrangement of the follicles can again be appreciated in the inset.(Bottom left) CD3 stains T cells in the interfollicular zones (inset); the T cells can also be seen percolating throughout the folliclesof RLH. (Bottom right) Follicular lymphoma manifests nearly identical CD3 staining, with CD3_ cells prominent in the interfollicular zones (inset) as well as scattered within the follicles. (Top left and top right, hematoxylin-eosin, 400, insets, 25;Middle left through Bottom right, immunoperoxidase reactions, diaminobenzidine chromogen, 200, insets 25) [42].

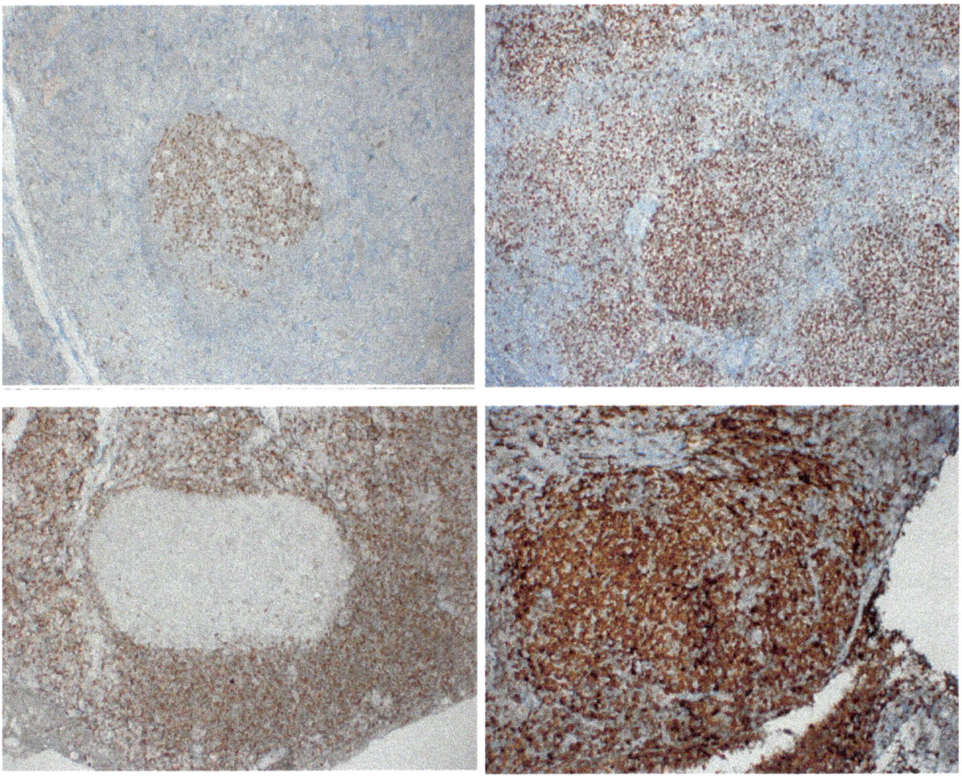

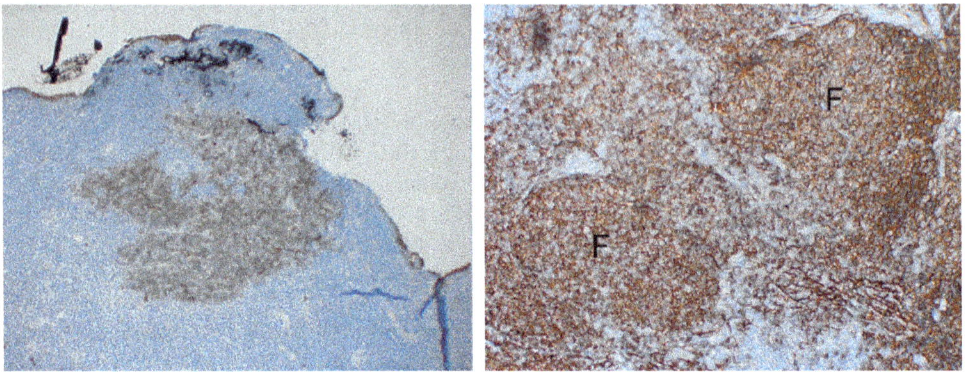

Fig. 2. Immunohistochemical characterization of reactive lymphoid hyperplasia and follicular lymphoma. (Top left) BCL-6stains B cells within follicles of reactive lymphoid hyperplasia (RLH). (Top right) Follicles of follicular lymphoma are also positivefor BCL-6. (Middle left) The follicles of RLH are negative for BCL-2. (Middle right) Follicles of follicular lymphoma are positivefor BCL-2. (Bottom left) Follicles in RLH are positive for CD10. (Bottom right) Follicles (F) of follicular lymphoma are also positive for CD10 but with more interfollicular staining than RLH. (Immunoperoxidase reactions, diaminobenzidine chromogen,200) [42].

8. Follicular lymphoma—How many grades?

The grading of FL was the subject of spirited discussion, both among the authors and the participants in the Clinical Advisory Committee. FL has traditionally been graded according to the proportion of centroblasts and into three Grades, 1-3 as detailed:

World Health Organization classification of follicular lymphoma (FL).

Follicular Lymphoma: Grading & Variants

Grade 1: 0–5 centroblasts/HPF
Grade 2: 6–15 centroblasts/HPF
Grade 3: > 15 centroblasts/HPF

3a: > 15 centroblasts, but centrocytes are still present
3b: centroblasts form solid sheets with no residual centrocytes [46].

Variants:

Primary cutaneous follicle center lymphoma
Pediatric follicle center lymphoma
Intestinal follicle center lymphoma
Diffuse follicle center lymphoma
Grade 1, 0–5 centroblasts/HPF
Grade 2, 6–15centroblasts/HPF[43]

Pediatric FL lacking an association with the t(14;18). Primary cutaneous follicle center lymphoma (PCFCL) may contain a high proportion of large B-cells including large

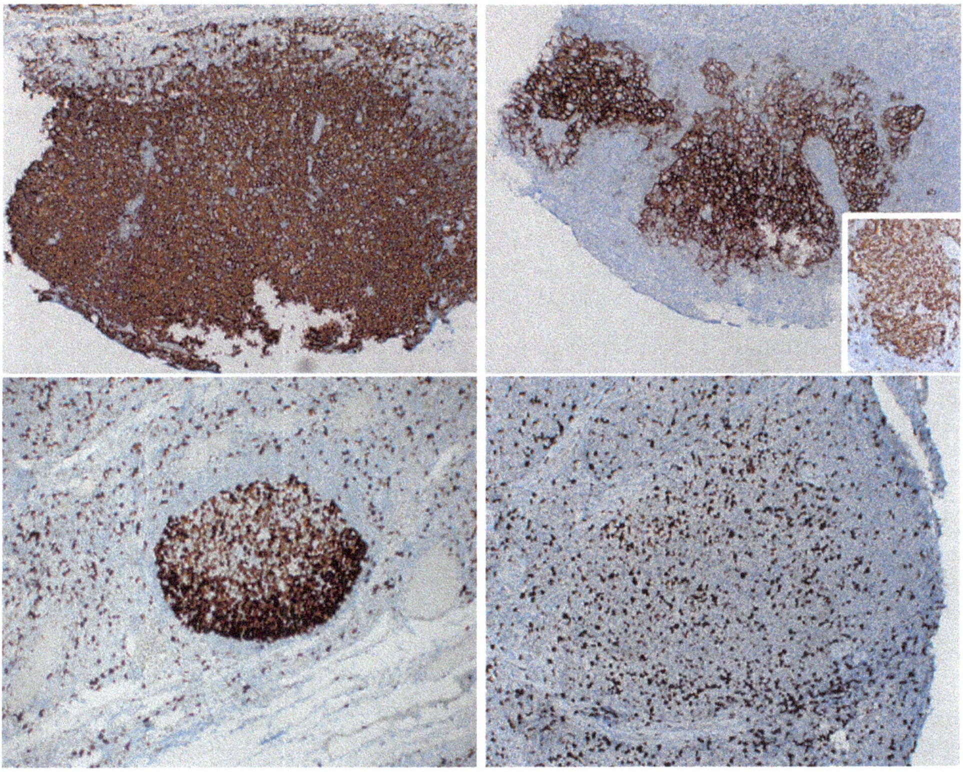

Fig. 3. Further immunohistochemical characterization of reactive lymphoid hyperplasia (RLH) and follicular lymphoma. (Topleft) CD20 densely stains this region of RLH without obvious follicular architecture. (Top right) CD23 highlights the dendritic cell scaffolding of the follicles in an adjacent section. The inset shows a similar dendritic architecture broughtout by CD23 in follicular lymphoma. (Bottom left) Ki-67 stains cells within follicles of RLH in an uneven distribution; staining is crescentic and more dense at the bottom of the follicle. (Bottom right) Follicular cells in follicular lymphoma are more evenly and diffusely positive for Ki-67.(Immunoperoxidase reactions, diaminobenzidine chromogen, 200, inset, 25) [42].

centrocytes and centroblasts. Evidence of the t(14;18) is uncommon and most cases are BCL2 negative. Dissemination beyond the skin is rare, and the prognosis is usually excellent [47].

However, most studies have shown poor interobserver and intraobserver reproducibility. Moreover, the clinical significance of the separation of Grades 1 and 2 has been questioned, with minimal differences seen in long term outcome. Thus, the 2008 WHO classification lumps cases with few centroblasts as "FL Grade 1-2 (low grade)" and does not require or recommend further separation. FL Grade 3 is divided into Grades 3A and 3B, based on the absence of centrocytes in the latter category. Several studies have identified biological differences between these two subtypes, with most cases of FL Grade 3B being more closely related to DLBCL at the molecular level [47].

However, in clinical practice the separation of Grades 3A and 3B can be challenging. Diffuse areas in any Grade 3 FL should be designated as DLBCL (with FL) and are more commonly observed in Grade 3B. Further studies are likely to lead to more precise delineation of the Grade 3 cases truly belonging within FL and those representing an intrafollicular variant of the GCB (germinal center B cell) type of DLBCL.

The presence of diffuse areas within a FL appears to confer more aggressive clinical behavior. In addition, unusual cytological variants can be encountered that are not included in the World Health Organization classification, including cases with large centrocytes and others with small centroblasts; in some cases the latter may resemble the cytomorphology of Burkitt lymphoma and may be associated with MYC oncogene translocations [43].

A truly diffuse form of FL may be rarely encountered, but on closer inspection, most cases demonstrate vaguely follicular architecture that is underappreciated without the routine use of immunostains for follicular dendritic cells. When a diagnosis of true diffuse follicle center lymphoma is considered, the pathologist is encouraged to demonstrate co-expression of CD10 and Bcl-6 as well as presumptive evidence of the t(14;18). Approximately 10% of FL cases reveal the presence of a zone of cells resembling marginal zone B cells, immediately surrounding neoplastic follicles. Importantly, a residual benign mantle zone is not seen, helping to distinguish FL from a marginal zone lymphoma. The area of marginal zone differentiation within a FL takes on a distinct morphology with cells having moderate amount of pale cytoplasm; moreover, the immunophenotype is also different, with downregulation of CD10 and Bcl-6 expression by cells within the marginal zone compartment [48].

Unresolved issues in FL pathology remain and to some extent contribute to problems with reproducibility. Diffuse areas in FL are often not identified, due to underutilization of follicular dendritic cell stains. Similarly, follicular areas in suspected de novo DLBCL are underappreciated. Variability in the cytology of cells within follicles contributes to inconsistent reporting of FL grade. Follicular dendritic are commonly misidentified as centroblasts, resulting in higher grade and, in general, there is poor interobserver reproducibility for the counting of centroblasts. All of these factors lead to inconsistencies in the diagnosis and grading of FL biopsies, and to some extent raise questions regarding the validity of grading and clinical decision making based on grade [43].

Finally, a rare form of FL may be seen referred to as "in-situ" FL. In these uncommon cases, scattered malignant follicles are identified within lymph nodes revealing mostly benign features. The malignant follicles show typically more monomorphic germinal centres (GCs). GCs involved in intrafollicular neoplasia/in situ follicular lymphoma are composed mainly of centrocytes with no evident atypia. A feature of these centres is the relative absence of macrophages with tingible bodies and the absence of polarization into light and dark zones. The paucity of large centroblasts reflects their low proliferation rate in insitu FLs. Intrafollicular neoplasia/in situ follicular lymphoma is characterized by strong co-expression of Bcl-2 and CD10 in the involved GCs [49].

9. Fine needle aspiration cytology

FNA is a useful tool for staging as well as evaluating recurrences in lymph nodes and extra nodal sites without subjecting patients to multiple excisional biopsies. Transformation can occur in some lymph nodes while low-grade lymphoma persists in others. An advantage of FNA is the ability to sample multiple lymph nodes, whereas open biopsy of different anatomic sites is not feasible

Grading FL is based on the proportion of centroblasts in neoplastic follicles; therefore, the ability to identify the various cellular components in a fine-needle aspirate is the first essential step to the grading process. In Papanicolaou stained preparations, centrocytes or cleaved follicular center cells are small to medium-sized cells with angulated, elongated, twisted, or cleaved nuclei with inconspicuous nucleoli and scant, pale cytoplasm.

Centroblasts are at least two times larger than a lymphocyte and usually are round or oval but occasionally have indented, irregular, or even lobulated nuclei. There is a narrow rim of cytoplasm, often basophilic to amphophilic. A large and central nucleolus with chromatin clearing around it is characteristic of immunoblasts. In more typical centroblasts, the chromatin generally is vesicular with one to three prominent, often peripherally located nucleoli. The cells also may be hyperchromatic. Centroblasts tend to be more fragile and, in some preparations, may not be preserved well [50].

It is important not to confuse centroblasts with follicular dendritic reticulum cells, which tend to aggregate within the center of the neoplastic follicles. Although dendritic cells have nuclei that are similar in size to centroblasts, the nuclei of dendritic cells are somewhat coffee bean-shaped with one side typically flattened and with fine, smooth nuclear membranes. The cytoplasm is indistinct, not basophilic, in contrast to that of centroblasts. In Papanicolaou-stained preparations, the chromatin is pale gray and finely granular with small, central, eosinophilic nucleoli. The cytoplasm of dendritic cells form long, dendritic processes that can be appreciated in cell blocks by IHC staining for CD21. Large cleaved cells also must be distinguished from centroblasts. Although there is an overlap in size with centroblasts, large centrocytes are more irregular in shape and lack the prominent nucleoli and chromatin pattern of centroblasts [50]

When it comes to differentiating individual cells, cytologic preparations are superior to hematoxylin and eosin-stained histologic sections, although cytologic preparations typically are less informative about architecture.

Cell blocks are complimentary to smears and provide additional architectural clues. The FNA process often aspirates intact follicular structures that can be appreciated in the cell block. The presence of intact follicles may be proven by special stains on sections of the cell block [50].

10. Grade versus pattern

All three grades of lymphoma can have varying proportions of follicular and diffuse areas. Grade 1 and 2 FL generally have a predominantly follicular pattern. Because they are better differentiated, they have retained the ability to recapitulate follicles [51].

Grade 3 FL occurs less frequently than Grade 1 and 2 FL, and a pure follicular pattern in Grade 3 FL is even more unusual. In Grade 3 FL, the presence of diffuse areas is more common, and most (but not all) studies show that this finding is associated with a worse prognosis.

In Grade 1 and 2 FL, there is conflicting evidence regarding whether the presence of large, diffuse areas or the degree of nodularity may alter prognosis significantly.

SO the WHO classification system recommends estimating the proportion of follicular and diffuse components in the pathology report

- Follicular (75% follicular),
- Follicular and diffuse (25–75% follicular),
- Minimally follicular (25% follicular).

Note, however, that the proportion of centroblasts within the neoplastic follicles is what determines the grade of a FL, not the degree of nodularity. Furthermore, the grade of FL, in combination with other clinical factors,ultimately is what influences treatment decisions [50].

11. Cytogenetics of follicular lymphoma

The t(14;18)(q32;q21) chromosome translocation represents the defining cytogenetic hallmark of FL and is encountered in 80%-90% of cases. Its molecular consequence is the juxtaposition of the B-cell lymphoma/leukemia 2 (BCL2) proto-oncogene with enhancer sequences of the immunoglobulin heavy chain gene (IGH) promoter region, thereby deregulating its expression and resulting in an overexpression of the BCL2 protein in the neoplastic follicles [52,53]. However, 10–15% of cases do not harbor the t(14;18)(q32;q21) and in these t(14;18)-negative cases, other mechanisms are thought to be involved in the pathogenesis [54]. Moreover, t(14;18)- positive B cells can be identified in the blood and lymphoid tissues of healthy individuals, and the number of t(14;18)-positive cells is influenced by gender, personal lifestyle and exposure to toxic substances [55].

The BCL2 proto oncogene, a potent anti-apoptotic molecule, is expressed in resting B cells in the perifollicular mantle zone and in post-follicular B cells, thereby promoting long-lived follicular precursor and memory B cells. Germinal center B cells, however, physiologically lack BCL2 expression and undergo apoptosis unless they are selected by specific antigens that drive them into processes termed somatic hypermutation and class switching. Due to the lack of BCL2 expression, amongst other factors, the large bulk of B-cells entering the GC microenvironment will be removed by apoptosis. The constitutive overexpression of BCL2 in germinal center B cells inferred by the t(14;18)(q32;q21) leads to an accumulation of inappropriately rescued B cells with a prolonged life span, allowing for the development of additional genetic hits to occur, that are required for the establishment of overt FL . Variant translocations of the t(14;18), such as the t(2;18) or t(18;22), juxtapose BCL2 to the loci of the immunoglobulin light chains (k,l) and, likewise, result in inappropriate and sustained BCL2 expression in GC B cells [56].

The occurrence of the t(14;18) in a pre-FL B cell can be viewed as a first hit in a multistep process that results in the clonal dysregulation of cell cycle control and apoptosis of the tumor cells. During process of lymphomagenesis, a number of additional genetic or epigenetic events occur in a non-random fashion that lead to overt FL .For example, constitutive expression of activation-induced cytidine deaminase (AID) in the GC environment in B cells overexpressing BCL2 may propagate continuous somatic hypermutation and class switch recombination activity that results in increased genomic instability. This may, in turn, foster the occurrence of secondary oncogenic hits and, finally, result in the malignant transformation to overt FL [57].

Cong and co-workers[58],described the phenomenon of what they termed follicular lymphoma in situ in otherwise reactive, hyperplastic lymph nodes possibly representing the morphological equivalent of early, pre-invasive FL.

12. Secondary chromosomal aberrations in follicular lymphoma

A number of secondary chromosomal alterations have been described in FL including: structural and numerical changes. The complexity of the secondary alterations correlates with the grade - the higher the grade, the more complex aberrations are usually encountered [59].

It has long been recognized that these alterations occur in a non-random fashion. Partial trisomies of chromosomes 1q, 7, 8 and 18q, and deletions in 1p and 6q have been described as the most common secondary alterations, and deletions in the long arm of chromosomes 1 and 6 and in the short arm of chromosome 17 have been associated with a worse prognosis [60]. Some of these alterations may occur early in the course of the disease, whereas others might represent late genetic events. In addition, some of the alterations are mutually exclusive, while alterations of other chromosomal regions frequently appear together possibly leading to a coordinated deregulation of genetic pathways [61].

Some of the secondary chromosomal alterations may cancel the effect of the t(14;18) that initially forms a low-grade neoplasia with a follicular growth pattern and subsequently enable the transformation to highgrade lymphoma. This process has been associated with three distinct secondary genetic alterations in FL that have a profound impact on the biological program and the clinical course in FL. These include an additional introduction of a t(8;14)/MYC rearrangement in the tumor cells [62], the inactivation of TP53 by mutation and deletion and, finally, the inactivation of p16, frequently occurring by biallelic deletion [63].

The occurrence of a secondary MYC rearrangement in FL deserves particular attention, because these cases frequently demonstrate a Burkitt-like appearance and may be detectable by virtue of this specific morphology in combination with an overexpression of the BCL2 protein caused by the t(14;18) that is usually not encountered in classical Burkitt's lymphomas. Some studies suggest that the detection of TP53 mutations in primary diagnostic specimens of FL without signs of transformation also characterizes a patient subgroup with worse prognosis [64].

13. BCL2-negative follicular lymphoma

From recent studies t(14;18)-negative FLs belong to the biologic spectrum of FL, but show distinct genetic features as well as gene expression and immunohistochemical profiles that differ from their t(14;18)-positive counterparts [65]. The t(14;18)-negative FL appears to harbor genetic rearrangements of the BCL6 gene in 3q27[66] or trisomy 3 [67] whereas others show BCL2 expression on the immunohistochemical level despite the lack of the t(14;18)[68]. Moreover, increased expression of IRF4/MUM1, a protein associated with plasma cell differentiation has been described in FL without BCL2 rearrangement [69].

14. Molecular genetics of follicular lymphoma

Immunoglobulin heavy and light chains are rearranged in FL with the variable region genes showing extensive and ongoing somatic hypermutation [70, 71]. As a result of these mutations in the CDR-regions, PCR primer annealing may be hampered and depending on the primers used, immunoglobulin-PCR may not yield monoclonal products in a proportion of FL cases (10-40%). Multiplex PCR reactions using BIOMED-2 expanded primer sets detect closer to 90% of complete *IGH* (VH-JH) gene rearrangements, and clonality detection approximates 100% when primers detecting incomplete *IGH* (DH-JH) and light chain gene rearrangements are included [72].

For amplification of complete *IGH* (VH-JH) gene rearrangement, BIOMED-2 developed three sets of VH primers corresponding to the three VH FR regions (FR1, FR2, and FR3). Each set of primers consisted of six or seven oligonucleotides capable of annealing to their corresponding VH segments (VH1–VH7) with no mismatches for most VH segments. These VH primer sets were used in conjunction with a single JH consensus primer. The JH primer is fluorescently labeled to allow the detection of PCR products by Gene Scanning [73].

For incomplete *IGH* (DH-JH) rearrangements, seven family-specific DH primers were designed based on the high degree of homology within each DH family in combination with the consensus JH primer. Primers were designed such that crossannealing to other DH family segments would be minimal or preferably absent [73].

Six family-specific Vk primers were designed by van Dongen et al [73], to recognize the various Vk gene segments of the seven Vk families. The family-specific Vk primers were designed to be used in combination with either a set of two Jk primers or a Kde primer.A single consensus primer recognizing both Vλ1 and Vλ2 gene segments, as well as a Vλ3 primer, were designed by van Dongen et al [73], in combination to a single consensus primer for the Jλ1, Jλ2, and Jλ3 gene segments.

The *t(14;18)* and *BCL2* gene rearrangements is one of the best characterized recurrent cytogenetic abnormalities in peripheral B-cell lymphoproliferative disease[74] . FL is genetically characterized by this translocation which is present in up to 90% of the grade 1-2 FL cases [75,76] but the proportion depends on the technique used [77, 78, 79]. BCL2 rearrangements are much less frequent in grade 3B FL [80]. As a consequence of the translocation, the *BCL2* gene (anti-apoptotic) from 18q21 is placed under the control of the strong enhancers of the *IGH* locus resulting in the deregulation of its normal pattern of expression [81,82]. The *BCL2/IGH* rearrangement is found in the PB of 25-75% of healthy donors, and also in reactive nodes, particularly if using sensitive nested or RT-PCR assays [83,84,85]. A recent study suggests that rather than being naive B-cells, these *BCL2*-rearranged cells are memory B-cells [86].

There is no single gold standard detection strategy for the *t(14;18)*, and a combination of cytogenetics and southern blotting have been generally used [87,88]. Interphase FISH detection strategies offer an applicable alternative that have the potential to pick up more translocations [89]. For molecular diagnostic laboratories PCR-based detection strategies offer rapid results, are generally applicable, and can be used for residual disease monitoring. However, the primers commonly used have not been designed to take into account recent information on the molecular anatomy of the breakpoints. As a consequence when compared to gold standard approaches, PCR-based techniques only detect up to 60% of translocations, which seriously impairs the diagnostic capability of PCR. However, BIOMED-2 primers have been developed using three multiplex tubes for detection of MBR-JH, 3'MBR- JH, and mcr-JH to maximize the detection of t(14;18) [73].). These data are supported by previous report from our molecular hematology laboratory. We found that FISH was superior to PCR in the detection of t(14'18) (q32'q21)-IGH-BCL-2 in formalin-fixed, paraffin-embedded tissue samples. Moreover, strong correlations between the FLIPI score and each of interphase FISH and CD10 expression were demonstrated [90].

Molecular profiling of many types of lymphoma using RQ-PCR and cDNA microarray has been used to predict survival by many researchers [91-94]. Genes involved in cell cycle control and DNA synthesis and metabolism (e.g. CXCL12, which is involved in signaling transduction and NEK2, which is involved in mitotic regulation, and MAPK1) are significantly up-regulated in the aggressive phase of FL[3]. MYC, as a known oncogene, and MYC-target genes (SFRS7, LDHA, MTHFD1, NME1, MSH2, and CKS2) are upregulated on transformation and may be implicated as a direct transforming factor [95-102].On the other hand, there is higher density of the T-cell infiltrate in low-grade FL as compared to high-grade disease and this is reflected by several T cell-related genes (CD3, CD2, CD69). However, genes related to T-cell and macrophage activation including several chemokine receptors (CCR1, CCL3, CCL5, CCL8, AKAP12, ILF3, GEM) are significantly upregulated on transformation, suggesting an important biologic role. Notably, specific antagonists to several of the above-mentioned chemokine receptors are available and offer an attractive possibility for therapeutic interventions [103].

15. Proposed algorithm for stratification of follicular lymphoma

The National Comprehensive Cancer Network(NCCN) has recently launched an algorithm for stratification of follicular lymphoma (Figure 4).

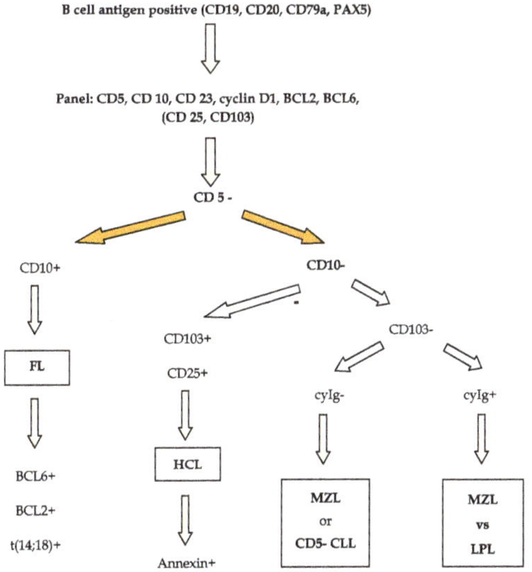

Fig. 4. Proposed algorithm for stratification of follicular lymphoma (NCCN)

16. References

[1] Anderson JR, Armitage JO, Weisenburger DD (1998): Epidemiology of the non-Hodgkin's lymphomas: distributions of the major subtypes differ by geographic locations. Non-Hodgkin's Lymphoma Classification Project. Ann Oncol9: 717-720.

[2] Reya T, Morrison SJ, Clarke MF, Weissman IL. Stem cells, cancer, and cancer stem cells.Nature. 2001;414(6859):105-11.

[3] Pardal R, Molofsky AV, He S, Morrison SJ.Stem cell self-renewal and cancer cell proliferation are regulated by common networks that balance the activation of proto-oncogenes and tumor suppressors. Cold Spring Harb Symp Quant Biol. 2005;70:177-85.

[4] Clarke MF, Fuller M. Stem cells and cancer(2006): two faces of eve. Cell (6):1111-5.

[5] Bruce WR, Van Der Gaag H (1963): A Quantitative assay for the number of murine lymphoma cells capable of proliferation in vivo. Nature. 199:79-80.

[6] Park CH, Bergsagel DE, McCulloch EA (1971).Mouse myeloma tumor stem cells: a primary cell culture assay. J Natl Cancer Inst.46(2):411-22.

[7] Hamburger AW, Salmon SE (1977): Primary bioassay of human tumor stem cells. Science.1977;197(4302):461-3.

[8] Lapidot T, Sirard C, Vormoor J, Murdoch B,Hoang T, Caceres-Cortes J, et al.(1994): A cell initiating human acute myeloid leukaemia after transplantation into SCID mice.Nature. 367(6464):645-8.

[9] Bonnet D, Dick JE (1997): Human acute myeloid leukemia is organized as a hierarchy that originates from a primitive hematopoietic cell. Nat Med.3(7):730-7.

[10] Al-Hajj M, Clarke MF (2004): Self-renewal and solid tumor stem cells. Oncogene.23(43):7274-82.

[11] Boman BM, Wicha MS (2008): Cancer stem cells:a step toward the cure. J Clin Oncol.26(17):2795-9.

[12] Martinez-Climent JA, Fontan L, Gascoyne RD, Siebert R, and Prosper F.(2010): Lymphoma stem cells: enough evidence to support their existence? Haematologica. 95:293-302.

[13] Salles GA (2007):Clinical Features, Prognosis and Treatment of Follicular Lymphoma. *Hematology* 216-25.

[14] Goodlad JR, MacPherson S, Jackson R, Batstone P, White J (2004):Extranodal follicular lymphoma: a clinicopathological and genetic analysis of 15 cases arising at non-cutaneous extranodal sites. Histopathology.44:268–276.

[15] Damaj G, Verkarre V, Delmer A, et al (2003): Primary follicular lymphoma of the gastrointestinal tract: a study of 25 cases and a literature review. Ann Oncol.14:623–629.

[16] Poggi MM, Cong PJ, Coleman CN, Jaffe ES (2002): Low-grade follicular lymphoma of the small intestine. J Clin Gastroenterol.34:155–159.

[17] Willemze R, Jaffe ES, Burg G, et al (2005): WHO-EORTC classification for cutaneous lymphomas. Blood.;105:3768–3785.

[18] Bacon CM, Ye H, Diss TC, et al (2007): Primary follicular lymphoma of the testis and epididymis in adults. Am J Surg Pathol. 31:1050–1058.

[19] Lorsbach RB, Shay-Seymore D, Moore J, et al (2002): Clinicopathologic analysis of follicular lymphoma occurring in children. Blood. 99:1959–1964.

[20] Yuen AR, Kamel OW, Halpern J, Horning SJ (1995): Long-term survival after histologic transformation of low-grade follicular lymphoma. J Clin Oncol. 13:1726–1733.
[21] Montoto S, Davies AJ, Matthews J, et al (2007): Risk and clinical implications of transformation of follicular lymphoma to diffuse large B-cell lymphoma. J Clin Oncol. 25:2426–2433.
[22] Federico M, Vitolo U, Zinzani PL, et al (2000): Prognosis of follicular lymphoma: a predictive model based on a retrospective analysis of 987 cases. Intergruppo Italiano Linfomi. Blood.95:783–9.
[23] Solal-Celigny P, Roy P, Colombat P, et al (2004): Follicular lymphoma international prognostic index. Blood. 104:1258–65.
[24] Conconi A, Motta M, Bertoni F, et al (2010): Patterns of survival of follicular lymphomas at a single institution through three decades. Leuk Lymphoma. 51:1028–34.
[25] Federico M, Bellei M, Marcheselli L, et al (2009): Follicular lymphoma international prognostic index 2: a new prognostic index for follicular lymphoma developed by the international follicular lymphoma prognostic factor project. J Clin Oncol. 27:4555–62 .
[26] Fisher R. , LeBlanc M. , Press O , Maloney D., Unger J, Miller T.(2005):New Treatment Options Have Changed the Survival of Patients With Follicular Lymphoma. JCO , 23 (33); 8447-8452
[27] Hitz F, Kettere N, Lohri A, Mey U, Pederiva S, Renner C, Taverna C, Hatmann A, Yeow K, Bodis S, Zucca E (2011):Diagnosis and treatment of follicular lymphoma Swiss Med Wkly. 141:w13247.
[28] Martinelli G, Hsu Schmitz SF, Utiger U, et al (2010): Long-Term Follow-Up of Patients With Follicular Lymphoma Receiving Single-Agent Rituximab at Two Different Schedules in Trial SAKK 35/98. J Clin Oncol. 28:4480–4.
[29] Ardeshna KM, Smith P, Qian W, et al (2010): An Intergroup Randomised Trial of Rituximab Versus a Watch and Wait Strategy In Patients with Stage II, III, IV, Asymptomatic, Non-Bulky Follicular Lymphoma (Grades 1, 2 and 3a). A Preliminary Analysis. Blood, ASH Annual Meeting Abstracts 116:Abstract 6.
[30] Horning SJ (1993): Natural history of and therapy for the indolent non-Hodgkin's lymphomas. Semin Oncol.20:75-88, (suppl 5.(
[31] Marcus R, Solal-Celigny P, Imrie K, et al (2006): Rituximab plus CVP improves survival in previously untreated patients with advanced follicular non-Hodgkin's lymphoma [abstract]. Blood. 108:481a
[32] Maloney DG, Press OW, Braziel RM, et al (2001): A phase II trial of chop followed by rituximab chimeric monoclonal anti-CD20 antibody for treatment of newly diagnosed follicular non-Hodgkin's lymphoma: SWOG 9800. Blood, 98:843a.
[33] Czuczman MS, Weaver R, Alkuzweny B, et al (2004): Prolonged clinical and molecular remission in patients with low-grade or follicular non-Hodgkin's lymphoma treated with rituximab plus CHOP chemotherapy: 9-Year follow-up. J Clin Oncol , 22:4711-4716
[34] Sacchi S,Pozzi S,Marcheselli L, Bari A,Stefano (2007): Introduction of rituximab in front-line and salvage therapies has improved outcome of advanced-stage follicular lymphoma patients. Cancer Volume 109, Issue 10, 2077–2082,

[35] Freedman A (2011): update on diagnosis and management. . Am. J. Hematol. 86:769-775, 2011.
[36] Vidal L, Gafter-Gvili A, Leibovici L, et al (2009) : Rituximab maintenance for the treatment of patients with follicular lymphoma: systematic review and meta-analysis of randomized trials. *J Natl Cancer Inst*;101:248-255.
[37] MacManus PM, Hoppe RT (1996): Is radiotherapy curative for stage I and II low grade follicular lymphoma? Results of a long term follow-up study of patients treated at Stanford University. *J Clin Oncol*;14:1282-1290.
[38] Advani R, Rosenberg SA, Horning SJ(2004): Stage I and II follicular non-Hodgkin's lymphoma: long-term follow-up of no initial therapy. *J Clin Oncol*;22:1454-1459.
[39] Kaminski MS, Tuck M, Estes J, et al (2005): ^{131}I-Tositumomab therapy as initial treatment for follicular lymphoma. *N Engl J Med*;352:441-449.
[40] Martinelli G, Schmitz SF, Utiger U, et al (2010): *Long-term follow-up of patients with follicular lymphoma receiving single-agent rituximab at two different schedules in trial SAKK 35/98 J Clin Oncol*;28:4480-4484.
[41] Hayashi D., Lee J.C., Devenney-Cakir B., Zaim S., Ounadjela S., Solal-Celigny P., Juweid M., Guermazi A (2010): Follicular non-Hodgkin's lymphoma. Clinical Radiology, (65): 408–420.
[42] Stacy R.C., Jakobiec F. A., Schoenfield L., Singh A. D (2010): Unifocal and Multifocal Reactive Lymphoid Hyperplasia vs Follicular Lymphoma of the Ocular Adnexa. American Journal of Ophthalmology. (150), NO. 3, 412-426.
[43] Winter J. N., Gascoyne R. D., Van Besien K (2004): Low-Grade Lymphoma. Hematology, 203-220.
[44] Klapper W (2011): Pathobiology and diagnosis of follicular lymphoma. Semin Diagn Pathol.28(2):146-60. Review
[45] Vitolo U., Ferreri A.J., Montoto S (2008): Follicular lymphoma. Crit Rev Oncol Hematol. Jun;66(3):248-61.
[46] Samsi S., Lozanski G., Shana'ah A., Krishanmurthy A. K., Gurcan M.N(2010): Detection of Follicles from IHC Stained Slides of Follicular Lymphoma Using Iterative Watersh.Trans Biomed Eng. October; 57(10): 2609–2612.
[47] Jaffe E.S (2009): The 2008 WHO classification of lymphomas: implications for clinical practice and translationalresearch, Hematology, 523-531.
[48] Gradowski J. F., Jaffe E. S., Warnke R. A., Pittaluga S., Surti U., Gole L. A., Swerdlow S. H (2010): Follicular lymphomas with plasmacytic differentiation include two subtypes . Modern Pathology. (23), 71–79.
[49] Montes-Moreno S., Garcı´a O. A., Santiago-Ruiz G., Ferreira J. A., Garcı´a J. F., Pinilla A. P (2010): Intrafollicular neoplasia in situ follicular lymphoma: review of a series of 13 cases., Histopathology, 56, 652–664.
[50] Young N. A (2006): Grading Follicular Lymphoma on Fine-Needle Aspiration Specimens—A Practical Approach (cancer cytopathology), Vol 108 no1
[51] Lejeune M, Álvaro T (2009): Clinicobiological, prognostic and therapeutic implications of the tumor microenvironment in follicular lymphoma. Haematologica, January; 94(1): 16–21.
[52] Bakhshi A, Jensen JP, Goldman P, Wright JJ, McBride OW, Epstein AL, Korsmeyer SJ (1985): Cloning the chromosomal breakpoint of t(14;18) human lymphomas:

clustering around JH on chromosome 14 and near a transcriptional unit on 18. Cell 41:899-906.

[53] Tsujimoto Y, Gorham J, Cossman J, Jaffe E, Croce CM (1985): The t(14;18) chromosome translocations involved in B-cell neoplasms result from mistakes in VDJ joining. Science; 229:1390-3.

[54] Keni Gu, Kai Fu, Smrati Jain, Zhongfen Liu, Javeed Iqbal, Min Li, Warren G Sanger, Dennis D Weisenburger, Timothy C Greiner, Patricia Aoun, Bhavana J Dave and Wing C Chan (2009): t(14;18)-negative follicular lymphomas are associated with a high frequency of BCL6 rearrangement at the alternative breakpoint region. Modern Pathology ; 22: 1251–1257.

[55] de Jong D (2005):. Molecular pathogenesis of follicular lymphoma: a cross talk of genetic and immunologic factors. J Clin Oncol;23:6358-63.

[56] German Ott and Andreas Rosenwald (2008): Molecular pathogenesis of follicular lymphoma. Haematologica; 93:1773-6.

[57] Pasqualucci L, Bhagat G, Jankovic M, Compagno M, Smith P, Muramatsu M, et al (2008): AID is required for germinal centerderived lymphomagenesis. Nat Genet; 40:108-12.

[58] Cong P, Raffeld M, Teruya-Feldstein J, Sorbara L, Pittaluga S, Jaffe ES (2002): In situ localization of follicular lymphoma: description and analysis by laser capture microdissection. Blood;99:3376-82.

[59] Ott G, Katzenberger T, Lohr A, Kindelberger S, Rudiger T, Wilhelm M, et al (2002): Cytomorphologic, immunohistochemical, and cytogenetic profiles of follicular lymphoma: 2 types of follicular lymphoma grade 3. Blood;99:3806- 12.

[60] Cheung KJ, Shah SP, Steidl C, Johnson N, Relander T, Telenius A, et al (2008): Genome-wide profiling of follicular lymphoma by array comparative genomic hybridization reveals prognostically significant DNA copy number imbalances. Blood.

[61] Hoglund M, Sehn L, Connors JM, Gascoyne RD, Siebert R, Sall T, et al (2004): Identification of cytogenetic subgroups and karyotypic pathways of clonal evolution in follicular lymphomas. Genes Chromosomes Cancer;39:195-204.

[62] Macpherson N, Lesack D, Klasa R, Horsman D, Connors JM, Barnett M, Gascoyne RD (1999):. Small noncleaved, non- Burkitt's (Burkit-Like) lymphoma: cytogenetics predict outcome and reflect clinical presentation. J Clin Oncol;17:1558-67.

[63] Elenitoba-Johnson KS, Gascoyne RD, Lim MS, Chhanabai M, Jaffe ES, Raffeld M (1998): Homozygous deletions at chromosome 9p21 involving p16 and p15 are associated with histologic progression in follicle center lymphoma. Blood;91:4677-85.

[64] O'Shea D, O'Riain C, Taylor C, Waters R, Carlotti E, Macdougall F, et al (2008): The presence of TP53 mutation at diagnosis of follicular lymphoma identifies a high-risk group of patients with shortened time to disease progression and a poorer overall survival. Blood;112:3126-9.

[65] Ellen Leich,Itziar Salaverria, Silvia Bea, Andreas Zettl, George Wright, Victor Moreno,Randy D. Gascoyne,Wing-Chung Chan,Rita M. Braziel,Lisa M. Rimsza, Dennis D. Weisenburger, Jan Delabie, Elaine S. Jaffe,Andrew Lister, Jude Fitzgibbon,Louis M. Staudt, Elena M. Hartmann,Hans-Konrad Mueller-Hermelink,Elias Campo,German Ott, and Andreas Rosenwald (2009): Follicular lymphomas with and without translocation t(14;18) differ in gene expression profiles and genetic alterations. Blood. 114: 826-834.

[66] Guo Y, Karube K, Kawano R, et al (2007): Bcl2-negative follicular lymphomas frequently have Bcl6 translocation and/or Bcl6 or p53 expression. Pathol Int.;57:148-152.

[67] Tagawa H, Karube K, Guo Y, et al (2007): Trisomy 3 is a specific genomic aberration of t(14;18) negative follicular lymphoma. Leukemia.;21:2549-2551.

[68] Horsman DE, Okamoto I, Ludkovski O, et al (2003): Follicular lymphoma lacking the t(14;18)(q32;q21): identification of two disease subtypes. Br J Haematol.;120:424-433.

[69] Karube K, Guo Y, Suzumiya J, et al (2007): CD10- MUM1- follicular lymphoma lacks BCL2 gene translocation and shows characteristic biologic and clinical features. Blood.;109:3076-3079.

[70] Cleary ML, Meeker TC, Levy S, Lee E, Trela M, Sklar J, Levy R(1986): clustering of extensive somatic mutations in the variable region of an immunoglobulin heavy chain gene from a human B cell lymphoma. Cell 44:97-106.

[71] Ottensmeier cCH,Thompesett AR, Zhu D,Wikins BS,Sweetenham JW,Stevenson FK,.(1998):Analysis of VH genes in follicular and diffuse lymphoma shows ongoing somatic mutation and multiple isotype transcriptsin early disease with changes during disease progression.Blood.91:4292-4299.

[72] Evans PA,PottC,GroenenPJ , SallesG, Davi F,Berger F,Garcia JF, Van Krieken JH, Pales S, Kluin P,Schuuring E et al.(2007):Significantly improved PCR based clonality testing in B cell malignancies by use of multiple immunoglobulin gene targets.Report of the Biomed -2 Concerted Action BHM4-CT983936.leukemia 21:207-214.

[73] van Dongen JJM, Langerak AW, Bruggemann M, Evans PAS, Hummel , Lavender FL, Delabesse E, Davi F, Schuuring E , Garcia-Sanz R, van Krieken JHJM, Droese J, Gonzalez D, Bastard C, White HE, Spaargaren M, Gonzalez M, Parreira A, Smith JL, Morgan GJ, Kneba M and Macintyre EA (2003):Design and standardization of PCR primers and protocols for detection of clonal immunoglobulin and T-cell receptor gene recombinations in suspect lymphoproliferations: Report of the BIOMED-2 Concerted Action BMH4-CT98-3936. Leukemia 17, 2257–2317.

[74] Fukuhara S, Rowley JD, Variakojis D, Golomb HM (1979): Chromosome abnormalities in poorly differentiated lymphocytic lymphoma. Cancer Res; 39: 3119–3128.

[75] Score J,CurtisC,Waghorn K,Stadler M,Jotterand M,Grand FH, Cross NC (2006): Identification of a novel imatinib responsive KIF5B-PDGFRA fusion gene following PDGFRA overexpression in patients with hyperoesinophilia .Leukemia 20:827-832.

[76] Rowley JD (1988):Chromosome studies in the hodgiken lymphomas:the role of t (14;18) translocation .J Clin Oncol6:919-925.

[77] Aster JC,Longtine JA (2002):Detection of BCL2 rearrangements in follicular lymphoma.Am J Path 160:759-763.

[78] Montolo S,Lopez Guillermo A,Colomer D, Esteve J, Bosh F, Ferrer A, Villamor N, Moreno C, Campo E, Montserrat E (2003): Incidence and clinical significance of bcl2/IgH rearrangements in follicular lymphoma.Leuk Lymphoma 44:71-76.

[79] Vaandrager JW,Schuuring E,RaapT,Phillipo K,Kleiverda K,Kluin P.2000. Interphase FISH detection of BCL2 rearrangement in follicular lymphoma using breakpoint flanking probes.Genes Chromosomes Cancer.27:85-94.

[80] Ott G, Katzenberger T,Lohr A,Kendelberger S, Rudgier T,Wihelm M, Kalla J, Rosenwald A, Muller JG ,Ott MM, Muller Hermlink HK

(2002):Cytomorphologic,immunohistochemical and cytogenetic profiles of follicular lymphoma :2 types of follicular lymphoma grade 3>Blood99:3806-3812.

[81] Bakhshi A, Jensen JP, Goldman P, Wright JJ, McBride OW, Epstein AL et al (1985): Cloning the chromosomal breakpoint of t(14;18) human lymphomas: clustering around JH on chromosome 14 and near a transcriptional unit on 18. Cell; 41: 899-906.

[82] Cleary ML, Sklar J (1985): Nucleotide sequence of a t(14;18) chromosomal breakpoint in follicular lymphoma and demonstration of a breakpoint-cluster region near a transcriptionally active locus on chromosome 18. Proc Natl Acad Sci USA; 82: 7439-7443.

[83] Rouland S,Lebality P, Roussel G,Briand M,Cappellen D,Pottier D,Hardouin A,Troussard X,Bastard C, Henery-Amar M,Gauduchon P(2003):BCL2/JH translocation in peripheral blood lymphocytes of unexposed individuals :lack of seasonal variations in frequency and molecular features.Int J Cancer 104:695-698.

[84] Schmitt C,Balogh B,Grudt A, Buchulotz C, Leo A,Benner A, Hensel M,Ho AD,Leo A(2006):The bcl2/IGH rearrangement in a population of 204 healthy individuals :occurance ,age,and gender distribution ,breakpoints and detection method validity.Leuk Res 30:745-750.

[85] Summers KE, Goff LK, Wilson AG, Gupta RK , Lister TA, Fitzgibbon J (2001): Frequency of BCL2/IgH rearrangement in Normal individuals :implications for the monitoring of disease in patients with follicular lymphoma .JClin Oncol 19 :420-424.

[86] Rouland S , Navaro JM, Grenot P, Milili M,Agopian J, Montpellier B, Gauduchon P, lebailly P, Sciff C,Nadel B (200):Follicular lymphoma like B cells in healthy individuals:a novel intermediate step in early lymphomagenesis .JExp Med 203:2425-2431.

[87] Pezzella F, Ralfkiaer E, Gatter KC, Mason DY (1990): The 14;18 translocation in European cases of follicular lymphoma: comparison of Southern blotting and the polymerase chain reaction. Br J Haematol; 76: 58–64.

[88] Turner GE, Ross FM, Krajewski AS (1995): Detection of t(14;18) in British follicular lymphoma using cytogenetics, Southern blotting and the polymerase chain reaction. Br J Haematol; 89: 223–225.

[89] Vaandrager JW, Schuuring E, Raap T, Philippo K, Kleiverda K, Kluin P (2000): Interphase FISH detection of BCL2 rearrangement in follicular lymphoma using breakpoint-?anking probes. Genes Chromosomes Cancer; 27: 85–94.

[90] Deghiedy H, Fouda M, Shahin D,shamaa S, El-Bedewy A, Abd El-Ghaffar H (2007): Diagnostic and prognostic utility of t(14;18) in follicular lymphoma. Acta Hematol. 118:231-236.

[91] Alizadeh AA, Eisen MB, Davis RE, Lossos IS, Rosenwald A, Boldrick JC, Sabet H, Tran T, Yu X, Powell JI, Yang L, Marti GE, Moore T, Hudson J Jr, Lu L, Lewis DB, Tibshirani R, Sherlock G, Chan WC, Greiner TC, Weisenburger DD, Armitage JO, Warnke R, Levy R, Wilson W, Grever MR, Byrd JC, Botstein D, Brown PO, Staudt LM (2000): Distinct types of diffuse large B-cell lymphoma identified by gene expression profiling. Nature.;403:503-511.

[92] Husson H, th G. Carideo EG, Neuberg D, Schultze J, Munoz O, Marks PW, Donovan JW, C. Chillemi AC, O'Connell P and Freedman AS (2002): Gene expression

profiling of follicular lymphoma and normal germinal center B cells using cDNA arrays. Blood, 99: 282-289
[93] 93 Rosenwald A, Wright G, Chan WC, Connors JM, Campo E, Fisher RI, Gascoyne RD, Muller-Hermelink HK, Smeland EB, Giltnane JM, Hurt EM, Zhao H, Averett L, Yang L, Wilson WH, Jaffe ES, Simon R, Klausner RD, Powell J, Duffey PL, Longo DL, Greiner TC, Weisenburger DD, Sanger WG, Dave BJ, Lynch JC, Vose J, Armitage JO, Montserrat E, López-Guillermo A, Grogan TM, Miller TP, LeBlanc M, Ott G, Kvaloy S, Delabie J, Holte H, Krajci P, Stokke T, Staudt LM (2002):. The use of molecular profiling to predict survival after chemotherapy for diffuse large-B-cell lymphoma. N Engl J Med.;346:1937-1947.
[94] Shipp MA, Ross KN, Tamayo P, Weng AP, Kutok JL, Aguiar RC, Gaasenbeek M, Angelo M, Reich M, Pinkus GS, Ray TS, Koval MA, Last KW, Norton A, Lister TA, Mesirov J, Neuberg DS, Lander ES, Aster JC, Golub TR (2002): Diffuse large B-cell lymphoma outcome prediction by gene-expression profiling and supervised machine learning. Nat Med.;8:68-74.
[95] Glas AM, Kersten MJ, Delahaye LJMJ, Witteveen AT, Kibbelaar RE, Velds A, Wessels LFA, Joosten P, Kerkhoven RM, Bernards R, van Krieken JHJM, Kluin PM, van't Veer LJ and de Jong D (2005): Gene expression profiling in follicular lymphoma to assess clinical aggressiveness and to guide the choice of treatment. Blood, 105: 301-307.
[96] Husson H, Carideo EG, Neuberg D, et al (2002): Gene expression profiling of follicular lymphoma and normal germinal center B cells using cDNA arrays. Blood.;99:282-289.
[97] de Vos S, Hofmann WK, Grogan TM, et al (2003): Gene expression profile of serial samples of transformed B-cell lymphomas. Lab Invest.;83:271-285.
[98] Elenitoba-Johnson KS, Jenson SD, Abbott RT, et al (2003):Involvement of multiple signaling pathways in follicular lymphoma transformation: p38-mitogen-activated protein kinase as a target for therapy. Proc Natl Acad Sci U S A.;100:7259-7264.
[99] Lossos IS, Alizadeh AA, Diehn M, et al (2002): Transformation of follicular lymphoma to diffuse large-cell lymphoma: alternative patterns with increased or decreased expression of c-myc and its regulated genes. Proc Natl Acad Sci U S A.;99:8886-8891.
[100] Adida C, Haioun C, Gaulard P, et al (2000): Prognostic signifcance of survivin expression in diffuse large B-cell lymphomas. Blood.;96:1921-1925.
[101] Akasaka T, Akasaka H, Ueda C, et al (2000): Molecular and clinical features of non-Burkitt's, diffuse large-cell lymphoma of B-cell type associated with the c-MYC/immunoglobulin heavy-chain fusion gene. J Clin Oncol.;18:510-518.
[102] Menssen A, Hermeking H (2002): Characterization of the c-MYC-regulated transcriptome by SAGE: identifcation and analysis of c-MYC target genes. Proc Natl Acad Sci U S A.;99:6274-6279.
[103] Homey B, Muller A, Zlotnik A (2002): Chemokines: agents for the immunotherapy of cancer? Nat Rev Immunol.;2:175-184).

5

MicroRNA Expression in Follicular Lymphoma

Charles H. Lawrie
[1]*Biodonostia Institute, San Sebastián*
[2]*IKERBASQUE, Basque Foundation for Science, Bilbao*
[3]*Nuffield Department of Clinical Laboratory Sciences, University of Oxford,*
[1,2]*Spain*
[3]*UK*

1. Introduction

Lymphoma is the fifth most common cancer type in the Western world, accounting for approximately 12,000 cases per annum in the UK alone. Moreover the occurrence of this type of cancer has been increasing. The age-adjusted incidence of non-Hodgkin's lymphoma (NHL) in the US for example has increased 74% between 1976 and 2001 (SEER 2005). Follicular lymphoma (FL) is the most common form of low grade B-cell lymphoma (75-80% of all cases) representing about a third of all NHL cases in the US, and a quarter of all cases in Europe (Anderson et al. 1998). FL is characterised by the presence of the t(14;18) translocation in 90% of patients associated with up-regulation of the anti-apoptotic protein BCL2. Whilst FL tumours are chemo-sensitive, the disease is essentially incurable, with patients following a relapsing-remitting clinical course, typically experiencing several episodes of disease before eventually becoming refractory to treatment.

Although indolent, with a median overall survival (OS) of ~10 years, about 30% of FL patients undergo high-grade transformation to an aggressive lymphoma that is histologically indistinguishable from diffuse large B-cell lympohoma (DLBCL). Transformed FL (tFL) patients have a particularly poor outcome with a median survival of <14 months (Wrench et al. 2010). The molecular basis of FL transformation is only poorly understood and importantly to date there are no reliable biomarkers that can identify FL patients at risk of transformation. In this chapter we will review the experimental evidence for the involvement of microRNAs in the pathology of FL with particular focus on the transformation process.

2. Follicular lymphoma

FL is a neoplasm of follicle center B cells (centrocytes) characterized by a (partially) follicular growth pattern. FL tumor cells are believed to arise from normal germinal centre–associated (GC) B cells as they express the same antigen profile as GC B cells (i.e. CD19, CD20, CD10, BCL6, and membrane-bound IgM or IgG), share many morphological features of normal GC cells, and are found within a follicular architecture embedded in a network of T cells and follicular dendritic cells. In contrast to normal GC cells however, FL tumour cells are characterised by the presence of t(14:18) translocation resulting in expression of the anti-apoptotic molecule BCL2. This translocation is detectable in approximately 75% of cases by traditional karyotyping techniques but in over 90% of cases measured by polymerase chain reaction (PCR) (Tsujimoto et al. 1985). Although considered to be an essential feature of FL pathology, this genetic insult appears not to be in itself sufficient to cause FL as *BCL2* transgenic mice do not readily develop lymphoma (McDonnell & Korsmeyer 1991; Strasser et al. 1993). Furthermore, the t(14;18) translocation is not an uncommon finding in normal B cells, being detectable in over 50% of healthy individuals (Roulland et al. 2006). Therefore, whilst the presence of t(14:18) is highly suggestive of FL, it is by no means diagnostic, and indeed may be found in other apparently unrelated cases of NHL including 15-30% of DLBCL cases (Iqbal et al. 2004). Furthermore about 5% of FL cases lack the t(14:18) translocation instead being characterised by a BCL6 translocation t(3;14) and displaying an almost exclusive centroblastic morphology (Jaffe et al. 2001).

FL predominantly affects adults with a median age of 59 years and a male:female ratio of 1:1.7 (Anderson et al. 1998). Most FL patients already have widespread disease at time of presentation, predominantly in the lymph nodes, but FL may also involve the spleen, bone marrow, and peripheral blood and occasionally extra-nodal sites such as the gastro-intestinal tract or skin. Patients may be asymptomatic with slowly progressive lymphadenopathy or present with symptomatic complications of advancing tumour growth that require treatment. In nearly all survival studies, despite initial responsiveness to treatment, most patients relapse, and will eventually die of their disease.

2.1 Histological transformation of FL tumors

A percentage of FL patients (10-60% depending on the study) will eventually undergo high grade transformation from indolent FL to a much more aggressive tumor that is histologically indistinguishable from DLBCL, and is associated with a much poorer prognostic outcome. A recent study of 325 patients (median follow-up 15 years) found the risk of transformation to be 28% (Montoto et al. 2007). Despite the use of high dose therapy for transformed FL (tFL) cases, response rates are still lower than histologically equivalent *de novo* cases of DLBCL with a median survival of just 1.2 years. The molecular mechanisms behind this phenomenon, however, are very poorly understood and consequently the identification of at-risk patients, who might benefit from up-front high dose treatment modalities, remains one of the greatest challenges facing onco-hematologists today.

Lossos *et al* identified 671 genes that were aberrantly expressed in at least three of twelve paired biopsy samples which fell into two distinct groups; those that had *c-myc* and its target genes up-regulated and those where these genes were down-regulated (Lossos et al. 2002). Another study of five paired samples identified 36 up-regulated and 66 down-regulated genes, seven of which were common with the study of Lossos *et al* (de Vos et al. 2003). Sixty-seven and 46 genes were found to be up-regulated and down-regulated respectively in a series of eleven paired samples analyzed by Elenitoba-Johnson *et al* (Elenitoba-Johnson et al. 2003). Up-regulation of p38BMAPK was confirmed immunohistochemically as it was detected in DLBCL cases but not FL or normal GC cells. Davies *et al* examined the gene expression profile of twenty paired lymphoma samples taken pre- and post-transformation (Davies et al. 2007). They found that transformation proceeded by at least two molecular pathways; one characterized by a cell proliferation signature that was associated with recurrent oncogenic abnormalities and a decrease in T cell and follicular dendritic cell genes, while the other group showed no increase in proliferation genes and followed an as yet undetermined route. In contrast a gene expression study of non-paired patients (24 FL patients who underwent transformation, 22 FL patients without transformation (after 7 years) and 24 DLBCL patients who had previously transformed from FL) found that gene expression was too heterogeneous to reliably predict transformation (Glas et al. 2007). They did however report a correlation by immunohistochemistry with the spatial distribution to neoplastic follicles and the activation of $CD4^+$ T cells and specifically T-helper 1 cells ($P>0.05$). They did not find any correlation with other infiltrating cell populations including $CD68^+$ macrophages or regulatory T cells.

Additionally, genomic alterations have been demonstrated to be associated with transformation of FL. The acquisition of novel mutations in PIM-1, PAX-5, RhoH/TTF and c-MYC genes, due to aberrant somatic hypermutation, was found in 5/9 cases that had undergone transformation (Rossi et al. 2006). Genomic aberrations were found to be more common in transformed cases of DLBCL than non-transformed FL and the alterations -6q16-21 and +7pter-q22 were only found in transformed DLBCL but not in follicular lymphoma whereas -4q13-21 was more common in transformed than *de novo* DLBCL (Berglund et al. 2007).

However, despite intensive research the molecular basis for transformation in FL patients remains largely unknown. Recently, ourselves and others, have raised the possibility that microRNAs may be important factors in both FL transformation and antecedent FL lymphogenesis (Roehle et al. 2008; Lawrie et al. 2009).

3. MicroRNAs

MicroRNAs are a recently discovered class of naturally occurring short non-coding RNA molecules that regulate eukaryotic gene expression post-transcriptionally. There are now more than 900 human microRNAs that have been identified through cloning and/or sequence analysis (miRBase- (Griffiths-Jones et al. 2006)), and it is believed some 60% of all human genes are a target for microRNA regulation (Friedman et al. 2009). MicroRNAs have been shown to play key regulatory roles in virtually every aspect of biology including developmental timing, cell differentiation, apoptosis, cell proliferation, metabolism organ development, and hematopoiesis (Kim 2005). The potential importance of microRNAs in cancer is implied by the finding that the majority of human microRNAs are located at cancer-associated genomic regions (Calin et al. 2004), and there is now overwhelming evidence that dysfunctional expression of microRNAs is a common, if not ubiquitous, feature of cancer in general and lymphoid malignancy in particular (Lawrie 2008; Iorio & Croce 2009).

Despite the fundamental role that microRNAs appear to play in biology, these molecules were unknown to the scientific world until 1993 when *lin-4*, a *C. elegans* developmental regulator was identified (Lee et al. 1993; Wightman et al. 1993). The significance of this finding was not however realised until seven years later when another worm microRNA, *let-7* was discovered (Reinhart et al. 2000). Unlike *lin-4*, the sequence of *let-7* was found to be highly conserved in almost all organisms (Pasquinelli et al. 2000). It was soon realised that similar sequences were scattered throughout eukaryotic genomes that were first called microRNAs in 2001 (Lee & Ambros 2001).

3.1 MicroRNA biosynthesis and function

The majority of human microRNAs are encoded within introns of coding or non-coding mRNAs whilst others are located exgenically, within the exons of non-coding mRNAs or within the 3′UTR sequence of mRNA (Rodriguez et al. 2004). MicroRNAs are transcribed as 5′-capped large polyadenylated transcripts (pri-microRNA) primarily in a Pol II-dependent manner (Figure 1), although the involvement of Pol-III transcription has also been postulated for microRNAs encoded within Alu repeat sequences (Borchert et al. 2006). Approximately 40% of human microRNAs are co-transcribed as clusters encoding up to eight distinct microRNA sequences in a single pri-microRNA transcript (Altuvia et al. 2005; Hertel et al. 2006). Pri-microRNAs are cleaved within the nucleus by Drosha, an RNaseIII-type nuclease, to form 60-70 nucleotide hairpin structures (pre-microRNA). Drosha by itself possesses little enzymatic activity and requires the cofactor DiGeorge syndrome critical region 8 gene (DGCR8) in humans (Pasha in *Drosophila*) to form the so-called microprocessor complex (Yeom et al. 2006). Once produced, the pre-microRNAs are

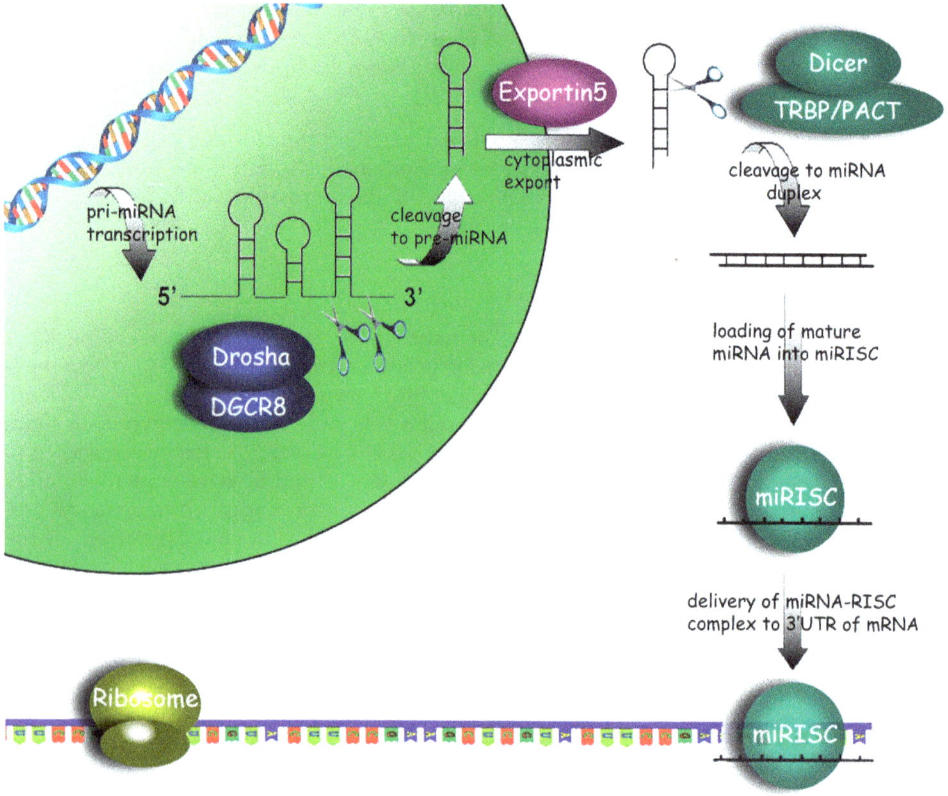

Fig. 1. **Schematic diagram of microRNA biosynthesis and function in animal cells.** Pri-microRNA precursor is transcribed in Pol-II dependent manner and then cleaved by microprocessor complex (Drosha/DGCR8) to form hairpin-structure pre-microRNA. Pre-microRNAs are exported from the nucleus by exportin-5 in a RAN-GTP dependent manner where they are cleaved into an asymmetric duplex by action of Dicer and accessory proteins. The mature microRNA is loaded into the miRISC complex which binds to cognate 3′UTR sequence of target mRNA resulting in either degradation of mRNA, or to blockage of translation without mRNA degradation.

exported from the nucleus to the cytoplasm by Exportin5 in a Ran-GTP dependent manner (Zeng 2006). The cytoplasmic pre-microRNA is further cleaved to form an asymmetric duplex intermediate (microRNA: microRNA*) by Dicer, another RNaseIII-type enzyme. Similar to Drosha, cofactors such as TRBP and PACT (in humans) are necessary for Dicer activity (Lee et al. 2006). The microRNA: microRNA* duplex is in turn loaded into the miRISC complex in which Argonaut (Ago) proteins appear to be the key effector molecules. The strand that becomes the active mature microRNA appears to be dependent upon which has the lowest free energy 5′ end and is retained by the miRISC complex whilst the other strand is usually degraded by an unknown nuclease (Khvorova et al. 2003; Schwarz et al. 2003).

The loaded miRISC is guided by the mature microRNA sequence (19-24 nucleotide) to partially complementary sequences within the 3′UTR (and probably coding sequences and 5′UTR as well) of the target mRNA, leading to inhibition of translation, transcript degradation, or both (Lawrie 2007; Lytle et al. 2007). Although repression of translation without mRNA degradation was originally believed to be the *modus operandi* of animal microRNAs, the situation appears to be more complex than previously thought, as there is now compelling evidence that microRNAs also effect transcriptional levels through de-adenylation and/or degradation (Giraldez et al. 2006) and may even positively affect translation in some instances (Vasudevan et al. 2007). How translational repression occurs remains unclear. It has been suggested that mRNA bound to the microRNA-miRISC complex may be sequestered away from the translational machinery in P-bodies that additionally act in concert with enzymes to remove the 5′-cap hence preventing translation (Liu et al. 2005; Sen & Blau 2005). Alternatively it has been suggested that microRNAs may prevent recognition of the 5′cap by translation factors (Pillai et al. 2005).

4. MicroRNA expression in FL

The following experimental details were taken in part from previously published research (Lawrie, CH et al., 2009). The only other study, as far we are aware, that considers microRNA expression in FL, was by Roehle *et al* which although it included 46 FL samples, only measured levels of 153 microRNA probes (compared with 464 microRNA probes in this study), and did not consider FL transformation (Roehle et al. 2008).

4.1 Materials and methods

4.1.1 Patient material

Formalin-fixed paraffin-embedded (FFPE) biopsy samples from 98 patients were obtained from the Pathology Department of the John Radcliffe Hospital, Oxford, UK. Eighty patients were diagnosed histologically and clinically as having DLBCL; 64 *de novo* (DLBCL-de novo) and 16 transformed cases with previously diagnosed FL (DLBCL-t). Of the 18 cases of FL used in this study, seven subsequently underwent high grade transformation (FL-t) with a median time to transformation of 24 months (range 10-96 months) from initial diagnosis. The remaining 11 FL cases (FL-nt) had no recorded transformation events (median follow-up time 60 months; range 52-132 months). The FL-t and DLBCL-t samples were not paired. All FL cases were grade 1 or 2 at time of original diagnosis. All samples were collected at time of initial diagnosis (i.e. prior to treatment) with the exception of DLBCL-t cases. Samples had >80% of tumor cells as determined by hematoxylin and eosin staining (not shown). Relevant ethical permission was obtained for the use of all samples.

4.1.2 RNA purification and microarray analysis

Total RNA was purified from four x 20 μm FFPE sections using the Recoverall kit from Ambion (Huntington, UK) in accordance with the manufacturers' instructions. RNA (3 μg) were labeled and hybridized to μRNA microarrays as previously described (Lawrie et al. 2008) using tonsillar material (pooled from twelve healthy individuals) as a common reference in a dye-balanced design.

Image analysis was carried out with BlueFuse software (BlueGnome, Cambridge, UK). Raw image data were global median-normalized within arrays and normalized between arrays using the LIMMA package (Smyth & Speed 2003). The normalized log ratios (average of four replicates per probe) were used for subsequent analysis in Genespring 7.2 (Agilent Technologies, CA, US). ANOVA analysis was used to identify microRNAs differentially expressed between sample types and P values were adjusted using the Benjamini-Hodgberg correction method. Differentially expressed genes were tested for their ability to predict sample class using the leave-one-out cross-validation support vector machine (SVM) function in Genespring.

4.2 Results & discussion

4.2.1 MicroRNA expression is distinct between DLBCL and FL

In order to investigate differences in microRNA expression between FL and DLBCL samples, and because *de novo* and transformed DLBCL are indistinguishable histologically, we initially compared expression in all DLBCL cases (n = 80) with that of all FL cases (n = 18). Thirty microRNAs were found to be differentially expressed ($P < 0.05$) (Table 1). Expression values of these microRNAs correctly predicted 95/97 (98%) of cases as DLBCL or FL by SVM, and clustered the cases distinctly (Fig. 2A).

The study by Roehle *et al* identified 10 microRNAs that were differentially expressed between FL and DLBCL cases (Roehle et al. 2008). Only two of these microRNAs (*miR-150* and *miR-135a*) were found to be differentially expressed ($P < 0.05$) in our patient cohort, although another two microRNAs, *miR-92* and *miR-125b*, had P values of < 0.1. These 10 microRNAs correctly predicted 74/97 (76%) of cases according to diagnosis.

Roehle's study, however, compared *de novo* cases of DLBCL with FL cases that did not undergo subsequent transformation. Therefore, in order to compare the data directly we used the same sample types (64 DLBCL-de novo and 11 FL-nt cases) to re-analyze the data. This resulted in 26 differentially expressed ($P < 0.05$) microRNAs (Table 2), 14 of which were also present in the previous list (Table 1). These microRNAs correctly predicted 73/75 (97%) of cases in this cohort (c.f. 60/75 (80%) with the 10 microRNA signature (Roehle et al. 2008)) and 92/97 (95%) of cases in the extended cohort. Again, the two sets of samples were found to cluster distinctly using the 26-microRNA signature (Fig. 2B).

microRNA	*P* value	Up	Fold change
hsa-miR-200c	8.20E-08	DLBCL	9.39
hsa-miR-518a	1.23E-03	DLBCL	3.15
hsa-miR-638	8.05E-04	DLBCL	3.09
hsa-miR-205	4.36E-02	DLBCL	2.85
hsa-miR-223	1.42E-02	DLBCL	2.75
hsa-miR-573	2.79E-02	DLBCL	2.35
hsa-miR-135b	3.83E-02	DLBCL	1.63
hsa-miR-133a	8.65E-03	DLBCL	1.38
hsa-miR-135a	3.72E-02	DLBCL	1.38
hsa-miR-451	3.67E-03	DLBCL	1.38
hsa-miR-27b	2.12E-06	DLBCL	1.21
hsa-miR-27a	4.62E-07	DLBCL	1.13
hsa-miR-18b	1.03E-02	DLBCL	0.93
hsa-miR-199b	3.23E-03	DLBCL	0.83
hsa-miR-19a	1.20E-02	DLBCL	0.80
hsa-miR-210	1.10E-02	DLBCL	0.75
hsa-miR-19b	7.60E-04	DLBCL	0.75
hsa-miR-99a	9.00E-05	DLBCL	0.72
hsa-miR-100	1.07E-02	DLBCL	0.51
hsa-miR-361	3.57E-02	FL	0.58
hsa-miR-29c	3.07E-02	FL	0.63
hsa-miR-26a	8.85E-03	FL	0.73
hsa-miR-29b	4.22E-03	FL	0.76
hsa-miR-26b	5.50E-03	FL	1.04
hsa-miR-655	4.76E-02	FL	2.32
hsa-miR-10b	3.10E-02	FL	2.38
hsa-miR-634	1.19E-02	FL	2.41
hsa-miR-593	3.30E-02	FL	2.43
hsa-miR-28	1.47E-02	FL	2.49
hsa-miR-150	1.45E-03	FL	3.37

Table 1. MicroRNAs differentially expressed ($P < 0.05$) between DLBCL (DLBCL-de novo and DLBCL-t) and FL (FL-nt and FL-t) diagnoses.

microRNA	*P* value	Up	Fold change
hsa-miR-200c	4.58E-06	DLBCL	10.03
hsa-miR-638	5.30E-04	DLBCL	3.31
hsa-miR-518a	3.85E-02	DLBCL	2.88
hsa-miR-199a	1.57E-02	DLBCL	2.67
hsa-miR-93	3.74E-02	DLBCL	2.64
hsa-miR-22	1.94E-02	DLBCL	2.46
hsa-miR-34a	3.92E-02	DLBCL	2.39
hsa-miR-362	4.68E-02	DLBCL	2.30
hsa-miR-206	3.93E-02	DLBCL	1.73
hsa-miR-451	3.23E-03	DLBCL	1.49
hsa-miR-636	8.55E-03	DLBCL	1.17
hsa-miR-92	4.05E-02	DLBCL	1.08
hsa-miR-27b	6.85E-04	DLBCL	1.04
hsa-miR-199b	1.15E-04	DLBCL	1.03
hsa-miR-27a	4.03E-04	DLBCL	0.97
hsa-miR-24	2.04E-02	DLBCL	0.75
hsa-miR-106a	1.16E-02	DLBCL	0.73
hsa-miR-20a	2.62E-02	DLBCL	0.67
hsa-miR-19b	4.95E-03	DLBCL	0.64
hsa-miR-99a	9.55E-03	DLBCL	0.56
hsa-miR-18b	3.27E-02	DLBCL	0.54
hsa-miR-100	1.95E-02	DLBCL	0.43
hsa-miR-26b	1.88E-02	FL	1.42
hsa-miR-217	2.84E-02	FL	2.44
hsa-miR-634	9.50E-04	FL	2.54
hsa-miR-150	4.55E-02	FL	3.46

Table 2. MicroRNAs differentially expressed ($P < 0.05$) between *de novo* DLBCL and non-transforming FL cases. Members of the *miR-17-92* cluster (and homologous clusters) are depicted in bold type.

Interestingly, six of the microRNAs that were identified as being up-regulated in DLBCL-*de novo* cases compared to FL-nt are encoded by the *miR-17-92* and/or homologous clusters (average fold-increase of 1.05 (range 0.54-2.64)) (He et al. 2005). The other four microRNAs encoded by these clusters, *miR-17-5p, miR-19a, miR-25* and *miR-106b,* had *P* values of 0.067, 0.087, 0.064 and 0.391 respectively. The *miR-17-92* cluster is encoded at the 13q31 locus, a region commonly amplified in lymphomas and ectopic expression of *miR-17-92* greatly accelerated lymphogenesis in a murine model (He et al. 2005). Moreover, direct binding of the c-myc protein up-regulates *miR*-17-92 expression (O'Donnell et al. 2005) and over-expression of c-myc has been demonstrated in the majority (66.6%) of DLBCL cases (Aref et al. 2004), which has also been associated with poorer outcome (Pagnano et al. 2001). An increased level of this cluster in DLBCL compared to FL is consistent with a more aggressive clinical phenotype of DLBCL.

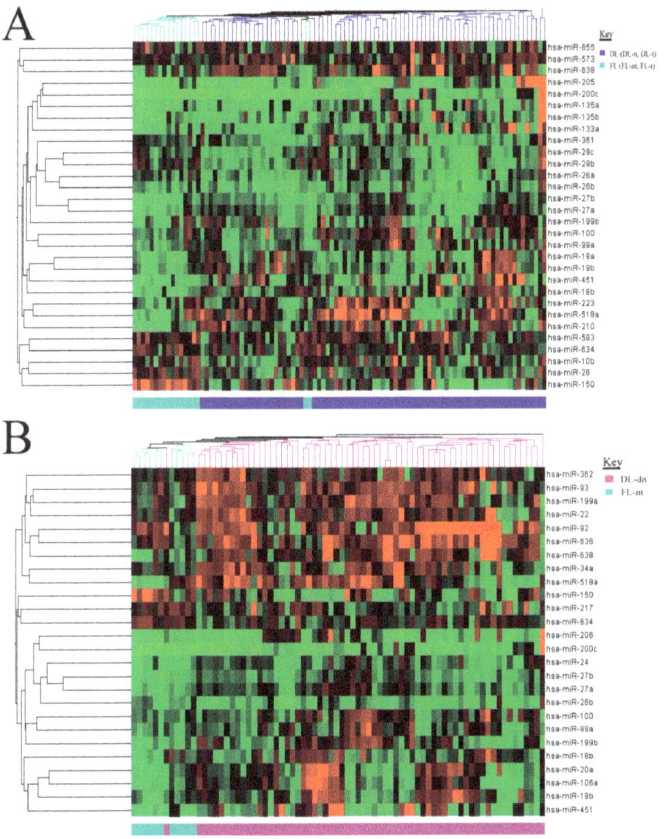

Fig. 2. **Cluster analysis of microRNAs differentially expressed between FL and DLBCL.** (A) All DLBCL cases (n = 80) and FL cases (n = 18). (B) Only *de novo* cases (DLBCL-de novo (n = 64)) and cases of FL that did not undergo transformation (FL-nt (n = 11)). Reproduced from (Lawrie et al. 2009).

4.2.2 Histological transformation of FL is associated with changes in microRNA expression

To investigate whether changes in microRNA expression were associated with transformation we first looked at differences between *de novo* (DLBCL-de novo (n = 64) and transformed (DLBCL-t (n = 16)) cases of DLBCL. Fourteen microRNAs (Table 3) were found to be differentially expressed ($P < 0.05$). These microRNAs correctly predicted transformation status in 73/80 (91%) of samples. Only one of these was up-regulated in DLBCL-t (*miR-491*). Four of the microRNAs down-regulated in DLBCL-t are encoded by the *miR-17-92* cluster suggesting an involvement of the cluster in high grade transformation. An alternative explanation is that because the cluster was also found to be down-regulated in FL compared with DLBCL-de novo (Table 2), the expression pattern of these microRNAs in DLBCL-t cases reflects that of antecedent FL. This latter hypothesis is consistent with gene expression profile studies that found that DLBCL-t cases were more closely related to FL than DLBCL-de novo cases (Lossos et al. 2002).

microRNA	***P* value**	**Up**	**Fold change**
hsa-miR-491	2.11E-02	trans	2.54
hsa-miR-27a	3.90E-02	*de novo*	0.47
hsa-miR-19b	3.77E-03	*de novo*	0.60
hsa-miR-25	3.84E-02	*de novo*	0.67
hsa-miR-18a	1.24E-02	*de novo*	0.72
hsa-miR-636	2.73E-02	*de novo*	1.06
hsa-miR-92	1.94E-02	*de novo*	1.14
hsa-miR-621	2.29E-02	*de novo*	1.98
hsa-miR-526c	2.44E-02	*de novo*	2.38
hsa-miR-766	2.75E-02	*de novo*	2.58
hsa-miR-299-5p	4.76E-02	*de novo*	2.61
hsa-miR-380-3p	5.94E-03	*de novo*	2.65
hsa-miR-129	2.98E-02	*de novo*	2.70
hsa-miR-588	9.05E-03	*de novo*	2.80

Table 3. MicroRNAs differentially expressed ($P < 0.05$) between DLBCL-de novo and DLBCL-t cases.

Next we compared FL cases that subsequently underwent high grade transformation (FL-t (n = 7)) with cases that did not (FL-nt (n = 11)). Six microRNAs were differentially expressed ($P < 0.05$) between these two groups (Table 4), whose expression levels correctly predicted 16/18 (89%) of cases.

microRNA	***P* value**	**Up**	
hsa-miR-223	1.43E-03	FL-nt	1.51
hsa-miR-217	5.56E-03	FL-nt	2.56
hsa-miR-222	1.41E-02	FL-t	1.26
hsa-let-7i	2.09E-02	FL-t	2.45
hsa-miR-221	2.34E-02	FL-t	3.14
hsa-let-7b	2.46E-02	FL-t	3.18

Table 4. MicroRNAs differentially expressed ($P < 0.05$) between FL cases that subsequently underwent high grade transformation (FL-t) and those that did not (FL-nt). Median follow-up time 60 months (range 52-132 months).

Let-7b, *let-7i*, *miR-221* and *miR-222* were up-regulated in FL-t whilst *miR-223* and *miR-217* were down-regulated (Fig. 3). Members of the *let-7* family have been shown to target c-myc expression in Burkitt lymphoma (Sampson et al. 2007) and decreased c-myc expression has been associated with high grade transformation of FL to DLBCL (Lossos et al. 2002). Interestingly, up-regulated microRNAs *miR-221* and *miR-222* target the tumor suppressor molecule p27(Kip1) (le Sage et al. 2007) whilst down-regulated *miR-223* has been shown to target Stathmin, a known oncogene (Alli et al. 2007). Although the number of cases in this analysis was small, and requires further validation, these data open up the exciting possibility that microRNA expression could be used to predict FL patients at risk of transformation that could benefit from an up-front aggressive therapy regimen.

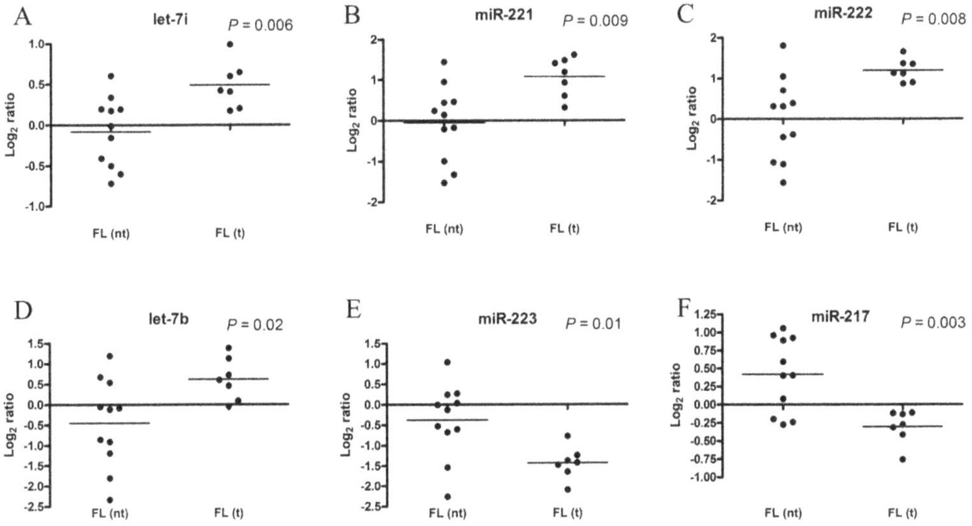

Fig. 3. **Expression levels of microRNAs differentially expressed between FL-t and FL-nt cases.** *P* values were calculated by independent *t*-test. Reproduced from (Lawrie et al. 2009).

5. Conclusion

In this chapter we have discussed some of the clinico-scientific issues pertaining to follicular lymphoma and the role that microRNAs may play in both its pathogenesis and in particular histological high grade transformation. As is outlined in this article there are in fact only two pieces of research published to date that have investigated microRNA expression in FL, and hence some caution should be applied when drawing conclusions about the role/potential of specific microRNAs in this disease, as clearly much more research is required. Nonetheless, these studies do present some interesting insights and offer the tantalizing possibility that microRNAs may deliver novel biomarkers that can identify FL patients at risk of transformation where other molecular techniques have failed.

6. Acknowledgments

CHL and his research are supported by grants from Ikerbasque- the Basque Foundation for Science and the Julian Starmer-Smith Memorial Fund.

7. References

Alli, E, Yang, JM & Hait, WN (2007). Silencing of stathmin induces tumor-suppressor function in breast cancer cell lines harboring mutant p53. *Oncogene*, 26(7), pp.1003-1012.

Altuvia, Y, Landgraf, P, Lithwick, G, Elefant, N, Pfeffer, S, Aravin, A, Brownstein, MJ, Tuschl, T & Margalit, H (2005). Clustering and conservation patterns of human microRNAs. *Nucleic Acids Res*, 33(8), pp.2697-2706.

Anderson, JR, Armitage, JO & Weisenburger, DD (1998). Epidemiology of the non-Hodgkin's lymphomas: distributions of the major subtypes differ by geographic locations. Non-Hodgkin's Lymphoma Classification Project. *Ann Oncol*, 9(7), pp.717-720.

Aref, S, Mabed, M, Zalata, K, Sakrana, M & El Askalany, H (2004). The interplay between c-Myc oncogene expression and circulating vascular endothelial growth factor (sVEGF), its antagonist receptor, soluble Flt-1 in diffuse large B cell lymphoma (DLBCL): relationship to patient outcome. *Leuk Lymphoma*, 45(3), pp.499-506.

Berglund, M, Enblad, G, Thunberg, U, Amini, RM, Sundstrom, C, Roos, G, Erlanson, M, Rosenquist, R, Larsson, C & Lagercrantz, S (2007). Genomic imbalances during transformation from follicular lymphoma to diffuse large B-cell lymphoma. *Mod Pathol*, 20(1), pp.63-75.

Borchert, GM, Lanier, W & Davidson, BL (2006). RNA polymerase III transcribes human microRNAs. *Nat Struct Mol Biol*, 13(12), pp.1097-1101.

Calin, GA, Sevignani, C, Dumitru, CD, Hyslop, T, Noch, E, Yendamuri, S, Shimizu, M, Rattan, S, Bullrich, F, Negrini, M & Croce, CM (2004). Human microRNA genes are frequently located at fragile sites and genomic regions involved in cancers. *Proc Natl Acad Sci U S A*, 101(9), pp.2999-3004.

Davies, AJ, Rosenwald, A, Wright, G, Lee, A, Last, KW, Weisenburger, DD, Chan, WC, Delabie, J, Braziel, RM, Campo, E, Gascoyne, RD, Jaffe, ES, Muller-Hermelink, K, Ott, G, Calaminici, M, Norton, AJ, Goff, LK, Fitzgibbon, J, Staudt, LM & Andrew Lister, T (2007). Transformation of follicular lymphoma to diffuse large B-cell lymphoma proceeds by distinct oncogenic mechanisms. *Br J Haematol*, 136(2), pp.286-293.

de Vos, S, Hofmann, WK, Grogan, TM, Krug, U, Schrage, M, Miller, TP, Braun, JG, Wachsman, W, Koeffler, HP & Said, JW (2003). Gene expression profile of serial samples of transformed B-cell lymphomas. *Lab Invest*, 83(2), pp.271-285.

Elenitoba-Johnson, KS, Jenson, SD, Abbott, RT, Palais, RA, Bohling, SD, Lin, Z, Tripp, S, Shami, PJ, Wang, LY, Coupland, RW, Buckstein, R, Perez-Ordonez, B, Perkins, SL, Dube, ID & Lim, MS (2003). Involvement of multiple signaling pathways in follicular lymphoma transformation: p38-mitogen-activated protein kinase as a target for therapy. *Proc Natl Acad Sci U S A*, 100(12), pp.7259-7264.

Friedman, RC, Farh, KK, Burge, CB & Bartel, DP (2009). Most mammalian mRNAs are conserved targets of microRNAs. *Genome Res*, 19(1), pp.92-105.

Giraldez, AJ, Mishima, Y, Rihel, J, Grocock, RJ, Van Dongen, S, Inoue, K, Enright, AJ & Schier, AF (2006). Zebrafish MiR-430 promotes deadenylation and clearance of maternal mRNAs. *Science*, 312(5770), pp.75-79.

Glas, AM, Knoops, L, Delahaye, L, Kersten, MJ, Kibbelaar, RE, Wessels, LA, van Laar, R, van Krieken, JH, Baars, JW, Raemaekers, J, Kluin, PM, van't Veer, LJ & de Jong, D (2007). Gene-expression and immunohistochemical study of specific T-cell subsets and accessory cell types in the transformation and prognosis of follicular lymphoma. *J Clin Oncol*, 25(4), pp.390-398.

Griffiths-Jones, S, Grocock, RJ, van Dongen, S, Bateman, A & Enright, AJ (2006). miRBase: microRNA sequences, targets and gene nomenclature. *Nucleic Acids Res*, 34(Database issue), pp.D140-144.

He, L, Thomson, JM, Hemann, MT, Hernando-Monge, E, Mu, D, Goodson, S, Powers, S, Cordon-Cardo, C, Lowe, SW, Hannon, GJ & Hammond, SM (2005). A microRNA polycistron as a potential human oncogene. *Nature*, 435(7043), pp.828-833.

Hertel, J, Lindemeyer, M, Missal, K, Fried, C, Tanzer, A, Flamm, C, Hofacker, IL & Stadler, PF (2006). The expansion of the metazoan microRNA repertoire. *BMC Genomics*, 7, pp.25.

Iorio, MV & Croce, CM (2009). MicroRNAs in cancer: small molecules with a huge impact. *J Clin Oncol*, 27(34), pp.5848-5856.

Iqbal, J, Sanger, WG, Horsman, DE, Rosenwald, A, Pickering, DL, Dave, B, Dave, S, Xiao, L, Cao, K, Zhu, Q, Sherman, S, Hans, CP, Weisenburger, DD, Greiner, TC, Gascoyne, RD, Ott, G, Muller-Hermelink, HK, Delabie, J, Braziel, RM, Jaffe, ES, Campo, E, Lynch, JC, Connors, JM, Vose, JM, Armitage, JO, Grogan, TM, Staudt, LM & Chan, WC (2004). BCL2 translocation defines a unique tumor subset within the germinal center B-cell-like diffuse large B-cell lymphoma. *Am J Pathol*, 165(1), pp.159-166.

Jaffe, ES, Harris, NL, Stein, H & Vardiman, J, Eds. (2001). World Health Organisation (WHO) Classification of Tumours-Pathology & Genetics-Tumours of Haematopoietic and Lymphoid Tissues. Lyon, IARC Press (International Agency for Research on Cancer).

Khvorova, A, Reynolds, A & Jayasena, SD (2003). Functional siRNAs and miRNAs exhibit strand bias. *Cell*, 115(2), pp.209-216.

Kim, VN (2005). MicroRNA biogenesis: coordinated cropping and dicing. *Nat Rev Mol Cell Biol*, 6(5), pp.376-385.

Lawrie, CH (2007). MicroRNAs and haematology: small molecules, big function. *Br J Haematol*, 137(6), pp.503-512.

Lawrie, CH (2008). microRNA expression in lymphoid malignancies: new hope for diagnosis and therapy? *J Cell Mol Med*, 12(5A), pp.1432-1444.

Lawrie, CH, Chi, J, Taylor, S, Tramonti, D, Ballabio, E, Palazzo, S, Saunders, NJ, Pezzella, F, Boultwood, J, Wainscoat, JS & Hatton, CS (2009). Expression of microRNAs in diffuse large B cell lymphoma is associated with immunophenotype, survival and transformation from follicular lymphoma. *J Cell Mol Med*, 13(7), pp.1248-1260.

Lawrie, CH, Saunders, NJ, Soneji, S, Palazzo, S, Dunlop, HM, Cooper, CD, Brown, PJ, Troussard, X, Mossafa, H, Enver, T, Pezzella, F, Boultwood, J, Wainscoat, JS & Hatton, CS (2008). MicroRNA expression in lymphocyte development and malignancy. *Leukemia*, 22(7), pp.1440-1446.

le Sage, C, Nagel, R, Egan, DA, Schrier, M, Mesman, E, Mangiola, A, Anile, C, Maira, G, Mercatelli, N, Ciafre, SA, Farace, MG & Agami, R (2007). Regulation of the p27(Kip1) tumor suppressor by miR-221 and miR-222 promotes cancer cell proliferation. *Embo J*, 26(15), pp.3699-3708.

Lee, RC & Ambros, V (2001). An extensive class of small RNAs in Caenorhabditis elegans. *Science*, 294(5543), pp.862-864.

Lee, RC, Feinbaum, RL & Ambros, V (1993). The C. elegans heterochronic gene lin-4 encodes small RNAs with antisense complementarity to lin-14. *Cell*, 75(5), pp.843-854.

Lee, Y, Hur, I, Park, SY, Kim, YK, Suh, MR & Kim, VN (2006). The role of PACT in the RNA silencing pathway. *Embo J*, 25(3), pp.522-532.

Liu, J, Valencia-Sanchez, MA, Hannon, GJ & Parker, R (2005). MicroRNA-dependent localization of targeted mRNAs to mammalian P-bodies. *Nat Cell Biol*, 7(7), pp.719-723.

Lossos, IS, Alizadeh, AA, Diehn, M, Warnke, R, Thorstenson, Y, Oefner, PJ, Brown, PO, Botstein, D & Levy, R (2002). Transformation of follicular lymphoma to diffuse large-cell lymphoma: alternative patterns with increased or decreased expression of c-myc and its regulated genes. *Proc Natl Acad Sci U S A*, 99(13), pp.8886-8891.

Lytle, JR, Yario, TA & Steitz, JA (2007). Target mRNAs are repressed as efficiently by microRNA-binding sites in the 5' UTR as in the 3' UTR. *Proc Natl Acad Sci U S A*, 104(23), pp.9667-9672.

McDonnell, TJ & Korsmeyer, SJ (1991). Progression from lymphoid hyperplasia to high-grade malignant lymphoma in mice transgenic for the t(14; 18). *Nature*, 349(6306), pp.254-256.

Montoto, S, Davies, AJ, Matthews, J, Calaminici, M, Norton, AJ, Amess, J, Vinnicombe, S, Waters, R, Rohatiner, AZ & Lister, TA (2007). Risk and clinical implications of transformation of follicular lymphoma to diffuse large B-cell lymphoma. *J Clin Oncol*, 25(17), pp.2426-2433.

O'Donnell, KA, Wentzel, EA, Zeller, KI, Dang, CV & Mendell, JT (2005). c-Myc-regulated microRNAs modulate E2F1 expression. *Nature*, 435(7043), pp.839-843.

Pagnano, KB, Vassallo, J, Lorand-Metze, I, Costa, FF & Saad, ST (2001). p53, Mdm2, and c-Myc overexpression is associated with a poor prognosis in aggressive non-Hodgkin's lymphomas. *Am J Hematol*, 67(2), pp.84-92.

Pasquinelli, AE, Reinhart, BJ, Slack, F, Martindale, MQ, Kuroda, MI, Maller, B, Hayward, DC, Ball, EE, Degnan, B, Muller, P, Spring, J, Srinivasan, A, Fishman, M, Finnerty, J, Corbo, J, Levine, M, Leahy, P, Davidson, E & Ruvkun, G (2000). Conservation of the sequence and temporal expression of let-7 heterochronic regulatory RNA. *Nature*, 408(6808), pp.86-89.

Pillai, RS, Bhattacharyya, SN, Artus, CG, Zoller, T, Cougot, N, Basyuk, E, Bertrand, E & Filipowicz, W (2005). Inhibition of translational initiation by Let-7 MicroRNA in human cells. *Science*, 309(5740), pp.1573-1576.

Reinhart, BJ, Slack, FJ, Basson, M, Pasquinelli, AE, Bettinger, JC, Rougvie, AE, Horvitz, HR & Ruvkun, G (2000). The 21-nucleotide let-7 RNA regulates developmental timing in Caenorhabditis elegans. *Nature*, 403(6772), pp.901-906.

Rodriguez, A, Griffiths-Jones, S, Ashurst, JL & Bradley, A (2004). Identification of mammalian microRNA host genes and transcription units. *Genome Res*, 14(10A), pp.1902-1910.

Roehle, A, Hoefig, KP, Repsilber, D, Thorns, C, Ziepert, M, Wesche, KO, Thiere, M, Loeffler, M, Klapper, W, Pfreundschuh, M, Matolcsy, A, Bernd, HW, Reiniger, L, Merz, H & Feller, AC (2008). MicroRNA signatures characterize diffuse large B-cell lymphomas and follicular lymphomas. *Br J Haematol*, 142(5), pp.732-744.

Rossi, D, Berra, E, Cerri, M, Deambrogi, C, Barbieri, C, Franceschetti, S, Lunghi, M, Conconi, A, Paulli, M, Matolcsy, A, Pasqualucci, L, Capello, D & Gaidano, G (2006). Aberrant somatic hypermutation in transformation of follicular lymphoma and chronic lymphocytic leukemia to diffuse large B-cell lymphoma. *Haematologica*, 91(10), pp.1405-1409.

Roulland, S, Navarro, JM, Grenot, P, Milili, M, Agopian, J, Montpellier, B, Gauduchon, P, Lebailly, P, Schiff, C & Nadel, B (2006). Follicular lymphoma-like B cells in healthy individuals: a novel intermediate step in early lymphomagenesis. *J Exp Med*, 203(11), pp.2425-2431.

Sampson, VB, Rong, NH, Han, J, Yang, Q, Aris, V, Soteropoulos, P, Petrelli, NJ, Dunn, SP & Krueger, LJ (2007). MicroRNA let-7a down-regulates MYC and reverts MYC-induced growth in Burkitt lymphoma cells. *Cancer Res*, 67(20), pp.9762-9770.

Schwarz, DS, Hutvagner, G, Du, T, Xu, Z, Aronin, N & Zamore, PD (2003). Asymmetry in the assembly of the RNAi enzyme complex. *Cell*, 115(2), pp.199-208.

SEER (2005). Cancer Statistics Review, 1975-2002. *National Cancer Institute*.

Sen, GL & Blau, HM (2005). Argonaute 2/RISC resides in sites of mammalian mRNA decay known as cytoplasmic bodies. *Nat Cell Biol*, 7(6), pp.633-636.

Smyth, GK & Speed, T (2003). Normalization of cDNA microarray data. *Methods*, 31(4), pp.265-273.

Strasser, A, Harris, AW & Cory, S (1993). E mu-bcl-2 transgene facilitates spontaneous transformation of early pre-B and immunoglobulin-secreting cells but not T cells. *Oncogene*, 8(1), pp.1-9.

Tsujimoto, Y, Cossman, J, Jaffe, E & Croce, CM (1985). Involvement of the bcl-2 gene in human follicular lymphoma. *Science*, 228(4706), pp.1440-1443.

Vasudevan, S, Tong, Y & Steitz, JA (2007). Switching from repression to activation: microRNAs can up-regulate translation. *Science*, 318(5858), pp.1931-1934.

Wightman, B, Ha, I & Ruvkun, G (1993). Posttranscriptional regulation of the heterochronic gene lin-14 by lin-4 mediates temporal pattern formation in C. elegans. *Cell*, 75(5), pp.855-862.

Wrench, D, Montoto, S & Fitzgibbon, J (2010). Molecular signatures in the diagnosis and management of follicular lymphoma. *Current Opinion in Hematology*, 17(4), pp.333-340.

Yeom, KH, Lee, Y, Han, J, Suh, MR & Kim, VN (2006). Characterization of DGCR8/Pasha, the essential cofactor for Drosha in primary miRNA processing. *Nucleic Acids Res*, 34(16), pp.4622-4629.

Zeng, Y (2006). Principles of micro-RNA production and maturation. *Oncogene*, 25(46), pp.6156-6162.

6

Animal Models of Lymphoproliferative Disorders Focusing on Waldenström's Macroglobulinemia

Anastasia S. Tsingotjidou
Laboratory of Anatomy and Histology,
Faculty of Veterinary Medicine,
Aristotle University of Thessaloniki
Greece

1. Introduction

Lymphoproliferative disorders (LPDs) represent a heterogeneous group of expanding, monoclonal or oligoclonal, lymphoid cells that occur in the setting of immune dysfunction. They are sometimes equated with "immunoproliferative disorders", but technically LPDs are a subset of immunoproliferative disorders, along with hypergammaglobulinemia and paraproteinemias. Several inherited gene mutations have been identified to cause lymphoproliferative disorders. Acquired and iatrogenic causes are also responsible for the appearance of these diseases.

The most common examples of LPDs are chronic lymphocytic leukemia, acute lymphoblastic leukemia, lymphomas/leukemias (including follicular lymphoma and hairy cell leukemia) and multiple myeloma, although less common LPDs such as post-transplant lymphoproliferative disorder, Waldenström's macroglobulinemia, Wiskott-Aldrich syndrome and Autoimmune LymphoProliferative Syndrome (ALPS) also belong to the same group of disorders.

A few basic current facts for the incidence rates, the prognosis and the treatment of the most common LPDs will be briefly mentioned in the beginning of this chapter. Following that, the recent advances in understanding the pathogenesis of these diseases coming from experimental animal studies will be reviewed in a greater detail. After all, understanding the mechanisms of neoplasia has always been a prerequisite for developing more effective treatments for cancer patients, and the sophisticated animal models available in our days have played a major role in enhancing this knowledge. We have developed an animal model for Waldenström's macroglobulinemia (WM), which is one of the less common LPDs. This will also be presented in detail as an example of the challenges met in developing an animal model that should emulate the human disease, or at least important aspects of it. By introducing core biopsies of WM patients into immunodeficient mice bearing human bone fragments, we established an animal model mimicking important aspects of the disease in humans.

2. Lymphoproliferative disorders

2.1 Chronic lymphocytic leukemia

Chronic lymphocytic leukemia (CLL) is the most common adult leukemia in North America and Europe; it is less frequent in Asia and Africa (Linet et al., 2006). The reported age-adjusted incidence rate of CLL in the United States between 1975 and 2006 was 4.43 per 100,000 persons (Horner et al., 2009). However, because of its long asymptomatic period, the incidence of CLL is under-reported in cancer registries (Dores et al., 2007).

Despite this uncertainty, it is clear that the incidence of CLL rises dramatically with age and that it is more common in men than women (Dores et al., 2007; Redaelli et al., 2004). As the proportion of older people has increased with improved life expectancy in the Western world, the CLL burden has also increased. The American Cancer Society projected 15,490 new cases for 2009, a substantial increase from the 11,168 new cases reported in 2005 (U.S. Cancer Statistics Working group, 2009). The disease burden is also significant in the European Union, with an estimated 46,000 individuals in 2006 living with CLL 5 years post-diagnosis (Watson et al., 2008).

CLL is characterized by a variable clinical course (Rozman & Montserrat, 1995) with some patients having an aggressive malignancy and others a slow, nonprogressive disease and a virtually normal life expectancy. Ideally, a detailed diagnostic workup of a CLL case should include the identification of standardized and reliable prognostic factors. Predicting the outcome of CLL with a statistically significant level of success will provide the basis for individualized therapeutic approaches and patient-adjusted disease management policies. Indeed, several prognostic factors, including serum (Hallek et al., 1999) and cytogenetic alteration markers (Dohner et al., 2000), have been used to assist individual CLL patient prognosis.

2.2 Acute lymphoblastic leukemia

There are two types of acute leukemia: acute myelogenous leukemia (AML) and acute lymphoblastic leukemia (ALL); (Ashfaq et al., 2010). Acute myelogenous leukemia (AML) is a clonal, malignant disease of hematopoietic tissue that is characterized by the proliferation of abnormal (leukemic) blast cells, principally in the marrow, and by impaired production of normal blood cells (Lichtman & Liesveld, 2001). It is the most common acute leukemia affecting adults, and its incidence increases with age. AML accounts for nearly one-third of all new cases of leukemia (Ashfaq et al., 2010).

Acute lymphoblastic leukemia is a neoplastic disease that results from somatic mutation in a single lymphoid progenitor cell at one of several discrete stages of development. The immunophenotype of the leukemic cells at diagnosis reflects the level of differentiation achieved by the dominant clone (Pui, 2001). At diagnosis the leukemic cells not only have replaced normal marrow cells but have disseminated to various extramedullary sites. Studies suggest that the activation of telomerase in leukemic cells contribute to their growth advantage and to disease progression (Ohyashiki et al., 1997; Shay et al., 1996).

ALL represents about 12 percent of all leukemias diagnosed in the US, and 60 percent of all cases occur in persons younger than 20 years (SEER, 1998). ALL is the most common malignancy diagnosed in patients under the age of 15 years, accounting for one-fourth of all cancers and 76 percent of all leukemias in this age group (Gurney et al., 1996). Data from UK showed that there were 691 new cases of ALL and 255 deaths from ALL in 2006 (Cancer Research U.K., 2010). Each year, around 3,250 children are diagnosed with leukemia, of which about 2,400 are ALL cases (Smith et al., 2000). In the USA, survival rate for children with ALL has improved markedly since the early 1970s and is now approximately 80%, but incidence rates have not decreased and have, in fact, increased by 0.8% annually from 1975 to 2007 (SEER, 2010). Worldwide, according to the World Health Organization (WHO), there were 33,142 deaths from leukemia among children under age 15 in 2004, and childhood (<15 years) leukemia caused 1,228,075 disability adjusted life years (WHO, 2010).

Identifying risk factors for childhood leukemia is an important step in the reduction of the overall burden of childhood diseases. Though it has been studied intensively, the etiology of childhood leukemia is not well established. A two-hit model was proposed by Greaves in which prenatal chromosome alterations and postnatal genetic alterations are necessary for childhood leukemia development (Greaves, 2002). Genetic susceptibility and environmental factors play potential roles in this process (Eden, 2010). Ionizing radiation has been significantly linked to childhood leukemia (Bailey et al., 2010). Evidence for an association with benzene exposure or with parental smoking and alcohol consumption is less convincing (Liu et al., 2011) .

Treatment for the majority of ALL subtypes consists of three phases: induction, intensification (consolidation) therapy, and continuation (maintenance) treatment. Although two-thirds of childhood cases are curable with only 12 months of treatment, the vast majority of patients undergo therapy for two years or more (Pui & Evans, 2006). Across medical institutions, chemotherapeutic agents used vary in type and amount, with the most common being methotrexate (MTX), cytosine arabinoside (cytarabine), anthracyclines (such as doxorubicin), asparaginase, mercaptopurine, vincristine, and corticosteroids, presented alone or in combination (Pui & Evans, 2006). Leukemic cells are transported by the circulatory system to nearly every organ system, including the Central Nervous System (CNS). The most common form of CNS prophylaxis was cranial irradiation, or cranial radiation therapy (CRT), which has largely been replaced by intrathecal (IT) and systemic chemotherapy. This change has been made in an effort to eliminate radiation-specific damage to the CNS (Stehbens et al., 1991). Recent regimens have tested whether CRT can be eliminated completely from standard treatment. To date, this has been successful, although alterations in long-term outcome are just beginning to unfold (Pui et al., 2009). Efforts like this are being made to eliminate the possible complications of any form of ALL treatment.

2.3 Lymphomas/leukemias

Despite remarkable advances in diagnosis and treatment, lymphoma continues to rank as a leading cause of cancer-related mortality. Recent cancer statistics for the United States project non-Hodgkin lymphoma (NHL) to be the sixth most commonly diagnosed cancer in 2010 in both men and women, and the eighth and sixth leading cause of cancer-related death in men and women, respectively (Jemal et al., 2010). Based on data from national cancer registries, 65,540 new cases of NHL and 20,210 deaths from NHL are estimated to occur in 2010. In contrast, Hodgkin lymphoma (HL) is less common (8,490 estimated new cases in 2010) and is associated with fewer deaths (1,320 estimated deaths in 2010) (Jemal et al., 2010). In the European Union, reported NHL estimates for the year 2006 were even higher, with 72,800 new cases and 33,000 deaths (Ferlay et al., 2007). In the US, on January 1, 2008, there were approximately 167,000 HL survivors and approximately 454,000 NHL survivors (Howlader et al., 2011). In the Nordic European Countries (NEC: Denmark, Faroe Islands, Finland, Iceland, Norway, Sweden), there were approximately 10,500 HL survivors and approximately 31,500 NHL survivors at the end of 2007 (Engholm et al., 2011). Although there are similarities between these subtypes of lymphoma, the incidence and age of onset are quite different.

Onset of the disease occurs most frequently between the ages of 20 and 35 years. Between 35 and 50 years, it occurs less often especially in females, but from the age of 50 onward there is again a rise in incidence with age (Howlader et al., 2011). The disease occurs predominantly in individuals aged over 45 years and the lifetime prevalence of NHL is one in 50 (Howlader et al., 2011). Due to chemotherapy, radiotherapy and stem cell transplantation, the survival of these patients has improved substantially in the seventies and eighties, but has nowadays leveled off. In effect, most trials focus on maintaining the high level of cure, while reducing the long-term effects of treatment. To date, more than 80% of patients diagnosed with HL are expected to live free of disease for 5 years or more after diagnosis (National Cancer Institute, 2009) The overall 5-year survival rate for all types of NHL (1999-2005) is 50-60%. The statistics vary depending on the cell type, stage of disease at diagnosis, treatment and age of the patient (National Cancer Institute, 2009).

Indolent Non-Hodgkin's lymphoma (NHL) represents a group of incurable slow growing lymphomas that are highly responsive to initial therapy but relapse with less responsive disease (Ardeshna et al., 2003; Horning, 1993; Johnson et al., 1995; Montoto et al., 2002). The landscape for treatment of indolent NHL has dramatically changed with the introduction of rituximab (Rituxan, Genetech, San Francisco, CA). Its greatest impact has been in follicular lymphoma (FL), which constitutes approximately 70% of indolent lymphomas and up to 25% of all cases of NHL (Marcus et al., 2005; The Non-Hodgkin's Lymphoma Classification Project, 1997). Although there are no defined first line therapies for indolent NHL, rituximab has become a standard component in treatment of Follicular Lymphoma (FL) (Friedberg et al., 2009). While indolent lymphoma remains an incurable disease, recent data from the Surveillance Epidemiology and End Results (SEER) database and retrospective analysis of clinical trials in indolent NHL suggest an improved overall survival with the use of rituximab (Fisher et al., 2005; Liu et al., 2006; Pulte et al., 2008). It is hoped that overall survival can be further improved with the use of extended rituximab dosing schedules.

2.4. Multiple Myeloma

Multiple Myeloma (MM) is a B cell malignancy characterized by the presence of bone marrow infiltration by clonal plasma cells that generally secrete a monoclonal component in the serum or urine (Kyle & Rajkumar, 2004). It is the second most frequent hematological malignancy, after non Hodgkin's lymphomas, and accounts approximately for a 10% of all hematological tumors and 1% of all cancers (Petrelli et al., 2009). MM is associated with a constellation of disease manifestations, including osteolytic lesions due to disrupted bone metabolism, anemia and immunosuppression due to loss of normal hematopoietic stem cell function, and end-organ damage due to monoclonal immunoglobulin secretion (Barlogie et al., 2001). The presence of somatic hypermutations of the immunoglobulin variable region genes in myeloma plasma cells suggests that malignant transformation occurs in a B cell that has traversed the germinal centers of lymph nodes. However, the hypoproliferative nature of myeloma has led to the hypothesis that the bulk of the tumor arises from a transformed B cell with the capacity for both self-renewal and production of terminally differentiated progeny (Billadeau et al., 1993; Corradini et al., 1993; Szczepek et al., 1998).

The clinical course of patients requiring therapy for myeloma varies markedly. Even with tandem autotransplants yielding complete remission (CR) rates in excess of 60%. Survival ranges from a few months to greater than 15 years. The extended time (almost 2 years) for those patients to achieve CR, and the even longer time to achieve magnetic resonance imaging (MRI)-CR, strongly suggests enormous tumor cell population heterogeneity in terms of drug responsiveness/resistance (Harousseau et al., 2004).

Differential expression of traditional prognostic factors, such as β2-microglobulin (β2M), albumin, and C-reactive protein (CRP), are thought to be responsible for only a 15%-20% of the outcome heterogeneity of MM. Abnormal metaphase karyotypes, present in one-third of newly diagnosed patients and reflecting stroma independence, have been consistently associated with a rapidly fatal outcome, and fewer than 10% of patients with these abnormalities survive > 5 years (Harousseau et al., 2004).

Advances in molecular cytogenetics have identified primary translocations involving the immunoglobulin heavy chain locus at 14q32 in 40% of patients (Kuehl & Bergsagel; 2002). According to a consensus report of a Paris workshop on myeloma genetics, hyperdiploid and t(11;14)(q13,q32)-positive myeloma are associated with a good prognosis, whereas non-hyperdiploidy, often associated with translocations other than t(11;14) and chromosome 13 deletion, imparts a strikingly dismal prognosis (Fonseca et al., 2004).

2.5 Other lymphoproliferative disorders

Along with Waldenström's macroglobulinemia, there are other LPDs, which are less frequently observed. From this group we will describe in more details the lymphoproliferative disorders detected after bone marrow and organ transplantation. Following this treatment and among patients infected with AIDS, LPDs are believed to result from uncontrolled proliferation of Epstein-Barr virus (EBV)-transformed B-lymphocytes in the setting of immune dysfunction (Cohen, 1991; Deeg & Socié, 1998; Goedert et al., 1998; Hoover, 1992; Kinlen, 1996; Newell et al., 1996; Opelz & Henderson, 1993; Swinnen et al., 1990). Allogeneic bone marrow transplantation, an effective treatment for leukemia and other disorders, produces profound immune deficiency in the early period after transplantation. Post-transplant lymphoproliferative disorders (PTLD) are an uncommon, but frequently fatal, complication of this defective immune function (Bhatia et al., 1996; Deeg & Socié, 1998; Witherspoon et al., 1989). PTLD typically develop in the first 6 months post-transplantantation as clinically aggressive lymphomas of donor origin; most are related to EBV (Deeg & Socié, 1998; Orazi et al., 1997; O'Reilly et al., 1996).

Post-transplant lymphoproliferative disorders are more common if donor and recipient are HLA-mismatched or if T-cell depletion is used for graft-versus-host disease (GVHD) prophylaxis (Curtis et al., 1999). The clinical diagnosis of PTLD may be difficult because it is a spectrum of heterogenous histologic and clinical entities. It may present as an infectious mononucleosis-like illness, with fatigue and lymphadenopathy, or as a febrile illness with leukopenia. Almost all organs may be affected by disease. Because of the progressive nature of PTLD, the key to management may be early or even preemptive treatment with either anti–B-cell monoclonal antibodies (Carpenter et al., 2002; Kuehnle et al., 2000; van Esser et al., 2002) or donor-derived EBV-specific cytotoxic T lymphocytes (CTLs) (Gustafsson et al., 2000; Heslop et al., 1996; Rooney et al., 1998).

3. Animal models of lymphoproliferative disorders

The bulk of LPD-related literature describes the different clinical manifestations encountered and evaluates treatment protocols. Fewer studies focus on dissecting the pathogenesis of LPD by developing animal models. Recent basic research is based on the development of genetically engineered mice or the use of immunodeficient mice as tumor transplant models. A few animal models other than mice have also been reported (miniature swine, zebrafish).

3.1 Chronic lymphocytic leukemia

Chronic lymphocytic leukemia cells require complex microenvironmental and immunologic interactions to survive and proliferate. Such interactions might be best studied in animal models; however, this needs extensive verification. Hofbauer et al. (2011) therefore investigated the composition of the T-cell compartment in the Eμ–*TCL1* transgenic mouse, currently the most widely used murine model for CLL. *TCL1* is a bona fide oncogene, developing a transgenic mouse model where ectopic expression driven by the *lck* promoter in the T cell compartment results in the development of mature T cell leukemias after a long latency period, in a pattern closely resembling human mature T cell leukemia (Virgilio et al., 1998). Immunophenotyping and transplant approaches were used to define T-cell subsets at various stages of CLL. Analogous to human CLL, they observed a skewing of T-cell subsets from naive to antigen-experienced memory T cells that was more pronounced in lymph nodes than in blood. Transplantation of CLL into non-transgenic recipients was feasible without immunosuppression in a pure C57BL/6 background and resulted in the prominent skewing of the T cells of the recipient mice. Both in spontaneously developed CLL and in the transplantation setting, a loss in T-cell receptor diversity was observed, with a relevant number of clonal T-cell populations arising. This suggests that antigen-dependent differentiation toward the T memory pool is initiated by murine CLL cells. In summary, this research team characterized the T-cell phenotypes in the *TCL1* transgenic mouse model and suggested a CLL-dependent antigen-driven skewing of T cells in these mice, making this model valuable for the research of the disease's pathogenesis, since murine CLL cells react similarly with human CLL cells.

The same transgenic mouse (Eμ–*TCL1* transgenic mouse,) was also used by Suljagic et al. (2010). They have investigated whether inhibition of BCR (antigen-dependent B-cell receptor) signaling with the selective Syk inhibitor fostamatinib disodium (R788) had an affect on the growth of the leukemias that develop in the Eμ–*TCL1* transgenic mouse model of CLL. Similarly to human CLL, these leukemias express stereotyped BCRs that react with autoantigens exposed on the surface of senescent or apoptotic cells, suggesting that they are antigen driven. They showed that R788 effectively inhibits BCR signaling *in vivo*, resulting in reduced proliferation and survival of the malignant B cells and significantly prolonged survival of the treated animals. The growth-inhibitory effect of R788 occurs despite the relatively modest cytotoxic effect *in vitro* and is independent of basal Syk activity, suggesting that R788 functions primarily by inhibiting antigen-dependent BCR signals. Importantly, the effect of R788 was found to be selective for the malignant clones, as no disturbance in the production of normal B lymphocytes was observed. Collectively, these data provide further rationale for clinical trials with R788 in CLL and establish the BCR-signaling pathway as an important therapeutic target in this disease.

In another approach, over-expression of human *TCL1*, leads to the development of mature CD19+/CD5+/IgM+ clonal leukemia with a murine disease phenotype similar to the human CLL. Herein, Chen et al. (2009) review their recent study using this *TCL1*-driven mouse model for CLL and corresponding human CLL samples in a cross-species epigenomics approach to address the timing and relevance of epigenetic events occurring during leukemogenesis. They demonstrated that the mouse model recapitulates the epigenetic events that have been reported for human CLL, affirming the power and validity of this mouse model to study early epigenetic events in cancer progression. Epigenetic alterations are detected as early as three months after birth, far before disease manifests at about 11 months of age. These mice undergo NFκ-B repressor complex-mediated inactivation of the transcription factor Foxd3, whose targets become aberrantly methylated and silenced in both mouse and human CLL. Overall, their data suggest the accumulated epigenetic alterations during CLL pathogenesis as a consequence of gene silencing through *TCL1* and NFκ-B repressor complex, suggesting the relevance for NFκ-B as a therapeutic target in CLL.

Another trangenic mouse model for CLL was generated by Santanam et al. (2010). They found that miR-29a is up-regulated in indolent human B-CLL as compared with aggressive B-CLL and normal CD19(+) B cells. To study the role of miR-29 in B-CLL, they generated Eμ-miR-29 transgenic mice overexpressing miR-29 in mouse B cells. Flow cytometric analysis revealed a markedly expanded CD5(+) population in the spleen of these mice starting at 2 months of age, with 85% (34/40) of miR-29 transgenic mice exhibiting expanded CD5(+) B-cell populations, a characteristic of B-CLL. On average, 50% of B cells in these transgenic mice were CD5 positive. At 2 years of age the mice showed significantly enlarged spleens and an increase in the CD5(+) B-cell population to approximately 100%. Of 20 Eμ-miR-29 transgenic mice followed to 24-26 mo of age, 4 (20%) developed frank leukemia and died of the disease. These results suggest that the dysregulation of miR-29 can contribute to the pathogenesis of indolent B-CLL, giving another opportunity to clarify all of its aspects.

The engraftment of cell lines into appropriate mice and/or the injection of fresh cells derived from patients have been used for the development of animal models in different disesases. Here, we describe one animal model where the researchers have developed a novel transplantable xenograft murine model of CLL by engrafting the CLL cell line MEC1 into Rag2(-/-)gamma(c)(-/-)mice. These mice lack B, T, and natural killer (NK) cells, and, in contrast to nude mice that retain NK cells, appear to be optimal recipient for MEC1 cells, which were successfully transplanted through either subcutaneous or intravenous routes. The result is a novel *in vivo* model that has systemic involvement, develops very rapidly, allows the measurement of tumor burden, and has 100% engraftment efficiency. This model closely resembles aggressive human CLL and could be very useful for evaluating both the biologic basis of CLL growth and dissemination as well as the efficacy of new therapeutic agents (Bertilaccio et al., 2010).

Another model has been developed by Aydin et al. (2011), and is exploring the role of CD38 and functionally associated molecular risk factors in a recently described CLL nonobese diabetic/severe combined immunodeficient xenograft model. Intravenous injection of peripheral blood mononuclear cells from 73 patients with CLL into 244 mice resulted in robust engraftment of leukemic cells into the murine spleens detected 4 weeks after transplantation. Leukemic cell engraftment correlated significantly ($P < 0.05$) with markers reflecting disease activity, e.g., Binet stage and lymphocyte doubling time, and the expression of molecular risk factors including CD38, CD49d, ZAP-70, and IgVH mutational status. Increased engraftment levels of CD38+ as compared to CD38- CLL cells could be attributed, in part, to leukemic cell proliferation as evidenced by simultaneous immunostaining of murine spleen sections for Ki-67 and CD20. In short-term (24 h) homing assays, CD38+ CLL cells migrated more efficiently to the bone marrow of the recipient animals than their CD38- counterparts. Finally, the expression of CD38 by the leukemic cells was found to be dynamic in that it was regulated not only by elements of the murine microenvironment but also by co-engrafting non-malignant human T cells. This model could be useful for evaluating the biological basis of CLL growth in the context of the hematopoietic microenvironment as well as for preclinical testing of novel compounds.

Last, but not least we describe the New Zealand Black (NZB) mouse model for CLL. Is a (*de novo)* mouse model of spontaneous CLL (Phillips et al., 1992), in contrast to all other models, which are induced by the expression of exogenous genes (Scaglione et al., 2007). Similar to a subset of human patients who progress from monoclonal B lymphocytosis (MBL) to CLL, NZB mice develop an age-associated progression to CLL. The murine disease is linked to a genetic abnormality in microRNA *mir-15a/16-1* locus, resulting in decreased mature miR-15a/16 (Salerno et al., 2010).

Similar to CLL, the disease in NZB mice is also an age-associated malignant expansion of poly-reactive CD5+ B-1 clones (Caligaris-Cappio & Ghia, 2007; Scaglione et al., 2007). The majority of B-1 clones are IgM+, B220 (CD45R)^{dim} and CD5^{dim} , increase with age, and often possess chromosomal abnormalities (Dang et al., 1996). NZB also seem to demonstrate an MBL-like stage at an early age, characterized by multiple clones, as seen in MBL cases reported by Lanasa et al. (2010). High levels of IL-10 are also correlated with the development of these malignant B-1 cells (Ramachandra et al., 1996). This MBL-like state in NZB precedes CLL, and although it exhibits similar manifestations to human MBL, NZB disease always progress to CLL, in contrast to humans who can have an indefinite state of indolent MBL disease (Lanasa et al., 2010). The NZB has also been studied as a model for autoimmunity (Theofilopoulos, 1996). Similar to the autoreactivity associated with CLL autoantibodies (Ghia et al., 2002), the NZB mouse develops a mild autoimmune reaction associated with B cell hyperactivity, resulting in autoimmune hemolytic anemia and antinuclear antibodies (Scaglione et al., 2007).

The diversity of exisitng animal models of CLL leads to multiple options for treatment approaches, which is the end-point of this research.

3.2 Acute lymphoblastic leukemia

The non-obese diabetic/severe combined immunodeficient (NOD/SCID) xenograft mouse model is currently one of the most successful models for studying haematological malignancies such as acute lymphoblastic leukaemia (ALL) (Macor et al., 2008). In this typical tumor transplant model patient bone marrow leukemia cells are directly transplanted into the recipient NOD/SCID mice (Lock et al., 2002). The kinetics of engraftment reflect the human disease, leading to bone marrow (BM) infiltration, followed by migration to the spleen, peripheral blood and other haematopoietic organs (Lock et al., 2002; Kamel-Reid et al., 1989; Nijmeijer et al., 2001). However, for this model to be effective for studying engraftment and therapy responses at the whole genome level, careful molecular characterization is essential.

In the ALL NOD/SCID xenograft model, Samuels et al. (2010) have combined all existing xenograft models and sought to validate species-specific gene expression. Using the human Affymetrix whole transcript platform they analyzed transcriptional profiles from engrafted tissues (e.g. bone marrow, spleen and/or peripheral blood) without prior cell separation of mouse cells and acquired highly reproducible profiles in xenografts from individual mice. The model was further tested with experimental mixtures of human and mouse cells, demonstrating that the presence of mouse cells does not significantly distort expression profiles when xenografts contain 90% or more human cells. In addition, they presented a novel *in silico* and experimental masking approach to identify probes and transcript clusters susceptible to cross-species hybridization. Hence, they demonstrated that species-specific transcriptional profiles can be obtained from xenografts when high levels of engraftment are achieved or with the application of transcript cluster masks. Importantly, this masking approach can be applied and adapted to other xenograft models where human tissue infiltration is lower. This model provides a powerful platform for identifying genes and pathways associated with ALL disease progression and response to therapy *in vivo*.

A genetically defined mouse retroviral transduction/bone marrow transplantation model was used by Medyouf et al. (2010) to investigate the possibility for NOTCH1 to act as a therapeutic target. This is based on the assumption that NOTCH1 is activated by mutation in more than 50% of human T-cell acute lymphoblastic leukemias (T-ALLs) and inhibition of Notch signaling causes cell-cycle/growth arrest. The tumor suppressor phosphatase and tensin homolog (PTEN) is also mutated or lost in up to 20% of cases. It was recently observed among human T-ALL cell lines that PTEN loss correlated with resistance to Notch inhibition, raising concern that patients with PTEN-negative disease may fail Notch inhibitor therapy. They observed primary murine leukemias to remain dependent on NOTCH1 signaling despite Pten loss, with or without additional deletion of p16(Ink4a)/p19(Arf). They also examined 13 primary human T-ALL samples obtained at diagnosis and found no correlation between PTEN status and resistance to Notch inhibition. Furthermore, they noted that Pten loss accelerated disease onset and produced multiclonal tumors, suggesting NOTCH1 activation and Pten loss may collaborate in leukemia induction. Thus, in contrast to previous findings with established cell lines, these results indicate that PTEN loss does not relieve primary T-ALL cells of their "addiction" to Notch signaling. They concluded that refractory/relapsed tumors that have undergone chemotherapy-induced mutation and/or selection may behave differently, but presumably will harbor many other genetic alterations besides PTEN loss. This conclusion, along others of the same research team provide new insight on the therapeutic management of ALL.

Introduction of cells into syngeneic mice is also useful tool for the investigation of ALL and its therapeutic approach. Cultured p185(BCR-ABL)-expressing (p185+) Arf (-/-) pre-B cells injected into healthy syngeneic mice induces aggressive acute lymphoblastic leukemia (ALL) that genetically and phenotypically mimics the human disease (Boulos et al., 2011).

They adapted the Philadelphia chromosome-positive (Ph(+)) ALL animal model for *in vivo* luminescent imaging to investigate disease progression, targeted therapeutic response, and ALL relapse in living mice. Mice bearing high leukemic burdens (simulating human Ph(+) ALL at diagnosis) entered remission on maximally intensive, twice-daily dasatinib therapy, but invariably relapsed with disseminated and/or central nervous system disease. Their research concluded that although non-tumor-cell-autonomous mechanisms can prevent full eradication of dasatinib-refractory ALL in this clinically relevant model, the emergence of resistance to BCR-ABL kinase inhibitors can be effectively circumvented by the addition of "conventional" chemotherapeutic agents with alternate antileukemic mechanisms of action. Thus, preclinical trials using multiple agents underscore the potential value of this murine Ph^{+} ALL model for efficiently and cheaply piloting combination therapies and for elucidating mechanisms of drug resistance, information that is much more difficult to extract from complex human clinical trials.

Other researchers have combined ALL models with exogenous factors, to test their influence in disease. For example, Yun et al. (2010) developed animal models of obesity and leukemia to test whether obesity could directly accelerate acute lymphoblastic leukemia (ALL) using BCR/ABL transgenic and AKR/J mice weaned onto a high-fat diet. Mice were observed until development of progressive ALL. Although obese and control BCR/ABL mice had similar median survival, older obese mice had accelerated ALL onset, implying a time-dependent effect of obesity on ALL. Obese AKR mice developed ALL significantly earlier than controls. The effect of obesity was not explained by WBC count, thymus/spleen weight, or ALL phenotype. However, obese AKR mice had higher leptin, insulin, and interleukin-6 levels than controls, and these obesity-related hormones all have potential roles in leukemia pathogenesis. In conclusion, obesity directly accelerates presentation of ALL, likely by increasing the risk of an early event in leukemogenesis. This is the first study to show that obesity can directly accelerate the progression of ALL. Thus, the observed associations between obesity and leukemia incidence are likely to be directly related to biological effects of obesity.

Smith et al. (2010) used another animal, zebrafish, where malignant cells can be transplanted into sibling animals without the need for immune suppression. Using cell-transplant zebrafish (Langenau et al., 2003) showed that self-renewing cells are abundant in T-ALL and comprise 0.1% to 15.9% of the T-ALL mass. Large-scale single-cell transplantation experiments established that T-ALLs can be initiated from a single cell and that leukemias exhibit wide differences in tumor-initiating potential. T-ALLs can also be introduced into clonal-outcrossed animals, and T-ALLs arising in mixed genetic backgrounds can be transplanted into clonal recipients without the need for major histocompatibility complex matching. Finally, high-throughput imaging methods are described that allow large numbers of fluorescent transgenic animals to be imaged simultaneously, facilitating the rapid screening of engrafted animals. These experiments show that large numbers of zebrafish can be experimentally assessed by cell transplantation and establish new high-throughput methods to functionally interrogate gene pathways involved in cancer self-renewal.

3.3 Lymphomas/leukemias

There are numerous studies utilizing mouse models to study different lymphomas/ leukemias. Here, only a few representative are mentioned, since the thorough report of these models is beyond the scope of this chapter. As with other LPDs, the use of knock-out and/or transgenic mice has been substantial to study lymphomas and leukemias.

The first animal model we describe studies the pathogenesis of multiple hematopoietic malignancies simultaneously. The researchers (Zhang et al., 2011) have generated inducible Pten/Myc double-knockout mice (Pten(-/-)/Myc(-/-)). By comparing the hematopoietic phenotypes of these double-knockout mice with those of Pten(-/-) mice, they found that both sets of animals developed myelo- and lympho-proliferative disorders. Their study suggests that the deregulation of phosphoinositide 3-kinase/Akt signaling in Pten(-/-) hematopoietic cells protects these cells from apoptotic cell death, resulting in chronic proliferative disorders. Since, none of the compound-mutant mice developed acute leukemia or lymphoma, it is concluded that Myc is absolutely required for the development of acute hematopoietic malignancies.

Other researchers (Mukherjee et al., 2011) managed to develop spontaneous T- and B-cell lymphomas, and leukemia in mice: Homozygous deletion of ESPL1 gene that encodes Separase protein (Cohesin protease Separase plays a key role in faithful segregation of sister chromatids by cleaving the cohesin complex at the metaphase to anaphase transition) results in embryonic lethality in mice and Separase overexpression lead to aneuploidy and tumorigenesis. By examining the ESPL1 heterozygosity using a hypomorphic mouse model that has reduced germline Separase activity, they reported that while ESPL1 mutant (ESPL1 (+/hyp)) mice have a normal phenotype, in the absence of p53, mice develop spontaneous T- and B-cell lymphomas, and leukemia with a significantly shortened latency as compared to p53 null mice. Their results indicate that reduced levels of Separase act synergistically with loss of p53 in the initiation and progression of B- and T- cell lymphomas, which is aided by increased chromosomal missegregation and accumulation of genomic instability. ESPL1(+/hyp), p53(-/-) mice provide a new animal model for mechanistic study of aggressive lymphoma and also for preclinical evaluation of new agents for its therapy.

An interesting murine model of diffuse large B-cell lymphoma (DLBCL) described by Yu et al. (2011), uses human DLBCL cell line LY8, to investigate its characteristics of growth pathogenesis and the effect of treatment protocols. LY8 cells were injected subcutaneously into the right flank of nude mice. Harvested tumor tissues were cut into small pieces of 1.5 mm × 1.5 mm × 1.5 mm and implanted subcutaneously into nude mice. Tumor growth was monitored and the histologic characteristics were documented. Expression of LCA, CD20, CD79α, Ki-67, CD3, CD45RO, bcl-6, MUM-1, CD10 and bcl-2 were examined by using immunohistochemistry. IgH clonal rearrangement and status of three microsatellite loci (D14S68, D18S69, D20S199) in the xenografted tumor samples and the parental cell line LY8 were detected using PCR amplification followed by PAGE. The subcutaneous xenograft DLBCL model was successfully established by using cell line LY8, and a stable growth was achieved up to the 9th generation. The tumor in each generation showed similar growth characteristics and the rate of subcutaneous tumor formation was 91.9% (114/124). The tumor growth was observed from the 2nd week after morphological characteristics with those of human DLBCL, and expressed LCA, CD20, CD79α, bcl-6, MUM-1, CD10 and bcl-2. The tumor of xenograft mice and cell line LY8 showed identical IgH rearrangement and microsatellite length. This mouse model recapitulates many features of human DLBCL with high stability and repeatability. Therefore, it provides an ideal animal model for in vivo studies of the biological characteristics and treatment of DLBCL.

Gaurnier-Hausser et al. (2011) set out to determine whether dogs with spontaneous DLBCL (diffuse large B-cell lymphoma) have comparative aberrant constitutive NF-κB activity and to determine the therapeutic relevance of NF-κB inhibition in dogs with relapsed, resistant DLBCL. Constitutive canonical NF-κB activity and increased NF-κB target gene expression were detected in primary DLBCL tissue. NF-κB essential modulator (NEMO)-binding domain (NBD) peptide inhibited this activity and induced apoptosis of primary malignant B cells *in vitro*. Intratumoral injections of NBD peptide to dogs with relapsed DLBCL inhibited NF-κB target gene expression and reduced tumor burden. This work shows that dogs with spontaneous DLBCL share therapeutic relevance of NF-κB inhibition in the treatment of ABC-DLBCL. These results have important translational relevance for ABC-DLBCL treatment in human patients, and dogs with spontaneous DLBCL may represent a clinically relevant, spontaneous, large animal model for human ABC-DLBCL.

Other findings suggest that increasing levels of human-derived IgG in peripheral blood from hu-PBL/SCID mice could be used to monitor EBV-related human B-cell lymphoma development in experimental animals (Tang et al., 2011). Epstein-Barr virus (EBV) has a close association with various types of human lymphomas. Tang et al. (2011) aimed to evaluate the association between human IgG concentration and EBV-associated lymphoma development in huPBL/SCID mice. For that, human peripheral blood lymphocytes (hu-PBL) from EBV-seropositive donors were inoculated intraperitoneally into SCID mouse. Twenty one out of 29 mice developed tumors in their body. Immunohistochemical staining showed that all induced tumors were LCA (leukocyte common antigen) positive, B-cell markers (CD20, CD79a) positive, and T-cell markers (both CD3 and CD45RO) negative. The tumors were diagnosed as human B-cell lymphomas by these morphological and immunohistochemical features. *In situ* hybridization exhibited resultant tumor cells with EBV encoded small RNA-1 (EBER-1). Human-derived IgG could be found in the serum of SCID mice on the 15th day following hu-PBL transplantation, and IgG levels increased as tumor grew in 6 hu-PBL/SCID chimeras. These data suggest that intraperitoneal transfer of hu-PBLs from EBV+ donors to SCID mice leads to high human IgG levels in mouse serum and B cell lymphomas.

3.4 Multiple Myeloma

Plasmacytoma or myeloma can be induced in BALB/c mice by pristane oil or can develop spontaneously in some mouse strains (Potter, 1982; Radl, 1981). In the former, pristane oil induces an oil granuloma cheracterized by a chemically-induced lymphoplasmacytic reaction. This progresses to an autonomously growing plasmacytoma with uncontrolled expression of c-MYC due to its rearrangement. Generally, these plasmacytomas secrete monoclonal immunoglobulin of the IgA isotype. Essential monoclonal gammopathies and a malignancy resembling human plasma cell myeloma may arise spontaneously in inbred mice (Radl et al., 1988; Radl, 1991).

Hence, the Radl model was produced using 5T myeloma cells that arose spontaneously in aged, inbred C57BL/KaLwRijHsd mice and is propagated by the inoculation of these myeloma cells into syngeneic mice. More specifically, in order to develop a better animal model of human myeloma bone disease, Garrett et al. (1997), have established and subcloned a cell line from this murine myeloma and found that it causes osteolytic bone lesions in mice characteristic of human myeloma bone disease. The cell line produces interleukin-6, but grows independent of exogenous interleukin-6. Mice inoculated intravenously with the cultured cells predictably develop an identical disease to the mice injected intravenously with fresh bone-marrow-derived myeloma cells, including monoclonal gammopathy and radiologic bone lesions. They found that some of the mice became hypercalcemic, and the bone lesions are characterized by increased osteoclast activity. They found identical results when they inoculated Nu/Bg/XID mice with cultured murine myeloma cells. Because they can inoculate mice with precise numbers of cells and predict accurately when the mice will develop bone lesions, become hypercalcemic, and die, they considered it as a convenient model for determining the mechanisms by which the myeloma cells cause osteoclast activation in this model of human myeloma bone disease (Garrett et al., 1997; Radl et al., 1979, 1988).

On another approach, researchers made use of two facts:

1. Human myeloma cell lines can survive and disseminate in mice with severe combined immunodeficiency (SCID; Feo-Zuppardi et al., 1992; Huang et al., 1993).
2. Fetal bone implants (SCID-hu) can sustain survival and expansion of primary human myeloma cells from untreated patients with a high success rate (Yaccoby et al., 1998).

Thus, the SCID-hu model is produced, which provides a suitable *in vivo* read out system to study human myeloma biology. Tumor self-renewal capacity can be examined in relation to maturation stage. The contributions of host accessory cells and cytokines to disease manifestation and progression can also be elucidated. It is anticipated that new treatment principles aiming, for example, to inactivate the marrow microenvironment (e.g. bisphosphonates: Aparicio et al., 1998; Shipman et al., 1997) and target neoangiogenesis (e.g. Thalidomide: D' Amato et al., 1994; Singhal et al., 1999) can be evaluated. Another animal model uses adult human bone engraftments into SCID mice. In these mice the engrafted human bone is injected and subsequently populated by fresh tumor cells. In that way a close resemblance to human multiple myeloma has been achieved (Sjak-Shie et al., 1999).

Similar to the extensively tested and validated SCID-hu system, which uses a human fetal bone (Yaccoby et al., 1998, 2002, 2006; Yaccoby & Epstein, 1999), MM cells from the majority of patients grow exclusively in the implanted bone and produce typical myeloma manifestations including stimulation of osteoclastogenesis, suppression of osteoblastogenesis, and induction of severe osteolytic bone disease (Fig. 1). Ethical and scientific concerns regarding the use of human fetal bones in the SCID-hu model of primary human myeloma prompted the researchers to develop a novel system that uses rabbit bones implanted subcutaneously in unconditioned SCID mice. Immunohistochemical analysis of the implanted bone revealed that the majority of bone marrow (BM) microenvironment cells such as blood vessels, osteoclasts and osteoblasts were of rabbit origin. The implanted bones were directly injected with myeloma cells from MM patients. Successful engraftment of unseparated BM cells from 85% of patients and CD138-selected myeloma plasma cells from 81% of patients led to the production of patients' M-protein isotypes and typical myelomamanifestations (osteolytic bone lesions and angiogenesis of rabbit origin; Fig. 1). Myeloma cells grew exclusively in the rabbit bone, but were able to metastasize into another bone at a remote site in the same mouse. Cells from patients with extramedullary disease also grew along the outer surface of the rabbit bones. This demonstrates the ability of SCID-rab model, marked by a nonmyelomatous, nonhuman, and nonfetal microenvironment, to support the growth of CD138-expressing myeloma cells. This system can now be widely used to study the biology of myeloma and its manifestations and to develop novel therapeutic approaches for this disease (Yata & Yaccoby, 2004).

Conclusively, the SCID-hu/rab xenograft model provides a system where primary human myeloma cells can be injected into either a fetal human bone or rabbit bone that is implanted subcutaneously into an immunocompromised mouse (Yaccoby et al., 1998; Yata &Yaccoby, 2004). This model (SCID-rab) has been used since its establishment for different studies, e.g. the effect of anti-DKK1 therapy on bone metabolism and tumor growth in a SCID-rab system, since DKK1 is a key player in MM bone disease and blocking DKK1 activity in myelomatous bones reduces osteolytic bone resorption, increases bone formation, and helps control MM growth (Yaccoby et al., 2007).

The most recent study from Fowler et al. (2009) describes a model of myeloma in which the host microenvironment could be modified genetically. They demonstrated 5T myeloma establishment in recombination activating gene 2 (RAG-2)-deficient mice, which have improper B- and T-cell development. Importantly, these mice can be easily bred with genetically modified mice to generate double knockout mice, allowing manipulation of the host microenvironment at a molecular level. Inoculation of 5TGM1 myeloma cells into RAG-$2^{-/-}$ mice resulted in myeloma development, which was associated with tumor growth within bone and an osteolytic bone disease, as assessed by microcomputed tomography (microCT), histology and histomorphometry. Myeloma-bearing RAG-$2^{-/-}$ mice displayed many features that were similar to both human myeloma and the original Radl 5T model. To demonstrate the use of this model, we have examined the effect of host-derived matrix metalloproteinase 9 (MMP-9) in the development of myeloma in vivo.

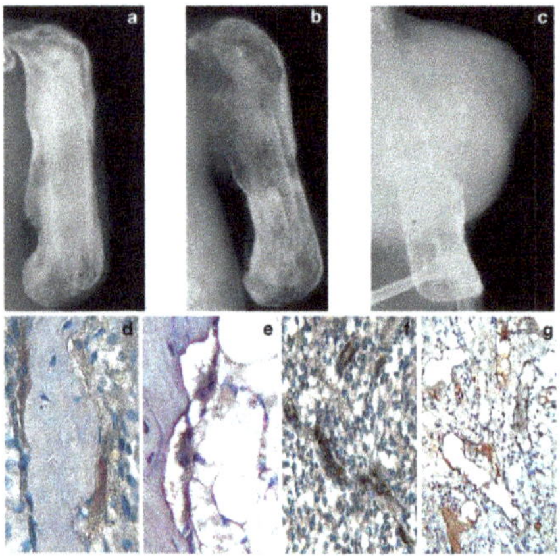

Fig. 1. Growth patterns and typical disease manifestations of myeloma cells in the SCID-rab model. (a, b) Myeloma cells from the majority ofpatients grew exclusively in the rabbit BM (medullary disease). Radiographs (a) before and (b) 12 weeks after myeloma PCs injection show severe resorption of the myelomatous rabbit bone. (c) Myeloma PCs taken from extramedullary disease grew also on the outer surface of the implanted rabbit bone. (d) Increased activity of mulinucleate osteoclasts was detected in myelomatous rabbit bone by staining sections for TRAP. (e) These osteoclasts were of rabbit origin, as revealed by their reactivity with anti-rabbit macrophage antibody. (f, g) Myelomatous rabbit bone sections immunostained with antibody to factor VIII (f) and rabbit CD141 (g) demonstrate increased numbers of tumor-associated microvessels of rabbit origin (From Yata & Yaccoby, 2004, permission pending).

Inoculation of 5TGM1 myeloma cells into mice that are deficient in RAG-2 and MMP-9 resulted in a reduction in both tumor burden and osteolytic bone disease when compared with RAG-2-deficient wild-type myeloma-bearing mice. The establishment of myeloma in RAG-$2^{-/-}$ mice permits molecular examination of the host contribution to myeloma pathogenesis in vivo.

3.5 Other lymphoproliferative disorders

Primates and swine have been used as experimental animals to develop animal models for post-transplant lymphoproliferative disorder (PTLD) one of the less frequently met LPDs.

As previously mentioned, PTLD has been shown to be associated with Epstein-Barr virus (EBV) infection. Although primate animal models of PTLD and the use of molecular markers in its diagnosis had not yet been reported, Schmidtko et al. (2002) designed a study to evaluate the frequency, pathology, and molecular characteristics of PTLD in cynomolgus monkey kidney allograft recipients. Of 160 consecutive primate renal transplants performed, 5.6% developed PTLD 28-103 days after transplantation. In all cases, the lymph nodes were involved and effaced by an atypical polymorphous lymphoid proliferation of EBER+ B cells, diagnostic for PTLD. Focal staining for EBNA-2 was noted in tumor cells. In 67% (six of nine) the PTLD infiltrates were present in extra nodal sites, notably liver (56%), lung (44%), heart (44%), renal allograft (44%), and native kidney (22%). The spleen was infiltrated by PTLD cells in all four animals that had not undergone a pre-transplant splenectomy. The PTLD morphology was similar in all cases and predominantly of the polymorphous type, however, some of these showed areas that appeared minimally polymorphous. No cases of monomorphic PTLD were seen. By *in situ hybridization,* expression of the RNA product, homologous for EBV-encoded RNA (EBER) was identified in the PTLD tumor cells of all cases, indicating latent primate EBV- related infection. This report identifies a novel animal model of EBV associated PTLD in the setting of kidney transplantation, with valuable implications for managing and understanding human PTLD and oncogenesis (Schmidtko et al., 2002).

Barth et al. (2009) developed another non-human primate facial composite tissue allotransplantation model to investigate strategies to achieve prolonged graft survival and immunologic responses unique to these allografts. For this reason, composite facial subunits consisting of skin, muscle, and bone were heterotopically transplanted to mixed lymphocyte reaction-mismatched Cynomolgus macaques. Tacrolimus monotherapy was administered via continuous intravenous infusion for 28 days then tapered to daily intramuscular doses. They concluded that Tacrolimus monotherapy provided prolonged rejection-free survival of composite facial allografts in this non-human primate model but was associated with the development of a high frequency of donor-derived PTLD tumors. The transplantation of a large volume of vascularized bone marrow in composite tissue allografts may be a risk factor for PTLD development.

A high incidence of a PTLD is observed in miniature swine conditioned for allogeneic hematopoietic cell transplantation using a protocol involving T-cell depletion and cyclosporine therapy. Cho et al. (2004), designed a study to assess contributing factors to disease development. Forty-six animals were studied including 12 (26%) that developed PTLD. A number of risk factors for PTLD were examined, including degree of immunosuppression, degree of MHC mismatch and infection by a porcine lymphotrophic herpesvirus (PLHV-1). Flow cytometry was used to measure host and donor T- and B-cell levels in the peripheral blood. Porcine lymphotrophic herpesvirus viral load was determined by quantitative PCR. Animals developing PTLD had significantly lower levels of T cells on the day of transplant. Cyclosporine levels did not differ significantly between animals with and without PTLD. Animals receiving transplants across a two-haplotype mismatch barrier showed an increased incidence of PTLD. All animals with PTLD had significant increases in PLHV-1 viral loads. Porcine lymphotrophic herpesvirus viral copy numbers remained at low levels in the absence of disease. The availability of a preclinical large-animal model with similarities to PTLD of humans may allow studies of the pathogenesis and treatment of that disorder.

Spleen transplantation (SpTx) was also performed in miniature swine across full major histocompatibility complex barriers to study the tolerogenic effect of the spleen (Dor et al., 2004). This study described the development of PTLD after allogeneic SpTx. Recipient pigs underwent whole body irradiation (100 cGy), thymic irradiation (700 cGy), and native splenectomy (day 0), and received a 45-day course of intravenous cyclosporine (trough level 400-800 ng/ml). After SpTx, two of seven pigs developed PTLD (1 donor-type, 1 host-type). These two pigs had greater T cell depletion and higher trough levels of cyclosporine. Early changes that occurred prior to the development of clinical features of PTLD were increased porcine lymphotropic herpesvirus-1 viral loads in blood and tissues, and increased numbers of leukocytes, B cells, and total serum IgM. PTLD can occur after allogeneic SpTx in swine. This model may be useful in studies of the pathogenesis of PTLD.

In another study using miniature swine (Doucette et al., 2007) the Porcine lymphotropic herpesvirus-1 (PLHV-1), a gamma-herpesvirus related to Epstein-Barr virus (EBV) was associated with development of PTLD following allogeneic stem cell or spleen transplantation. Oligonucleotide microarrays were designed based on known open reading frames (ORFs) of PLHV-1. Expression was compared by cohybridization of cDNA from lymph nodes of PLHV-1+ swine after allogeneic spleen transplantation between either: 1) PTLD-affected and PTLD-unaffected swine; or 2) PTLD-affected swine vs. samples from the same animal prior to diagnosis. In PTLD-affected animals, consistent upregulation (nine ORFs) and downregulation (four ORFs) of PLHV-1 mRNA was observed in comparison to those without PTLD. No differences in gene expression were discovered at the time of clinical PTLD diagnosis compared to six to nine days prior to diagnosis in the same animals. This model provides insights into the pathogenesis of PTLD and, by extension, potential diagnostic and therapeutic tools for human EBV-associated PTLD.

4. Waldenström's macroglobulinemia

This disease was first identified by J. Waldenström when he reported two patients with a syndrome of oronasal bleeding, lymphadenopathy, an elevated sedimentation rate, hyperviscosity, normal bone films, cytopenias and a bone marrow with a predominantly lymphoid infiltrate (Waldenström, 1944).

In the Revised European-American Lymphoma (REAL) classification, Waldenström macroglobulinemia (WM) has become viewed as a distinct clinicopathological entity, and is defined largely as a lymphoplasmacytic lymphoma (LPL); (Harris et al, 1994). The Second International Workshop on Waldenström macroglobulinemia attempted to refine further the working definition of the disease within the context of a LPL (Owen et al., 2003). For review, see Ansell et al., 2010.

Despite these efforts, the debate remains within the hematological and hematopathological communities with respect to nosology. These issues of definition have and continue to affect the interpretation of results within and across clinical trials as well as in basic and epidemiological research (Fonseca & Hayman, 2007). The same researchers (Fonseca & Hayman, 2007) used the definition of WM as proposed at the Second International Workshop on WM, with the exception that the original criterion of the presence of any degree of marrow involvement with a lymphoplasmacytoid infiltrate has been modified to allow a distinction to be made between an immunoglobulin (Ig) M monoclonal gammopathy of undetermined significance (MGUS) and WM. This change is based on analyses that have established the prognostic relevance and statistically significant survival differences among IgM MGUS (<10% marrow lymphoplasmacytic infiltrate) and symptomatic/smouldering WM and symptomatic/active WM(≥10% lymphoplasmacytic marrow infiltrate; usually intertrabecular).

Thus, Waldenström macroglobulinemia is a B-cell lymphoproliferative disorder characterized by a lymphoplasmacytic infiltration in the bone marrow or lymphatic tissue and a monoclonal immunoglobulin M protein (IgM) in the serum (Dimopoulos et al., 2005; Owen et al., 2003). Is a rare hematological neoplasm with an overall incidence of approximately 5 cases per 1 million persons per year, accounting for 1-2% of haematological malignancies (Groves et al., 1998; Herrinton & Weiss, 1993).

The median age at diagnosis varies between 63 and 68 years, and most patients (55%-70%) with newly diagnosed disease are men (Dimopoulos et al., 2000). The incidence of Waldenström macroglobulinemia is highest among white people and is rare in other population groups (Benjamin et al., 2003). More specifically, WM is rare in Blacks, who represent only 5% of cases, and it is also rare in those of Mexican-Mestizo descent (Groves et al, 1998; Herrinton & Weiss, 1993; Ruiz-Arguelles et al, 2000). To date, there is no compelling evidence to link WM to specific occupational or environmental exposures, tobacco or alcohol use (Linet et al., 1993).

The aetiology of WM remains unknown. It appears to be primarily a sporadic disease, although there are multiple reports of familial clustering (Blattner et al., 1980; Brown et al., 1967; Elves & Brown, 1968; Getaz & Staples, 1977; McMaster et al., 2005; Ogmundsdottir et al., 1999; Renier et al., 1989; Treon et al., 2006). McMaster et al. (2006) performed a genomewide linkage analysis in 11 high-risk families with WM that were informative for linkage (including a total of 122 individuals with DNA samples). The strongest evidence of linkage was found on chromosomes 1q and 4q (McMaster et al., 2006). Treon et al. (2006) evaluated 257 patients with previously untreated WM and found that 18,7% had at least one first-degree relative with either WM or another B-cell disorder. In addition, those with a familial history had higher percentages of bone marrow involvement, were diagnosed at a younger age, and were more likely to have higher IgM levels upon initial presentation (Treon et al., 2006).

The greatest risk factor for the development of WM is that of having an IgM MGUS. These patients have 46 times greater risk of developing WM than the general population (Kyle et al., 2002). Factors affecting the progression from IgM MGUS to WM are unknown. Infiltration of the bone marrow and extramedullary sites by malignant B cells and elevated IgM levels account for the symptoms associated with this disease. Patients may develop constitutional symptoms, pancytopenia, organomegaly, neuropathy, and symptoms associated with immunoglobulin deposition or hyperviscosity (Dimopoulos et al., 2000; Vijay & Gertz, 2007). However, symptoms vary considerably in individual patients. Although some patients present with the aforementioned symptoms, many are asymptomatic at the time of diagnosis.

Waldenström macroglobulinemia is incurable with current therapy, and half of the patients die of disease progression; median survival is approximately 5 years (Dimopoulos et al., 1999). This disease is diagnosed in many patients at an advanced age, and thus approximately half of the patients die of causes unrelated to Waldenström macroglobulinemia. Because the disease is incurable and the clinical presentations, comorbidities, and causes of death vary substantially, the decision to treat patients and the choice of treatment can be complex. A number of consensus meetings have listed reasonable treatment options (Gertz et al., 2003; Treon et al., 2006; Dimopoulos et al., 2009) but the physician is still faced with a difficult treatment decision in a patient with an uncommon disease.

5. Animal models of Waldenström's macroglobulinemia

In 2003, the Wayne State University Waldenstrom's Macroglobulinemia xenograft model in mice with severe combined immune deficiency (WSU-WM-SCID) was developed (Al-Katib et al., 2003). The WSU-WM-SCID is a model of a more aggressive and resistant WM usually seen toward the late stages of disease. It is, therefore, a particularly useful tool in developing new therapeutic strategies for the more aggressive WM, including targeted therapy, which exploits unique molecular characteristics of tumor cells. The WSU-WM-SCID is the first preclinical animal model available for this disease. It is based on a permanent, EBV-IgMlambda cell line (WSU-WM) established from a patient with a 10-year history of Waldenstrom's macroglobulinemia. These cells are CD5(-)CD10(+)CD19(+)CD20(+)CD22(+) and have t(8;14) (q24;32), t(12;17) (q24;q21), 2p-. WSU-WM cells also express DNA topoisomerase II (alpha and beta), and are bcl(2)(+)bcl(XL)(+)bax(-). Although the tumor has aggressive biological behavior with c-myc-IgH rearrangement, it has retained the salient features of WM. The breakpoint on 8q24 is downstream of c-myc exon 3, which is not usual for Burkitt-type breakpoints. WSU-WM cells also express both secretory (s(u)) and membrane (m(u)) IgM mRNA and secrete IgM in culture supernatant. Histiologically, WSU-WM-SCID xenograft tumors have lymphoplasmacytoid morphology. These features indicate biological, but not histological evolution.

In 2005, Tassone et al., developed a novel *in vivo* model of human WM in severe combined immunodeficient (SCID) mice implanted with human fetal bone chips (SCID-hu mice) into which WM cells from patient bone marrow are engrafted directly into the human bone marrow (huBM) microenvironment. WM cells in SCID-hu mice produced human monoclonal paraprotein (immunoglobulin M [IgM] and/or kappa or lambda chain) detectable in mice sera. Immunohistochemical analysis of human bone retrieved from SCID-hu mice showed infiltration with CD20+, IgM+, and monotypic light chain+ lymphoplasmacytic cells. Mast cells were observed to be associated with the infiltrate in these sections. Treatment of SCID-hu mice bearing WM with rituximab induced tumor regression, associated with a decrease in serum paraprotein. This model, therefore, recapitulates the in vivo biology of WM and allows the study of novel investigational drugs targeting WM cells in the huBM milieu.

Model cell lines are essential tools for investigating the biology and therapeutics of cancer. Approximately 1500 human hematopoietic neoplastic cell lines have been described, covering most major disease entities. Waldenström's macroglobulinemia (WM) is a rare incurable hematological neoplasm from which four cell lines have been derived.

In 2007 a cell line, the BCWM.1 cell line (Ditzel Santos et al., 2007), which was derived from the long-term culture of CD19(+) selected bone marrow lymphoplasmacytic cells isolated from an untreated patient with WM. BCWM.1 cells morphologically resemble lymphoplasmacytic cells (LPC) and propagate in RPMI-1640 medium supplemented with 10% fetal bovine serum. Phenotypic characterization by flow cytometric analysis demonstrated typical WM LPC characteristics: CD5(-), CD10(-), CD19(+), CD20(+), CD23(+), CD27(-), CD38(+), CD138(+), CD40(+), CD52(+), CD70(+), CD117(+), cIgM(+), cIgG(-), cIgA(-), ckappa(-), clambda(+), as well as the survival proteins APRIL and BLYS, and their receptors TACI, BCMA and BAFF-R. Enzyme-linked immunosorbent assay studies demonstrated secretion of IgMlambda and soluble CD27. Karyotypic and multicolor fluorescence in situ hybridization studies did not demonstrate cytogenetic abnormalities. Molecular analysis of BCWM.1 cells confirmed clonality by determination of IgH rearrangements. Inoculation of BCWM.1 cells in human bone marrow chips implanted in severe combined immunodeficient-hu mice led to rapid engraftment of tumor cells and serum detection of human IgM, lambda, and soluble CD27. These studies support the use of BCWM.1 cells as an appropriate model for the study of WM, which in conjunction with the severe combined immunodeficient-hu mouse model may be used as a convenient model for studies focused on both WM pathogenesis and development of targeted therapies for WM.

In 2008, Drexler et al., summarized on the existence of three cell lines, that although are currently used as *in vitro* models, none convincingly pass muster. Mindful that candidate tumor cell lines sometimes arise spuriously by viral immortalization of bystander cells, they reviewed the extent to which WM cell lines portray established disease features in vitro. At closer inspection, it seems that none convincingly displays morphological, immunophenotypic, genotypic or biological features characteristic of WM. Rather it appears that two cell lines (WM1 and BCWM.1) are most probably Epstein-Barr virus-immortalized B-lymphoblastoid cell lines, derived from bystander B-cells. The third cell line (WSU-WM) carries the most common cytogenetic hallmark of Burkitt lymphoma, namely t(8;14)(q24;q32), while none have been shown to carry chromosome 6 deletions recently demonstrated as indicative of disease progression in this entity.

Recently, Hodge et al. (2011) described the establishment of a new WM cell line, MWCL-1. Comprehensive genetic analyses have unequivocally confirmed a clonal relationship between this novel cell line and the founding tumor. MWCL-1 cells exhibit an immunophenotype consistent with a diverse, tumor clone composed of both small B lymphocytes and larger lymphoplasmacytic cells and plasma cells: $CD3^-$, $CD19^+$, $CD20^+$, $CD27^+$, $CD38^+$, $CD49D^+$, $CD138^+$, $cIgM^+$, and κ^+. Cytogenetic studies identified a monoallelic deletion of 17p13 (TP53) in both the cell line and the primary tumor. Direct DNA resequencing of the remaining copy of TP53 revealed a missense mutation at exon 5 (V143A, GTG>GCG). In accordance with primary WM tumors, MWCL-1 cells retain the ability to secrete high amounts of IgM protein in the absence of an external stimulus. The genetic, immunophenotypic, and biologic data presented here confirm the validity of the MWCL-1 cell line as a representative model of WM.

Dr. Janz at Department of Pathology at University of Iowa is currently developing a mouse model of Waldenström's macroglobulinemia. An immunocompetent, transgenic mouse model of human WM that will be useful for preclinical testing of WM drug candidates. Transgenic mouse models of human cancer are experimental model systems that rely on laboratory mice that have been genetically manipulated to render them prone to neoplasms that accurately recapitulate important features of their human cancer counterparts. Model systems of this sort: enable researchers to study the onset and progression of cancer in ways that cannot be pursued in human beings; advance our understanding of the molecular genetic and biological events that contribute to the development and spread of cancer cells; and provide a valuable preclinical platform for evaluating new approaches to treat and prevent cancer in patients. The latter is particularly important in circumstances in which drug testing requires an intact, immunocompetent animal that is able to produce the same kind of tumor microenvironment and recruit the same types of tumor bystander cells commonly found in human patients. To give but one example, therapeutic antibodies target cancer cells by recruiting normal immune cells to the site of attack; thus, the preclinical testing of these antibodies requires strains of laboratory mice that have a normal, fully functioning immune system. To that end, Janz and collaborators are generating a designer model of human WM designated C.IL6/BCL2/AID^{null}. This model combines three crucial pathogenetic factors of human WM - namely the B-lymphocyte growth, differentiation and survival factor IL-6, the cellular oncoprotein BCL-2, and the inability of WM cells to perform immunoglobulin isotype switching (AID^{null}) - on the genetic backgroud of BALB/c (abbreviated as C). Strain C mice are highly susceptible to malignant B-lymphocyte transformation (Diagram 1; http://www.medicine.uiowa.edu Pathology/site/research/ janz/res_projects.html; selected publications of Dr.Janz: de Jong & Janz, 2010; Park et al., 2005).

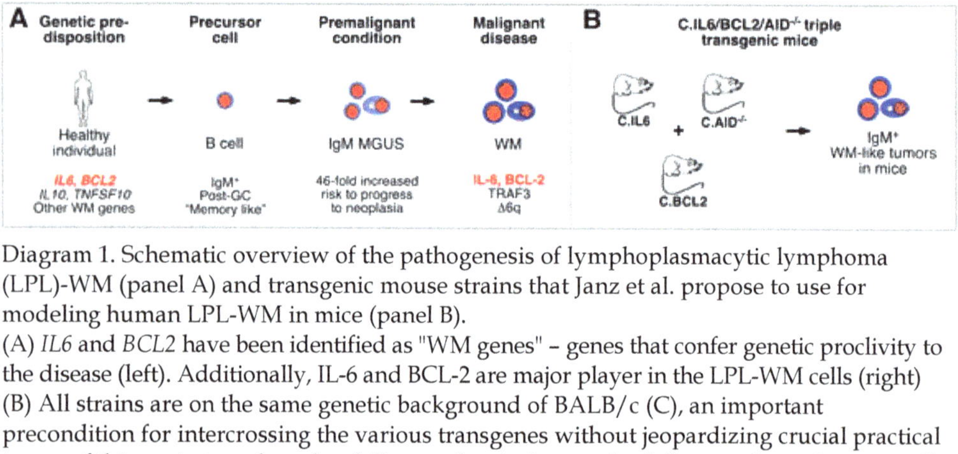

Diagram 1. Schematic overview of the pathogenesis of lymphoplasmacytic lymphoma (LPL)-WM (panel A) and transgenic mouse strains that Janz et al. propose to use for modeling human LPL-WM in mice (panel B).
(A) *IL6* and *BCL2* have been identified as "WM genes" – genes that confer genetic proclivity to the disease (left). Additionally, IL-6 and BCL-2 are major player in the LPL-WM cells (right)
(B) All strains are on the same genetic background of BALB/c (C), an important precondition for intercrossing the various transgenes without jeopardizing crucial practical issues of this project, such as the ability to adoptively transfer fully transformed tumor cells or premalignant B-lineage cells from transgenic mice. We hypothesize that strain C.IL6/BCL2/AID$^{-/-}$ mice will develop IgM$^+$ WM-like tumors.

5.1 Waldenström's macroglobulinemia in NOD/SCID mice

Although important advances have been made in the classification of lymphomas, the remaining discrepancies in WM definition reflect the fact that the pathogenesis of this disease remains largely unknown.

As stated in the previous paragraph, the establishment of reliable animal models will significantly enhance research in dissecting the complicate pathogenesis of WM. In addition, suitable animal models may be used to assess the efficacy of existing treatments and develop novel therapeutic strategies (Al-Katib et al., 1993; 2003). Severe combined immunodeficient (SCID) mice injected with subcutaneous xenografts of neoplastic cells were originally used to study WM. However, the usefulness of these models is limited because they do not recapitulate typical features of WM, such as bone marrow localization. Recently developed SCID mouse WM models overcome this drawback, by utilizing subcutaneous implants of human fetal bone chips. The subsequent injection of bone marrow (BM) aspirates from WM patients directly into the fetal bone implants resulted in successful WM cell engraftment in 69% of animals (Tassone et al., 2005). Although this model offers a potential advantage in that human bone is used, fetal bone, which is at a state of rapid growth, clearly differs from adult bone. It is apparent that there are differences between the bone marrow of a newborn and an adult bone marrow, including apoptotic cells, T cells, B cells and macrophages, developing the microenvironment where the WM cells are being hosted. Not to mention the fact that human bone is made of cells forming temporary anatomical structures, called basic multicellular units that execute bone remodeling, which change with ageing of humans (Seeman, 2008).

Our study was undertaken with the aim to develop a novel non-obese SCID (NOD-SCID) mouse model of WM. For that, pairs of bone particles derived from adult humans were successfully implanted intramuscularly in mice. Each mouse was implanted with a bone fragment taken from a neoplastic disease-free individual in the one hind limb and with a different biopsy taken from a WM patient, in the other. IgM producing neoplastic cells not only retained viability in the bone marrow of the WM bone biopsy but also metastasized to the normal bone marrow of the distant bone implant. The mouse model reported here improves on existing models of WM by recapitulating the adult human bone marrow microenvironment of abnormal WM neoplastic cells.

For this reason, twenty-nine NOD-SCID mice (Charles River Laboratories, France) were used. The animals were housed in static microisolator cages at the bio-containment animal Research Facility of the G. Papanicolaou General Hospital. All experimental procedures and protocols were in accordance with the European Council Directive 86/609 as well as the national and institutional guidelines for animal care.

Cancellous bone core fragments ranging from 16 to 22 mm^3 in size were obtained from the femoral head of neoplastic disease-free adult humans during hip arthroplasty or hemiarthroplasty. Bone fragments were subsequently implanted into the right or left hindlimb muscles of 6 to 8 weeks-old mice (n=23), weighing 25 - 30 grams, as previously described (Tsingotjidou et al., 2001). To test viability of implanted tissue, implants were retrieved from 9 mice that were sacrificed at 4 (n=3), 8 (n=3) and 12 (n=3) weeks post-implantation. Based on previous studies (Boynton et al., 1996) in order to detect hematopoietic cells of human origin mouse anti-human CD45 antibody (1:500; Dako, Carpinteria, CA) was used. Eight to twelve weeks following first bone implantation, the non-implanted hindlimb of the remaining 12 mice was also engrafted with a human bone biopsy taken from WM patients (see flow chart; Diagram 2). For that, bone marrow core needle biopsies (bone biopsies) were obtained from the posterior iliac crest of five patients with active WM during scheduled clinical visits. The biopsy was maintained in RPMI medium until its use. Typically, two implants were produced from each bone biopsy. In one case, however, a single WM bone biopsy was large enough to be the source of 6 implants. All human bone biopsy donors signed Institutional Review Board-approved informed consent forms. Control mice received no implant (n=3) or were implanted only, either with non-WM (n=2) or with WM (n=3) human bone fragments (Diagram 2).

To detect human IgM in the serum of mice, thus providing evidence for presence of human IgM-secreting B-cells or WM cells, mouse blood was collected from the orbital sinus of each mouse monthly during the experiment. Blood serum was serially tested for circulating IgM by ELISA (Diagnostic automation Inc., Calabasas, CA, USA).

Mice were sacrificed at different time points ranging from 1 to 5 months following the implantation of WM bone biopsies (Diagram 2). At necropsy, tissues including femur, tibia, brain, liver, spleen, lungs, kidneys and the WM and non-WM bone grafts were collected and fixed in formalin. Decalcified bones together with other formalin-fixed tissues were processed routinely, embedded in paraffin, sectioned at 5 μm, and stained with haematoxylin and eosin (HE) or immunohistochemistry (IHC). The latter was performed with mouse monoclonal antibodies directed against human CD20 (Biogenex, San Ramon, CA, USA), IgM (Cell Marque, Rocklin, CA, USA), and κ and λlight chains (Novocastra Laboratories, Newcastle-upon-Tyne, UK). Antigens were retrieved with microwave heating in citrate buffer (pH 6) for CD20, or with proteinase K (DAKO, Carpinteria, CA, USA) digestion for 6 minutes at room temperature for IgM and κ or λ chains. Poly-HRP goat anti-mouse IgG (Chemikon, Temecula, CA, USA) was used as secondary antibody. Signal was detected with diaminobenzidine and tissues were counterstained with haematoxylin. Wild type mouse colon along with mesenteric lymph nodes sections were used as negative tissue controls, whereas positive controls were procured from bone biopsy of WM patients not involved in the study. Irrelevant mouse antibodies were used instead of primary antibodies for negative staining controls.

We (Tsingotjidou et al., 2001) and others (Yonou et al., 2001) have previously shown that adult human bone retains viability after engraftment subcutaneously or within the skeletal muscles of immunocompromised mice. In the present study, we first sought to determine whether the above-mentioned model of bone engraftment was successfully reproduced. For that, adult human cancellous bone intramuscular implants were recovered from control SCID mice at 4, 8 or 12 weeks post-implantation for histological evaluation. At four weeks, specimens showed multifocal necrosis and fibrosis. The surface of the human bone was lined by small numbers of osteoblast-like cells and minute amount of newly synthesized osteoid. In contrast, all human bone implants from intramuscularly implanted mice were largely normal at the 8-week time-point. Viable osteocytes and increased numbers of osteoblasts forming adequate amounts of osteoid were evident. However, rare foci of remaining osteonecrotic and fibrotic changes were noticed. At 12 weeks after implantation, the histology of intramuscularly implanted bone was completely restored. The population and spatial distribution of osteoblasts, the amounts of newly formed bone matrix, the restored numbers of viable osteocytes (Fig. 2A) and the presence of active bone marrow cavities (Fig. 2B) were all consistent with normal bone histology. The human origin of haematopoietic cells populating the bone marrow of implants was confirmed by IHC using an antibody against human CD45 that shows no cross-reactivity with mouse CD45 protein (Tsingotjidou et al., 2001; Boynton et al., 1996). No human lymphoid cell was found in murine tissues examined. These results suggest that human bone implant was maintained and thrived in the mouse skeletal muscle environment.

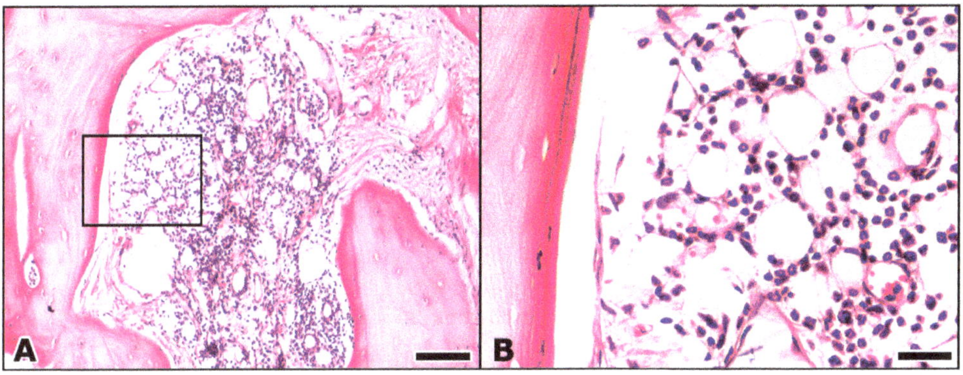

Fig. 2. Non-WM human bone implanted in the hind limb muscles of a NOD-SCID mouse at 12 weeks post-implantation. Higher magnification of the boxed area in A is shown in B. Histology of the human bone is restored. Note new bone formation with viable osteoblasts and bone marrow reconstitution. Haematoxylin & Eosin. Bars, A: 100 μm; B: 25 μm.

Three animals bearing WM bone biopsy alone were sacrificed at 1 (*n*=1), 2 (*n*=1) and 3 (*n*=1) months post implantation (Diagram 2). In all three animals, the bone marrow was diffusely infiltrated by neoplastic cells that had lymphocytic, plasma cell or lymphoplasmacytic phenotype. Tumor cells were often arranged in discrete nodules. Reactive hyperplasia of tumor-associated mast cells was common. Necrotic areas were evident at 1 month post implantation, feature that was diminished afterwards (at 2 and 3 months post implantation).

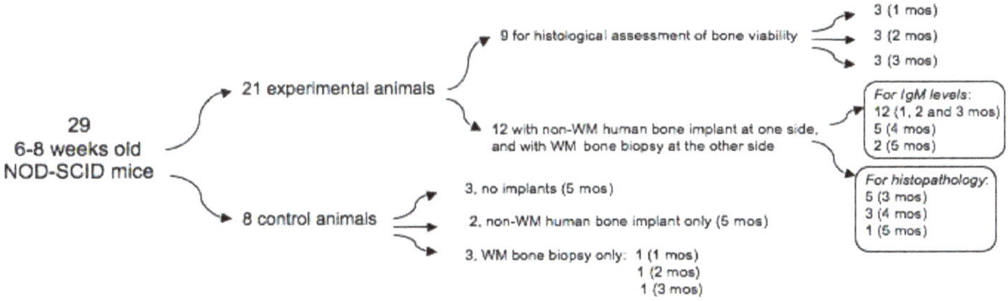

Diagram 2. Flow chart of the experimental design; Time at parentheses indicates the sacrifice point, mos=months

Immunohistochemically, neoplastic cells were CD20 positive. IgM-positive neoplastic cells were also identified in large numbers. Both CD20 and IgM antibodies used for this purpose was against human lymphocytes and IgM. These mice also had elevated IgM in serum at one month following the intramuscular implantation of the biopsy. However, two months post-implantation, blood IgM was moderately-to-markedly reduced. In a single mouse IgM fell to non-detectable levels, while in the remaining moderately elevated IgM was detectable up to three months following the WM bone biopsy implantation, without reaching, however, the high IgM levels encountered at one month post-implantation (Tsingotjidou et al., 2009). Control animals that received no implant (n=3) or were implanted only with non-WM (n=2) showed no elevation in serum IgM throughout the duration of experiment. Upon histological and IHC examination control mice had no detectable lymphocytes or plasma cells in all tissues examined.

Twelve animals (*n*=12) implanted with both WM and non-WM bones were monitored for serum IgM levels throughout the experiment. Necropsies were performed in nine of those (9/12) at 3 (*n*=5), 4 (*n*=3) and 5 (*n*=1) months following implantation of WM bone biopsies (Diagram 2). Histopathological and immunohistochemical analysis of WM implants in these mice (*n*=9) yielded similar results as those described in the control mice bearing WM bone biopsy alone (*n*=3), namely a CD20+, IgM+ neoplastic cell infiltrate. These results indicated that survival of neoplastic cells in this experimental model could be prolonged for at least 5 months post implantation. Interestingly, histopathology and IHC analysis of the controlateral, non-WM implant of 4 out 9 mice revealed that the bone marrow was infiltrated by large numbers of neoplastic cells (Fig. 3). In order to confirm the validity of our findings, clonality by staining against κ- and λ- light chains was documented in two, randomly selected animals (W6 and W10). Cytoplasmic immunolabelling for κ- but not for λ-light chains was evident and restricted specifically and exclusively within the plasmacytic component of the tumor (Fig. 4). Thus, light chain predominance confirmed the clonality of neoplastic cells. Sparsely dispersed IgM positive cells were found in the bone marrow of tibia and femur of one animal (W10). Diffuse infiltration of WM cells was also seen in the liver and kidney of another animal (W44).

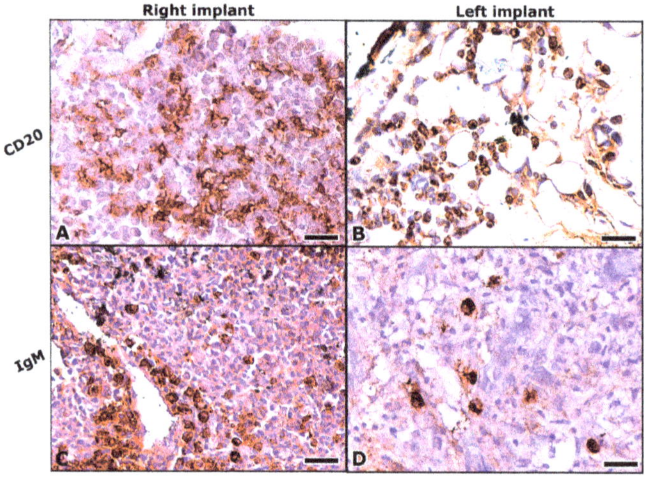

Fig. 3. CD20-specific (A and B) and IgM-specific (C and D) immunohistochemistry of human bone implants. Large numbers of human CD20-positive (A) and IgM-positive (C) WM cells remain viable in the bone marrow of the WM bone biopsy implanted in NOD-SCID mice. CD20-positive (B) and IgM-positive (D) cells could also be detected at the non-WM human bone that was distantly implanted in the same mice. Haematoxylin counterstain, DAB chromogen. Bars: 25 μm.

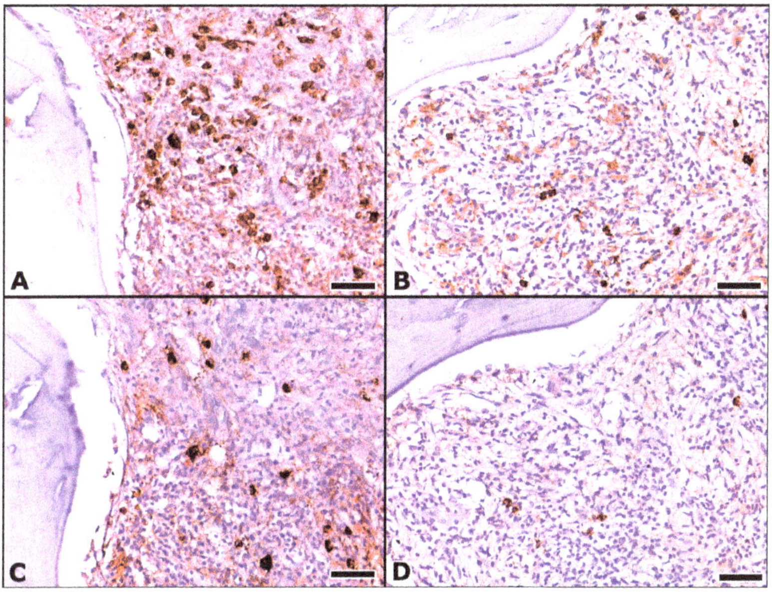

Fig. 4. κ (A and B) and λ (C and D) chain immunophenotyping of neoplastic cells performed in consecutive histological sections taken from both WM (A and C) and non-WM (B and D) bone implants of the same mouse. κ-chain-positive cell predominance in both implants provided evidence for the clonality of neoplastic cells. Haematoxylin counterstain, DAB chromogen. Bars: 50 μm

Serum IgM values in all mice implanted with both WM and non-WM bone biopsies (*n*=12) correlated with histopathological observations and IHC analysis for neoplastic cell density and metastatic growth. Indeed, mice with increased neoplastic cell burden and controlateral bone implant metastasis (W10, W44, W52 and W6) had increased IgM values in their blood serum (Tsingotjidou et al., 2009). In contrast, mice with sparse neoplastic cells in the WM implant and no evidence of metastasis (W45, W51 and W50) had low or non-detectable levels of serum IgM. It is interesting that 2 out of these 3 mice received implants originating from patients that had the two lowest percentages of bone marrow infiltration by neoplastic cells (20% and 33%) among human bone biopsy donors in this study. In a single mouse (W46), a sudden abolishment of serum IgM levels was observed at the 4th month post implantation of the WM bone (Tsingotjidou et al., 2009). Histological evidence of necrosis found in both implanted bone fragments examined, however, explained this abnormality.

Overall analysis of the monthly records of serum IgM values of mice used in this study reveals that after the second month, there is an overall progressive rise of IgM during months 3 and 4 post implantation of the WM biopsy (Tsingotjidou et al., 2009).

Taken together these results suggest that the WM neoplastic cells in the bone marrow of adult human bone implanted in SCID mice not only survive and grow but also are capable of producing IgM and metastasize (Tsingotjidou et al., 2009). The relatively high value of IgM obtained one month after implantation is considered an artifact attributable to cell damage, as discussed below.

This study described a novel NOD-SCID mouse model of WM. Using the SCID mouse as a vehicle of two human adult bone intramuscular implants we demonstrated that IgM producing WM neoplastic cells retain viability in the bone marrow of the implant originating from WM patients. Interestingly, neoplastic cells not only grew but also metastasized to the normal bone marrow of the second distant bone implant (Fig. 3).

A significant drawback in understanding pathogenesis of WM and developing novel therapeutics is the lack of animal models that recapitulate most features of human WM. Hence, several studies have focused in the development of animal models to study this rare but incurable neoplastic disease. In the past, attempts to grow WM cells *in vitro* or engraft them in immunocompromised mice have failed (Al-Katib et al., 2003). This probably was due to the lack of human bone marrow stromal cells, which are important elements of tumor microenvironment and facilitate both survival and proliferation of WM cells. Recently, however, important advances have been made utilizing SCID mice that were implanted with human fetal bone chips. The bone marrow of fetal bone implants successfully supported the survival and growth of WM cells derived either directly from patients (Tassone et al., 2005) or from a WM cell line that was established for that purpose (Santos et al., 2007). Both those experimental models are important, since they recapitulate a typical feature of the human disease, which is the bone marrow microenvironment-depended growth of WM cells. However, the natural niche of WM cells is the adult and not the fetal bone marrow that both these studies utilized for the engraftment of malignant cells. Adult and fetal bone marrow may differ in the pattern of growth stimuli imparted to WM cells. Although these differences cannot be elucidated, without elaborate research, the murine model of WM proposed in the present study overcomes this skepticism by simply using adult human bone implants.

An interesting observation of this study was that mice implanted with a WM bone fragment, showed elevation of blood IgM one month following the implantation. This peak in IgM levels observed at the first month coincided with the period of maximum damage to the implanted bone particle (Tsingotjidou et al., 2001). This particular elevation, however, may not reflect an active secretion of IgM from WM cells, but rather be due to an initial phase of ischaemic injury leading to WM cell necrosis and subsequent IgM leak. Indeed, histological studies of the human bone implants performed in the present study matched our previous observations (Tsingotjidou et al., 2001), which indicated that 8-12 weeks are needed before implanted bones become adequately vascularized, and restore their pre-transplant normal histology. A similar phenomenon of IgM release is well characterized in human patients following effective anti-neoplastic treatment, due to WM cell damage (Treon et al., 2004). For that reason, only IgM serum values obtained from the second month onwards were taken into consideration and were used as reliable indicators of disease burden of the implanted mice.

The wide range of IgM levels observed in mice of our experiments mimic analogous findings in humans. Accumulated data suggest that the levels of IgM production are highly variable among WM patients. Therefore, such data are valuable for follow-up examinations of individual patients and do not represent a universal indicator of WM burden. Irrespectively of initial IgM levels, however, most mice used in this study showed a similar pattern of IgM fluctuation over time. Following an elevation of IgM at the first month and a subsequent reduction at the second month, which can be considered baseline, there was a progressive rise of IgM during months 3 and 4 post implantation of the WM biopsy.

An interesting feature of the WM murine model presented here is the observed metastasis of the malignant cells. In approximately half of mice implanted with both WM and non-WM bone implants, WM cells metastasized from the affected implant to the healthy one, which was located in the contralateral hindlimb. Human bone, albeit from unrelated individual, was colonized preferentially, since metastasis to murine bone was observed only in a single mouse. Accordingly, existing murine models of WM show either no (Santos et al., 2007) or rare (Tassone et al., 2005) metastases to murine tissues. It is possible, that WM cells engrafted in mice could infrequently acquire novel properties that allow them to traffic, home and survive in murine bone marrow or other tissues. Obviously, accumulated genetic abnormalities driven by a physical selection process, may result in WM cells able to survive in the murine microenvironment. However, these genetic alterations render these cells less appropriate to model metastatic phenomena occurring in human WM, which is predominately an indolent disease. The murine model developed in the present study overcomes inherited disadvantages of existing WM *in vivo* models and better recapitulates metastasis, since it is supporting relocation of primary WM cells derived from patients from one human bone implant to another.

6. Conclusion

The use of bone biopsies taken from different WM patients as implants in SCID mice appears as highly attractive biological system to study aspects of the human disease. The quantitative limitation of harvesting BM particles from patients restricts the possibility to produce large highly homogeneous experimental groups of mice, given the variability of biological behaviour of WM among patients. This fact is exemplified by the results of the present study. Indeed, high levels of serum IgM and infiltration of the contralateral non-WM bone biopsy, by WM cells did not occur consistently in all mice. Hence, we reason that this model may not be suitable for screening specific therapeutic factors of WM. For such studies, the adult bone implant approach might still be considered if the healthy bone was artificially populated with WM cell line. On the other hand, the experimental design used in the present study may be useful for studying the pathogenesis of WM and particularly the interaction with the bone marrow stroma as it exists in the adult bone marrow. It may also be an ideal setting for studying the disease in long term, since the model allows indolent growth in mice, and consequently to assess the pathophysiology of epiphenomena such as neuropathy (work in progress). It is believed that the experimental setting as presented here will contribute to the unraveling of the etiology and pathogenesis of WM to the benefit of the patients.

7. Acknowledgments

This research was supported by the International Waldenström's Macroglobulinemia Foundation (IWMF) grant to A.S.T. We would like to thank Dr. Theofilos Poutahidis for his critical review of the manuscript, and Stergios J. Emmanouilides for his secretarial help.

8. References

Al-Katib, A.R., Mohammad, R., Hamdan, M., Mohamed, A.N., Dan, M. & Smith, M.R. (1993). Propagation of Waldenström's macroglobulinemia cells in vitro and in severe combined immune deficient mice: utility as a preclinical drug screening model. *Blood,* Vol. 81, No. 11, (June, 1993), pp. 3034-3042, ISSN 0006-4971

Al-Katib, A.M., Mensah-Osman, E., Aboukameel, A. & Mohammad, R. (2003). The Wayne State University Waldenstrom's Macroglobulinemia preclinical model for Waldenstrom's macroglobulinemia. *Seminars in Oncology.*, Vol. 30, No. 2, (April, 2003), pp. 313-317, ISSN 0093-7754

Ansell, S.M., Kyle, R.A., Reeder, C.B., Fonseca, R., Mikhael, J.R., Morice, W.G., Bergsagel, P.L., Buadi, F.K., Colgan, J.P., Dingli, D., D,ipenzieri, A., Greipp, P.R., Habermann, T.M., Hayman, S.R., Inwards, D.J., Johnston ,P.B., Kumar, S.K., Lacy, M.Q., Lust, J.A., Markovic, S.N., Micallef, I.N., Nowakowski, G.S., Porrata, L.F., Roy. V., Russell, S.J., Short, K.E., Stewart, A.K,. Thompson, C.A., Witzig, T.E., Zeldenrust, S.R., Dalton, R.J., Rajkumar, S.V. & Gertz, M.A. (2010). Diagnosis and management of Waldenström macroglobulinemia: Mayo stratification of macroglobulinemia and risk-adapted therapy (mSMART) guidelines. *Mayo Clinic Proceedings.*, Vol. 85, No.9, (September, 2010), pp. 824-33, ISSN 0025-6196

Aparicio, A., Gardner, A., Tu, Y., Savage, A., Berenson, J. & Lichtenstein, A. (1998). In vitro cytoreductive effects on multiple myeloma cells induced by bisphosphonates. *Leukemia.*, Vol. 12, No. 2, (February, 1998), pp. 220-229, ISSN 0887-6924

Ardeshna, K.M., Smith, P., Norton, A., Hancock, B.W., Hoskin, P.J., MacLennan, K.A., Marcus, R.E., Jelliffe, A., Vaughan, G., Hudson & Linch, D.C.; British National Lymphoma Investigation. (2003). Long-term effect of a watch and wait policy versus immediate systemic treatment for asymptomatic advanced-stage non-Hodgkin lymphoma: a randomised controlled trial. *Lancet,* Vol. 362, No. 9383, (August, 2003), pp. 516–522, ISSN 0140-6736

Ashfaq, K., Yahaya, I., Hyde, C., Andronis, L., Barton, P., Bayliss, S. & Chen, Y.F. (2010). Clinical effectiveness and cost-effectiveness of stem cell transplantation in the management of acute leukaemia: a systematic review. *Health Technology Assessment,.* Vol. 14, No. 54:iii-iv, ix-xi, pp. 1-141, ISSN 1366-5278

Aydin, S., Grabellus, F., Eisele, L., Möllmann, M., Hanoun, M., Ebeling, P., Moritz, T., Carpinteiro, A., Nückel, H., Sak, A., Göthert, J.R., Dührsen, U. & Dürig, J. (2011). Investigating the role of CD38 and functionally related molecular risk factors in the CLL NOD/SCID xenograft model. *European Journal of Haematology.*, Vol. 87, No. 1, (July, 2011), pp. 10-19:10-9. doi: 10.1111/j.1600-0609.2011.01626.x, ISSN 0902-4441

Bailey, H. D., Armstrong, B. K., De Klerk, N. H., Fritschi, L., Attia, J., Lockwood, L., Milne, E.; Aus-ALL Consortium. (2010). Exposure to diagnostic radiological procedures and the risk of childhood acute lymphoblastic leukemia. *Cancer Epidemiology Biomarkers and Prevention,* Vol. 19, No. 11, (November, 2010), pp. 2897–2909, ISSN 1055-9965

Barlogie, B., Shaughnessy, J., Munshi, N. & Epstein, J. (2001). Plasma cell myeloma. In: *Williams Hematology,* E. Beutler, M. Lichtman, B. Coller, T. Kipps, & U. Seligsohn, (Eds.; ed 6). New York: McGraw-Hill; pp. 1279-1304, ISBN 0-07-116293-3

Barth, R.N., Nam, A.J., Stanwix, M.G., Kukuruga, D., Drachenberg, C.I., Bluebond-Langner, R., Hui-Chou, H., Shipley, S.T., Bartlett, S.T. & Rodriguez, E.D. (2009). Prolonged survival of composite facial allografts in non-human primates associated with posttransplant lymphoproliferative disorder. *Transplantation.*, Vol. 88, No. 11, (December, 2009), pp. 1242-1250, ISSN 0041-1337

Benjamin, M., Reddy, S. & Brawley, O.W. (2003). Myeloma and race: a review of the literature. *Cancer Metastasis Reviews*, Vol. 22, No. 1, (March, 2003), pp. 87-93, ISSN 1573-7233

Bertilaccio, M.T., Scielzo, C., Simonetti, G., Ponzoni, M., Apollonio, B., Fazi, C., Scarfò, L., Rocchi, M., Muzio, M., Caligaris-Cappio, F. & Ghia, P. (2010). A novel Rag2-/-gammac-/--xenograft model of human CLL. *Blood.,* Vol. 115, No. 8, (February, 2010), pp. 1605-1609, ISSN 0006-4971

Bhatia, S., Ramsay, N.K., Steinbuch, M., Dusenbery, K.E., Shapiro, R.S., Weisdorf, D.J., Robison, L.L., Miller, J.S. & Neglia, J.P. (1996). Malignant neoplasms following bone marrow transplantation. *Blood,* Vol. 87, No. 9, (May, 1996), pp. 3633-3639, ISSN 0006-4971

Billadeau, D., Ahmann, G., Greipp, P. & Van Ness, B. (1993). The bone marrow of multiple myeloma patients contains B cell populations at different stages of differentiation that are clonally related to the malignant plasma cell. *Journal of Experimental Medicine,* Vol. 178, No. 3, (September, 1993), pp. 1023-1031, ISSN 0022-1007

Blattner, W.A., Garber, J.E., Mann, D.L., McKeen, E.A., Henson, R., McGuire, D.B., Fisher, W.B., Bauman, A.W., Goldin, L.R. & Fraumeni, Jr, J.F. (1980). Waldenstrom's macroglobulinemia and autoimmune disease in a family. *Annals of Internal Medicine,* Vol. 93, No. 6, (December, 1980), pp. 830–832, ISSN 0003-4819

Boulos, N., Mulder, H.L., Calabrese, C.R., Morrison, J.B., Rehg, J.E., Relling, M.V., Sherr, C.J., & Williams, R.T. (2011). Chemotherapeutic agents circumvent emergence of dasatinib-resistant BCR-ABL kinase mutations in a precise mouse model of Philadelphia chromosome-positive acute lymphoblastic leukemia. *Blood,* Vol. 117, No. 13, (March, 2011), pp. 3585-3595, ISSN 0006-4971

Boynton, E., Aubin, J., Gross, A., Hozumi, N. & Sandhu, J. (1996). Human osteoblasts survive and deposit new bone when human bone is implanted in SCID mouse. *Bone,* Vol. 18, No. 4, (April, 1996), pp. 321-326, ISSN 8756-3282

Brown, A.K., Elves, M.W., Gunson, H.H. & Pell-Ilderton, R. (1967). Waldenstroms macroglobulinaemia. A family study. *Acta Haematologica,* Vol. 38, No. 3, pp. 184–192, ISSN 0001-5792

Caligaris-Cappio, F. & Ghia, P. (2007). The normal counterpart to the chronic lymphocytic leukemia B cell. *Best Practice & Research: Clinical Haematology,* Vol. 20, No. 3 (September, 2007), pp. 385–397, ISSN 1521-6926

Cancer Research, U.K. (2010). Latest UK cancer incidence and mortality summary–numbers. Available from:
http://info. cancerresearchuk.org/cancerstats/incidence/index. htm

Carpenter, P.A., Appelbaum, F.R., Corey, L., Deeg, H.J., Doney, K., Gooley, T., Krueger, J., Martin, P., Pavlovic, S., Sanders, J., Slattery, J., Levitt, D., Storb, R., Woolfrey, A. & Anasetti, C. (2002). A humanized non-FcR–binding anti-CD3 antibody, visilizumab, for treatment of steroid-refractory acute graft-versus-host disease. *Blood,* Vol. 99, No. 8, (April, 2002), pp. 2712-2719, ISSN 0006-4971

Chen, S.S., Sherman, M.H., Hertlein, E., Johnson, A.J, Teitell, M.A., Byrd, J.C. & Plass, C. (2009). Epigenetic alterations in a murine model for chronic lymphocytic leukemia. *Cell Cycle.,* Vol. 8, No. 22, (November, 2009), pp. 3663-3667, ISSN 1538-4101

Cho, P.S., Mueller, N.J., Cameron, A.M., Cina, R.A., Coburn, R.C., Hettiaratchy, S., Melendy, E., Neville, D.M. Jr, Patience, C., Fishman, J.A., Sachs, D.H. & Huang, C.A. (2004).

Risk factors for the development of post-transplant lymphoproliferative disorder in a large animal model. *American Journal of Transplantation*, Vol. 4, No. 8, (August, 2004), pp. 1274-1282, ISSN 1600-6135

Cohen, J.I. (1991). Epstein-Barr virus lymphoproliferative disease associated with acquired immunodeficiency. *Medicine (Baltimore)*, Vol. 70, No. 2, (March, 1991), pp. 137-160, ISSN 0025-7974

Corradini, P., Boccadoro, M., Voena, C. & Pileri, A. (1993). Evidence for a bone marrow B cell transcribing malignant plasma cell VDJ joined to C mu sequence in immunoglobulin (IgG)- and IgA secreting multiple myelomas. *Journal of Experimental Medicine*, Vol. 178, No. 3, (September, 1993), pp. 1091-1096, ISSN 0022-1007

Curtis, R.E., Travis, L.B., Rowlings, P.A., Socié, G., Kingma, D.W., Banks, P.M., Jaffe, E.S., Sale, G.E., Horowitz, M.M., Witherspoon, R.P., Shriner, D.A., Weisdorf, D.J., Kolb, H.J., Sullivan, K.M., Sobocinski, K.A., Gale, R.P., Hoover, R.N., Fraumeni, J.F. Jr, & Deeg, H.J. (1999). Risk of lymphoproliferative disorders after bone marrow transplantation: a multi-institutional study. *Blood*, Vol. 94, No. 7, (October, 1999), pp. 2208-2216, ISSN 0006-4971

D'Amato, R.J., Loughnan, M.S., Flynn, E. & Folkman, J. (1994). Thalidomide is an inhibitor of angiogenesis. *Proceedings of the National Academy of Sciences U S A*, Vol. 91, No. 9, (April, 1994), pp. 4082-4085, ISSN 0027-8424

Dang, A.M., Phillips, J.A., Lin, T. & Raveche, E.S. (1996). Altered CD45 expression in malignant B-1 cells. *Cellular Immunology*, Vol. 169, No. 2, (May, 1996), pp. 196–207, ISSN 0008-8749

Deeg, H.J. & Socié, G. (1998). Malignancies after hematopoietic stem cell transplantation: Many questions, some answers. *Blood*, Vol. 91, No. 6, (March, 1998), pp. 1833-1844, ISSN 0006-4971

Dimopoulos, M.A., Galani, E. & Matsouka, C. (1999). Waldenström's macroglobulinemia. *Hematology/Oncology Clinics of North America*, Vol. 13, No. 6, (December, 1999), pp. 1351-1366, ISSN 0889-8588

Dimopoulos, M.A., Panayiotidis, P., Moulopoulos, L.A., Sfikakis, P. & Dalakas, M. (2000). Waldenström's macroglobulinemia: clinical features, complications, and management. *Journal of Clinical Oncology*, Vol. 18, No. 1, (January, 2000), pp. 214-226, ISSN 0732-183X

Dimopoulos, M.A., Kyle, R.A., Anagnostopoulos, A. & Treon, S.P. (2005). Diagnosis and management of Waldenström's macroglobulinemia. *Journal of Clinical Onco*logy, Vol. 23, No. 7, (March, 2005), pp. 1564-1577, ISSN 0732-183X

Dimopoulos, M.A., Gertz, M.A., Kastritis, E., Garcia-Sanz, R., Kimby, E.K., Leblond, V., Fermand, J.P., Merlini. G., Morel, P., Morra, E., Ocio, E.M., Owen, R., Ghobrial, I.M., Seymour, J., Kyle, R.A. & Treon, S.P. (2009). Update on treatment recommendations from the Fourth International Workshop on Waldenström's Macroglobulinemia. *Journal of Clinical Oncology*, Vol. 27, No. 1, (January, 2009), pp. 120-126, ISSN 0732-183X

Ditzel Santos, D., Ho, A.W., Tournilhac, O., Hatjiharissi, E., Leleu, X., Xu, L., Tassone, P., Neri, P., Hunter, Z.R., Chemaly, M.A., Branagan, A.R., Manning, R.J., Patterson, C.J., Moreau, A.S., Ciccarelli, B., Adamia, S., Kriangkum, J., Kutok, J.L., Tai, Y.T., Zhang, J., Pilarski, L.M., Anderson, K.C., Munshi, N., Treon, S.P. (2007).

Establishment of BCWM.1 cell line for Waldenström's macroglobulinemia with productive in vivo engraftment in SCID-hu mice. *Experimental Hematology.*, Vol. 35, No. 9, (September, 2007), pp. 1366-1375, ISSN 0301-472X

Dohner, H., Stilgenbauer, S., Benner, A., Leupolt, E., Kröber, A., Bullinger, L., Döhner, K., Bentz, M. & Lichter, P. (2000). Genomic aberrations and survival in chronic lymphocytic leukemia. *New England Journal of Medicine,* Vol. 343, No. 26, (December, 2000), pp. 1910-1916, ISSN 0028-4793

Dor, F.J., Doucette, K.E., Mueller, N.J., Wilkinson, R.A., Bajwa, J.A., McMorrow, I.M., Tseng, Y.L., Kuwaki, K., Houser, S.L., Fishman, J.A., Cooper, D.K., Huang, C.A. (2004). Posttransplant lymphoproliferative disease after allogeneic transplantation of the spleen in miniature swine. *Transplantation,* Vol. 78, No. 2, (July, 2004), pp: 286-291, ISSN 0041-1337

Dores, G.M., Anderson, W.F., Curtis, R.E., Landgren, O., Ostroumova, E., Bluhm, E.C., Rabkin, C.S., Devesa, S.S. & Linet, M.S. (2007). Chronic lymphocytic leukaemia and small lymphocytic lymphoma: Overview of the descriptive epidemiology. *British Journal of Haematology,* Vol.139, No. 5, (December, 2007), pp. 809–819, ISSN 0007-1048

de Jong, D. & Janz, S. (2010). Anaplastic plasmacytoma of mouse--establishing parallels between subtypes of mouse and human plasma cell neoplasia. *Journal of Pathology,* Vol. 221, No. 3, (July, 2010), pp. 242-247, ISSN 1096-9896

Doucette, K., Dor, F.J., Wilkinson R.A., Martin, S.I., Huang, C.A., Cooper, D.K., Sachs, D.H. & Fishman, J.A. (2007). Gene expression of porcine lymphotrophic herpesvirus-1 in miniature Swine with posttransplant lymphoproliferative disorder. *Transplantation.,* Vol. 83, No. 1, (January, 2007), pp. 87-90, ISSN 0041-1337

Drexler, H.G. & MacLeod, R.A. (2008). Malignant hematopoietic cell lines: in vitro models for the study of Waldenström's macroglobulinemia. *Leukemia Research.,* Vol. 32, No. 11, (November, 2008), pp. 1669-1673, ISSN 0887-6924

Eden, T. (2010). Aetiology of childhood leukaemia, *Cancer Treatment Reviews,* Vol. 36, No. 4, (June, 2010), pp. 286–297, ISSN 0305-7372

Elves, M.W. & Brown, A.K. (1968). Cytogenetic studies in a family with Waldenstrom's macroglobulinaemia. *Journal of Medical Genetics,* Vol. 5, No. 2, (June, 1968), pp. 118–122, ISSN 0022-2593

Engholm, G., Ferlay, J., Christensen, N, Bray, F., Gjerstorff, M.L., Klint, A., Kotlum, J.E., Olafsdottir, E., Pukkala, E. & Storm, H.H. (2010). NORDCAN—Cancer Incidence, Mortality, Prevalence and Prediction in the Nordic Countries, version 3.6. Association of the Nordic Cancer Registries. Danish Cancer Society. Available from: http://www.ancr.nu

Feo-Zuppardi, F.J., Taylor, C.W., Iwato, K., Lopez, M.H., Grogan, T.M., Odeleye, A., Hersh, E.M. & Salmon, S.E. (1992). Long-term engraftment of fresh human myeloma cells in SCID mice. *Blood,* Vol. 80, No. 11, (December, 1992), pp. 2843-2850, ISSN 0006-4971

Ferlay, J., Autier, P., Boniol, M., Heanue, M., Colombet, M. & Boyle, P. (2007). Estimates of the cancer incidence and mortality in Europe in 2006. *Annals in Oncology,* Vol. 18, No. 3, (March, 2007), pp. 581-592, ISSN 0923-7534

Fisher, R.I., LeBlanc, M., Press, O.W., Maloney, D.G., Unger, J.M. & Miller, T.P. (2005). New treatment options have changed the survival of patients with follicular lymphoma.

Journal of Clinical Oncology, Vol. 23, No. 33 (November, 2005), pp. 8447–8452, ISSN 0732-183X

Fonseca, R. & Hayman, S. (2007). Waldenström macroglobulinaemia. *British Journal of Haematology.*, Vol. 138, No. 6 (September, 2007), pp. 700-720, ISSN 0007-1048

Fonseca, R., Barlogie, B., Bataille, R., Bastard, C., Bergsagel, P.L., Chesi, M., Davies, F.E., Drach. J., Greipp, P.R., Kirsch, I.R., Kuehl, W.M., Hernandez, J.M., Minvielle, S., Pilarski, L.M., Shaughnessy, J.D. Jr, Stewart A.K. & Avet-Loiseau, H. (2004). Genetics and cytogenetics of multiple myeloma: a workshop report. *Cancer Research,* Vol. 64, No. 4, (February, 2004), pp.1546-1558, ISSN 0008-5472

Fowler, J.A., Mundy, G.R., Lwin, S.T., Lynch, C.C. & Edwards, C.M. (2009). A murine model of myeloma that allows genetic manipulation of the host microenvironment. *Disease Models & Mechanisms.,* (Vol. 2), No. 11-12, (Nov-Dec, 2009), pp. 604-611, ISSN 1754-8403

Friedberg, J.W., Taylor, M.D., Cerhan, J.R., Flowers, C.R., Dillon, H., Farber, C.M., Rogers, E.S., Hainsworth, J.D., Wong, E.K., Vose, J.M., Zelenetz, A.D. & Link, B.K. (2009). Follicular lymphoma in the United States: first report of the national LymphoCare study. *Journal of Clinical Oncology,* Vol. 27, No. 8, (March, 2009), pp. 1202–1208, ISSN 0732-183X

Garrett, I.R., Dallas, S., Radl, J., & Mundy, G. R. (1997). A murine model of human myeloma bone disease. *Bone.,* Vol. 20, No. 6, (June, 1997), pp. 515-520, ISSN 8756-3282

Gaurnier-Hausser, A., Patel, R., Baldwin, A.S., May, M.J. & Mason, N.J. (2011). NEMO-binding domain peptide inhibits constitutive NF-κB activity and reduces tumor burden in a canine model of relapsed, refractory diffuse large B-cell lymphoma. *Clinical Cancer Research.,* Vol. 17, No. 14, (July, 2011), pp. 4661-4671, ISSN 1078-0432

Gertz, M.A., Anagnostopoulos, A., Anderson, K., Branagan, A.R., Coleman, M., Frankel, S.R., Giralt, S., Levine, T., Munshi, N., Pestronk, A., Rajkumar, V. & Treon, S.P. (2003). Treatment recommendations in Waldenstrom's macroglobulinemia: consensus panel recommendations from the Second International Workshop on Waldenström's Macroglobulinemia. *Seminars in Oncology,* Vol. 30, No. 2, (April, 2003), pp. 121-126, ISSN 0093-7754

Getaz, E.P. & Staples, W.G. (1977). Familial Waldenstrom's macroglobulinaemia: a case report. *South African Medical Journal,* Vol. 51, No. 24, (June, 1977), pp. 891–892, ISSN 0038-2469

Ghia, P., Scielzo, C., Frenquelli, M., Muzio, M., & Caligaris-Cappio, F. (2007). From normal to clonal B cells: Chronic lymphocytic leukemia (CLL) at the crossroad between neoplasia and autoimmunity. *Autoimmunity Reviews,* Vol. 7, No. 2, (December, 2007), pp. 127–131, ISSN 1568-9972

Goedert, J.J., Cote, T.R., Virgo, P., Scoppa, S.M., Kingma, D.W., Gail. M.H., Jaffe, E.S. & Biggar. R.J. (1998). Spectrum of AIDS-associated malignant disorders. *Lancet,* Vol. 351, No. 9119, (June, 1998), pp. 1833-1839, ISSN 0140-6736

Greaves, M. (2002). Science, medicine, and the future: childhood leukaemia. *British Medical Journal,* Vol. 324, No. 7332, pp. 283–287, ISSN 0959-8138

Groves, F.D., Travis, L.B., Devesa, S.S., Ries, L.A. & Fraumeni, J.F. Jr. (1998). Waldenström's macroglobulinemia: incidence patterns in the United States, 1988-1994. *Cancer,* Vol. 82, No. 6, (March, 1998), pp. 1078-1081, ISSN 0008-543X

Gurney, J.G., Davis, S., Severson, R.K., Fang, J.Y., Ross, J.A. & Robison, L.L. (1996). Trends in cancer incidence among children in the U.S. *Cancer*, Vol. 78, No. 3, (August, 1996), pp. 532-541, ISSN 0008-543X

Gustafsson, A., Levitsky, V., Zou, J.Z., Frisan, T., Dalianis, T., Ljungman, P., Ringden, O., Winiarski, J., Ernberg, I., & Masucci, M.G. (2000). Epstein-Barr virus (EBV) load in bone marrow transplant recipients at risk to develop posttransplant lymphoproliferative disease: prophylactic infusion of EBV-specific cytotoxic T cells. *Blood*, Vol. 95, No. 3, (February, 2000), pp. 807-814, ISSN 0006-4971

Hallek, M., Langenmayer, I., Nerl, C., Knauf, W., Dietzfelbinger, H., Adorf, D., Ostwald, M., Busch, R., Kuhn-Hallek, I., Thiel, E. & Emmerich, B. (1999). Elevated serum thymidine kinase levels identify a subgroup at high risk of disease progression in early, nonsmoldering chronic lymphocytic leukemia. *Blood*, Vol. 93, No. 5, (March, 1999), pp.1732-1737, ISSN 0006-4971

Harousseau, J.L., Shaughnessy, J.Jr & Richardson, P. (2004). Multiple myeloma. *Hematology, American Society of Hematology Educational Program*, pp. 237-256, ISSN 1520-4391

Harris, N.L., Jaffe, E.S., Stein, H., Banks, P.M., Chan, J.K., Cleary, M.L., Delsol, G., De Wolf-Peeters, C., Falini, B. & Gatter, K.C. (1994). A revised European-American classification of lymphoid neoplasms: a proposal from the International Lymphoma Study Group [see comments; Review; 296 refs]. *Blood*, Vol. 84, No. 5, (September, 1994), pp. 1361-1392, ISSN 0006-4971

Herrinton, L.J. & Weiss, N.S. (1993). Incidence of Waldenström's macroglobulinemia. *Blood*, Vol. 82, No. 10, (November, 1993), pp. 3148-3150, ISSN 0006-4971

Heslop, H.E., Ng, C.Y.C., Li, C., Smith, C.A., Loftin, S.K., Krance, R.A., Brenner, M.K. & Rooney, C.M. (1996). Long-term restoration of immunity against Epstein-Barr virus infection by adoptive transfer of gene-modified virus- specific T lymphocytes. *Nature Medicine*, Vol. 2, No. 5, (May, 1996), pp. 551-555, ISSN 1078-8956

Hodge, L.S., Novak, A.J., Grote, D.M., Braggio, E., Ketterling, R.P., Manske, M.K., Price Troska, T.L., Ziesmer, S.C., Fonseca, R., Witzig, T.E., Morice, W.G., Gertz, M.A. & Ansell, S.M. (2011). Establishment and characterization of a novel Waldenstrom macroglobulinemia cell line, MWCL-1. *Blood.*, Vol. 117, No. 19, (May, 2011), e190-197, ISSN 0006-4971

Hofbauer, J.P., Heyder, C., Denk, U., Kocher, T., Holler, C., Trapin, D., Asslaber, D., Tinhofer, I., Greil, R. & Egle, A. (2011). Development of CLL in the TCL1 transgenic mouse model is associated with severe skewing of the T-cell compartment homologous to human CLL. *Leukemia*, Vol. 25, No. 9, (September, 2011):1452-1458. doi: 10.1038/leu.2011.111. Epub 2011 May 24, ISSN 0887-6924

Hoover, R.N. (1992). Lymphoma risks in populations with altered immunity—A search for mechanism. *Cancer Research*, Vol. 52, No. suppl. 19, (October, 1992), pp. 5477s-5478s, ISSN 0008-5472

Horner, M.J., Ries, L.A.G., Krapcho, M., Neyman, N., Aminou, R., Howlader, N., Altekruse, S.F., Feuer, E. J., Huang, L., Mariotto, A., Miller, B. A., Lewis, D.R., Eisner, M.P., Stinchcomb, D.G. & Edwards, B.K. (Ed.); (2009). In: *SEER Cancer Statistics Review 1975–2006*. Bethesda, MD: National Cancer Institute; Available from http://seer.cancer.gov/csr/1975_2006/ (based on November 2008 SEER data submission, posted to the SEER web site, 2009)

Horning, S.J. (1993). Natural history of and therapy for the indolent non-Hodgkin's lymphomas. *Seminars in Oncology*, Vol. 20, No. 5, Suppl. 5, (October, 1993), pp. 75–88, ISSN 0093-7754

Howlader, N., Noone, A.M., Krapcho, M., Neyman, N., Aminou, R., Waldron, W., Altekruse, S.F., Kosary, C.L., Ruhl, J., Tatalovich, Z., Cho, H., Mariotto, A., Eisner, M.P., Lewis, D.R., Chen, H.S., Feuer, E.J., Cronin, K.A. & Edwards, B.K. (2010). In: *SEER Cancer Statistics Review, 1975–2008,* National Cancer Institute, Bethesda, MD. Available from: http://seer.cancer.gov/csr/1975_2008/

Huang, Y.W., Richardson, J.A., Tong, A.W., Zhang, B.Q., Stone, M.J. & Vitetta, E.S. (1993). Disseminated growth of a human multiple myeloma cell line in mice with severe combined immunodeficiency disease. *Cancer Research,* Vol. 53, No. 6, (March, 1993), pp. 1392-1396, ISSN 0008-5472

Jemal, A., Siegel, R., Xu, J. & Ward, E. (2010). Cancer statistics, 2010. *CA: A Cancer Journal for Clinicians,* Vol. 60, No. 5, pp. 277-300, ISSN 0007-9235

Johnson, P.W., Rohatiner, A.Z., Whelan, J.S., Price, C.G., Love, S., Lim, J., Matthews, J., Norton, A.J., Amess, J.A. & Lister, T.A. (1995). Patterns of survival in patients with recurrent follicular lymphoma: a 20-year study from a single center. *Journal of Clinical Oncology,* Vol. 13, No. 1, (January, 1995), pp. 140–147. ISSN 0732-183X

Kamel-Reid, S., Letarte, M., Sirard, C., Doedens, M., Grunberger, T., Fulop, G., Freedman, M.H., Phillips, R.A. & Dick, J.E. (1989). A model of human acute lymphoblastic leukemia in immune-deficient SCID mice. *Science,* Vol. 246, No. 4937, (December, 1989), pp. 1597-1600, ISSN 0036-8075

Kinlen, L.J. (1996). Immunologic factors, including AIDS, In: *Cancer Epidemiology and Prevention,* D. Schottenfeld & J.F. Fraumeni Jr, (Eds): (Ed 2), pp. 532-545, ISBN 978-0-19-514961-6, Oxford University Press, New York, NY, USA

Kuehl, W.M. & Bergsagel, P.L. (2002). Multiple myeloma: evolving genetic events and host interactions. *Nature Reviews Cancer,* Vol. 2, No. 3, (March, 2002), pp. 175-187, ISSN 1474-175X

Kuehnle, I., Huls, M.H., Liu, Z., Semmelmann, M., Krance, R.A., Brenner, M.K., Rooney, C.M. & Heslop, H.E. (2000). CD20 monoclonal antibody (rituximab) for therapy of Epstein-Barr virus lymphoma after hemopoietic stem-cell transplantation. *Blood,* Vol. 95, No. 4, (February, 2000), pp. 1502-1505, ISSN 0006-4971

Kyle, R.A., Therneau, T.M., Rajkumar, S.V., Offord, J.R., Larson, D.R., Plevak, M.F. & Melton, III, L.J. (2002). A long-term study of prognosis in monoclonal gammopathy of undetermined significance. *New England Journal of Medicine,* Vol. 346, No. 8, (February, 2002), pp. 564–569, ISSN 0028-4793

Kyle, R.A. & Rajkumar, S.V. (2004). Multiple myeloma. *New England Journal of Medicine,* Vol. 351, No. 18, (October, 2004), pp. 1860–1873, ISSN 0028-4793

Lanasa, M.C., Allgood, S.D., Volkheimer, A.D., Gockerman, J.P., Whitesides, J.F., Goodman, B.K., Moore, J.O., Weinberg, J.B. & Levesque, M.C. (2010). Single-cell analysis reveals oligoclonality among 'low-count' monoclonal B-cell lymphocytosis. *Leukemia,* Vol. 24, No. 1, (January, 2010), pp. 133–140, ISSN 0887-6924

Langenau, D.M., Traver, D., Ferrando, A.A., Kutok, J.L., Aster, J.C., Kanki, J.P., Lin, S., Prochownik, E., Trede, N.S., Zon, L.I. & Look, A.T. (2003). Myc-induced T cell leukemia in transgenic zebrafish. *Science.,* Vol. 299, No. 5608, (February, 2003), pp. 887-890, ISSN 0036-8075

Lichtman, M.A. & Liesveld, J.L. (2001). Acute Myelogenous Leukemia. In: *Williams Hematology,* E. Beutler, M. Lichtman, B. Coller, T. Kipps, & U. Seligsohn, (Eds.; ed 6), pp. 1047-1083, McGraw-Hill, ISBN 0-07-116293-3, New York, NY, USA

Linet, M.S., Humphrey, R.L., Mehl, E.S., Brown, L.M., Pottern, L.M., Bias, W.B. & McCaffrey, L. (1993). A case-control and family study of Waldenstrom's macroglobulinemia. *Leukemia,* Vol. 7, No. 9 (September, 1993), pp. 1363–1369, ISSN 0887-6924

Linet, M.S., Devesa, S.S. & Morgan, G.J. (2006). The leukemias, In: *Cancer Epidemiology and Prevention. 3rd edition,* D. Schottenfeld, & J.F. Fraumeni, (Ed.), 841-871, Oxford University Press, ISBN 978-0-19-514961-6, New York, USA

Liu, Q., Fayad, L., Cabanillas, F., Hagemeister, F.B., Ayers, G.D., Hess, M., Romaguera, J., Rodriguez, M.A., Tsimberidou, A.M., Verstovsek, S., Younes, A., Pro, B., Lee, M,S., Ayala, A., McLaughlin, P. (2006). Improvement of Overall and Failure-Free Survival in Stage IV Follicular Lymphoma: 25 Years of Treatment Experience at The University of Texas M.D. Anderson Cancer Center. *Journal of Clinical Oncology,* Vol. 24, No. 10, (April, 2006), pp. 1582–1589, ISSN 0732-183X

Liu, R., Zhang, L., McHale, C.M. & Hammond, S.K. (2011). Paternal smoking and risk of childhood acute lymphoblastic leukemia: systematic review and meta-analysis. *Journal of Oncology,* 2011:854584. Epub 2011 May, 29, doi:10.1155/2011/854584, ISSN 1687-8450

Lock, R.B., Liem, N., Farnsworth, M.L., Milross, C.G., Xue, C., Tajbakhsh, M., Haber, M., Norris, M.D., Marshall, G.M. & Rice, A.M. (2002). The nonobese diabetic/severe combined immunodeficient (NOD/SCID) mouse model of childhood acute lymphoblastic leukemia reveals intrinsic differences in biologic characteristics at diagnosis and relapse. *Blood,* Vol. 99, No. 11, (June, 2002), pp. 4100-4108, ISSN 0006-4971

Macor, P., Secco, E., Zorzet, S., Tripodo, C., Celeghini, C. & Tedesco, F. (2008). An update on the xenograft and mouse models suitable for investigating new therapeutic compounds for the treatment of B-cell malignancies. *Current Pharmaceutical Design,* Vol. 14, No. 21, pp. 2023-2039, ISSN 1381-6128

Marcus, R., Imrie, K., Belch, A., Cunningham, D., Flores, E., Catalano, J., Solal-Celigny, P., Offner, F., Walewski, J., Raposo, J., Jack, A. & Smith P. (2005). CVP chemotherapy plus rituximab compared with CVP as firstline treatment for advanced follicular lymphoma. *Blood,* Vol. 105, No. 4, (February, 2005), pp. 1417–1423, ISSN 0006-4971

McMaster, M.L., Giambarresi, T., Vasquez, L., Goldstein, A.M. & Tucker, M.A. (2005). Cytogenetics of familial Waldenstrom's macroglobulinemia: in pursuit of an understanding of genetic predisposition. *Clinical Lymphoma,* Vol. 5, No. 4, (March, 2005), pp. 230–234, ISSN 1526-9655

McMaster, M.L., Goldin, L.R., Bai, Y., Ter-Minassian, M., Boehringer, S., Giambarresi, T.R., Vasquez, L.G. & Tucker, M.A. (2006). Genomewide linkage screen for Waldenstrom macroglobulinemia susceptibility loci in high-risk families. *American Journal of Human Genetics,* Vol. 79, No. 4 (October, 2006), pp. 695-701, ISSN 0002-9297

Medyouf, H., Gao, X., Armstrong, F., Gusscott, S., Liu, Q., Gedman, A.L., Matherly, L.H., Schultz, K.R., Pflumio, F., You, M.J. & Weng, A.P. (2010). Acute T-cell leukemias remain dependent on Notch signaling despite PTEN and INK4A/ARF loss. *Blood.,* Vol. 115, No. 6, (February, 2010), pp. 1175-1184, ISSN 0006-4971

Montoto, S., López-Guillermo, A., Ferrer, A., Camós, M., Alvarez-Larrán, A., Bosch, F., Bladé, J., Cervantes, F., Esteve, J., Cobo, F., Colomer, D., Campo, E. & Montserrat, E. (2002). Survival after progression in patients with follicular lymphoma: analysis of prognostic factors. *Annals of Oncology,* Vol. 13, No. 4, pp. 523–530, ISSN 0923-7534

Mukherjee, M., Ge, G., Zhang, N., Huang, E., Nakamura, L.V., Minor, M., Fofanov, V., Rao, P.H., Herron, A. & Pati, D. (2011). Separase loss of function cooperates with the loss of p53 in the initiation and progression of T- and B-cell lymphoma, leukemia and aneuploidy in mice. *PLoS One.,* Vol. 6, No. 7:e22167. Epub 2011 Jul 25, ISSN 1932-6203

National Cancer Institute (2009). General information about adult non-Hodgkin's lymphoma, Available from: http://www.cancer.gov.libproxy.lib.unc.edu/cancertopics/pdq/treatment/adult-non-Hodgkins

Newell, K.A., Alonso, E.M., Whitington, P.F., Bruce, D.S., Millis, J.M., Piper, J.B., Woodle, E.S., Kelly, S.M., Koeppen, H., Hart, J., Rubin, C.M. & Thistlethwaite, J.R. Jr. (1996). Posttransplant lymphoproliferative disease in pediatric liver transplantation. Interplay between primary Epstein-Barr virus infection and immunosuppression. *Transplantation,* Vol. 62, No. 3, (August, 1996), pp. 370-375, ISSN 0041-1337

Nijmeijer, B.A., Mollevanger, P., van Zelderen-Bhola, S.L., Kluin-Nelemans, H.C., Willemze, R. & Falkenburg, J.H. (2001). Monitoring of engraftment and progression of acute lymphoblastic leukemia in individual NOD/SCID mice. *Experimental Hematology,* Vol. 29, No. 3, (March, 2001), pp. 322-329, ISSN 0301-472X

Ohyashiki, J.H., Ohyashiki, K., Iwama, H., Hayashi, S., Toyama, K. & Shay, J.W. (1997). Clinical implications of telomerase activity levels in acute leukemia. *Clinical Cancer Research,* Vol. 3, No. 4, (April, 1997), pp. 619-625, ISSN 0008-5472

Ogmundsdottir, H.M., Sveinsdottir, S., Sigfusson, A., Skaftadottir, I., Jonasson, J.G. & Agnarsson, B.A. (1999). Enhanced B cell survival in familial macroglobulinaemia is associated with increased expression of Bcl-2. *Clinical & Experimental Immunology,* Vol. 117, No. 2, (August, 1999), pp. 252–260, ISSN 0009-9104

Opelz, G. & Henderson, R (1993). Incidence of non-Hodgkin's lymphoma in kidney and heart transplant recipients. *Lancet,* Vol. 342, No. 8886-8887, (December, 1993), pp. 1514-1516, ISSN 0140-6736

Orazi, A., Hromas, R.A., Neiman, R.S., Greiner, T.C., Lee, C.H., Rubin, L., Haskins, S., Heerema, N.A., Gharpure, V., Abonour, R. Srour, E.F., & Cornetta, K. (1997). Posttransplantation lymphoproliferative disorders in bone marrow transplant recipients are aggressive diseases with a high incidence of adverse histologic and immunobiologic features. *American Journal of Clinical Pathology,* Vol. 107, No. 4, (April, 1997), pp. 419-429, ISSN 0002-9173

O'Reilly, R.J., Lacerda, J.F., Lucas, K.G., Rosenfield, N.S., Small, T.N. & Papadopoulos, E.B. (1996). Adoptive cell therapy with donor lymphocytes for EBV-associated lymphomas developing after allogeneic marrow transplants. In: *Important Advances in Oncology,* T.D. De Vita, S. Helman & S.A. Rosenberg (Eds), pp. 149-166, Lippincott-Raven, ISBN 0-7020-1546-6, Philadelphia, PA, USA

Owen, R.G., Treon, S.P., Al-Katib, A., Fonseca, R., Greipp, P.R., McMaster, M.L., Morra, E., Pangalis, G.A., San Miguel, J.F., Branagan, A.R., & Dimopoulos, M.A. (2003). Clinicopathological definition of Waldenstrom's macroglobulinemia: consensus panel recommendations from the Second International Workshop on Waldenström's Macroglobulinemia. *Seminars in Oncology,* Vol. 30, No. 2, (April, 2003), pp. 110-115, ISSN 0093-7754

Park, S.S., Kim, J.S., Tessarollo, L., Owens, J.D., Peng, L., Han, S.S., Tae, Chung, S., Torrey, T.A., Cheung, W.C., Polakiewicz, R.D., McNeil, N., Ried, T., Mushinski, J.F., Morse, H.C. 3rd & Janz, S. (2005). Insertion of c-Myc into Igh induces B-cell and plasma-cell neoplasms in mice. *Cancer Research,* Vol. 65, No. 4 (February, 2005), pp. 1306-1315, ISSN 0008-5472

Petrelli, N.J., Winer, E.P., Brahmer, J., Dubey, S., Smith, S., Thomas, C., Vahdat, L.T., Obel, J., Vogelzang, N., Markman, M., Sweetenham, J.W., Pfister, D., Kris, M.G., Schuchter, L.M., Sawaya, R., Raghavan, D., Ganz, P.A. & Kramer, B. (2009). Clinical Cancer Advances 2009: major research advances in cancer treatment, prevention, and screening–a report from the American Society of Clinical Oncology. *Journal of Clinical Oncology,* Vol. 27, No. 35, (December, 2009), pp. 6052–6069, ISSN 0732-183X

Phillips, J.A., Mehta, K., Fernandez, C. & Raveche, E.S. (1992). The NZB mouse as a model for chronic lymphocytic leukemia. *Cancer Research,* Vol. 52, No. 2, (January, 1992), pp. 437–443, ISSN 0008-5472

Potter, M. (1982). Pathogenesis of plasmacytomas in mice, In: *Cancer: A Comprehensive Treatise,* F. F. Becker, (Ed.), 139, Plenum, New York, NY, USA

Pui, C.-H. (2001). Acute Lymphoblastic Leukemia. In: *Williams Hematology,* E. Beutler, M. Lichtman, B. Coller, T. Kipps, & U. Seligsohn, (Eds.; ed 6), McGraw-Hill; pp. 1141-1161, ISBN 0-07-116293-3, New York, USA

Pui, C. & Evans, W.E. (2006). Treatment of acute lymphoblastic leukemia. *New England Journal of Medicine,* Vol. 354, No. 2, (January, 2006), pp. 166-178, ISSN 0028-4793

Pui, C., Campana, D., Pei, D., Bowman, W.P., Sandlund, J.T., Kaste, S.C., Ribeiro, R.C., Rubnitz, J.E., Raimondi, S.C. Onciu, M., Coustan-Smith, E., Kun, L.E., Jeha, S., Cheng, C., Howard, S.C., Simmons, V., Bayles, A., Metzger, M.L., Boyett, J.M., Leung, W., Handgretinger, R., Downing, J.R., Evans, W.E. & Relling, M.V. (2009). Treating childhood acute lymphoblastic leukemia without cranial irradiation. *New England Journal of Medicine,* Vol. 360, No. 26, (January, 2009), pp. 2730-2741, ISNN 0028-4793

Pulte, D., Gondos, A. & Brenner, H. (2008). Ongoing improvement in outcomes for patients diagnosed as having Non-Hodgkin lymphoma from the 1990s to the early 21st century. *Archives of Internal Medicine,* Vol. 168, No. 5, (March, 2008), pp. 469–476, ISSN 0003-9926

Radl, J., De Glopper, E.D., Schuit, H.R., & Zurcher, C. (1979). Idiopathic paraproteinemia. II. Transplantation of the paraprotein-producing clone from old to young C57BL/KaLwRij mice. *Journal of Immunology,* Vol. 122, No. 2, (February, 1979), pp. 609-613, ISSN 0022-1767

Radl, J. (1981). Animal model of human disease. Benign monoclonal gammopathy (idiopathic paraproteinemia). *American Journal of Pathology,* Vol. 105, No. 1, (October, 1981), pp. 91-93, ISSN 0002-9440

Radl, J., Croese, J.W., Zurcher, C. Van den Enden-Vieveen, M. H. & de Leeuw, A. M. (1988). Animal model of human disease. Multiple myeloma. *American Journal of Pathology,* Vol. 132, No. 3, (September, 1988), pp. 593-597, ISSN 0002-9440

Radl, J. (1991). Four major mechanisms in the development of monoclonal gammopathies. Postulations and facts, *Proceedings of the Third EURAGE Symposium on Monoclonal Gammopathies: Clinical Significance and Basic Mechanisms,* pp. 5, ISBN 907-1021-14-9, Brussels, Belgium, September 18-20, 1991

Ramachandra, S., Metcalf, R.A., Fredrickson, T., Marti, G.E. & Raveche, E. (1996). Requirement for increased IL-10 in the development of B-1 lymphoproliferative disease in a murine model of CLL. *Journal of Clinical Investigation,* Vol. 98, No. 8, (October, 1996), pp. 1788–1793, ISSN 0021-9738

Redaelli, A., Laskin, B.L., Stephens, J.M., Botteman, M.F. & Pashos, C.L. (2004). The clinical and epidemiological burden of chronic lymphocytic leukaemia. *European Journal of Cancer Care (Engl),* Vol.13, No, 3, (July, 2004), pp. 279–287, ISSN 0961-5423

Renier, G., Ifrah, N., Chevailler, A., Saint-Andre, J.P., Boasson, M. & Hurez, D. (1989). Four brothers with Waldenstrom's macroglobulinemia. *Cancer,* Vol. 64, No. 7, (October, 1989), pp. 1554–1559, ISSN 0008-543X

Rooney, C.M., Smith, C.A., Ng, C.Y.C., Loftin, S.K., Sixbey, J.W., Gan, Y., Srivastava, D.K., Bowman, L.C., Krance, R.A., Brenner, M.K. & Heslop, H.E. (1998). Infusion of cytotoxic T cells for the prevention and treatment of Epstein-Barr virus–induced lymphoma in allogeneic transplant recipients. *Blood,* Vol. 92, No. 5, (September, 1998), pp. 1549-1555, ISSN 0006-4971

Rozman, C. & Montserrat, E. (1995). Chronic lymphocytic leukemia. *New England Journal of Medicine,* Vol. 333, No. 16, (October, 1995), pp.1052-1057, ISSN 0028 4793

Ruiz-Arguelles, G.J., Ramirez-Cisneros, F.J., Flores-Martinez, J. & Cernuda-Graham, M.C. (2000). Waldenstrom's macroglobulinemia is infrequent in Mexican Mestizos: experience of a hematological diseases referral center. Revista de Investigación Clínica, Vol. 52, No. 5, (September, 2000), pp. 497–499, ISSN 0034-8376

Salerno, E., Yuan, Y., Scaglione, B.J., Marti, G., Jankovic, A., Mazzella, F., Laurindo, M.F., Despres, D., Baskar, S., Rader, C. & Raveche, E. (2010). The New Zealand black mouse as a model for the development and progression of chronic lymphocytic leukemia. *Cytometry Part B Clinical Cytometry,* Vol. 78, No. Suppl 1, pp. S98-109, ISSN 1552-4949

Samuels, A.L., Peeva, V.K., Papa, R.A., Firth, M.J., Francis, R.W., Beesley, A.H., Lock, R.B. & Kees U.R. (2010). Validation of a mouse xenograft model system for gene expression analysis of human acute lymphoblastic leukaemia. *BMC Genomics.,* Vol. 21, No. 11 (April, 2010), pp. 256, ISSN 1471-2164

Santanam, U., Zanesi, N., Efanov, A., Costinean, S., Palamarchuk, A., Hagan, J.P., Volinia, S., Alder, H., Rassenti, L., Kipps, T., Croce, C.M. & Pekarsky, Y. (2010). Chronic lymphocytic leukemia modeled in mouse by targeted miR-29 expression. *Proceedings of the National Academy of Sciences U S A.,* Vol. 107, No. 27, (July, 2010), pp. 12210-12215, ISSN 0027-8424

Santos, D.D., Ho, A.W., Tournilhac, O., Hatjiharissi, E., Leleu, X., Xu, L., Tassone, P., Neri, P., Hunter, Z.R., Chemaly, M.A., Branagan, A.R., Manning, R.J., Patterson, C.J., Moreau, A.S., Ciccarelli, B., Adamia, S., Kriangkum, J., Kutok, J.L., Tai, Y.T., Zhang, J., Pilarski, L.M., Anderson, K.C., Munshi, N. & Treon, S.P. (2007). Establishment of BCWM.1 cell line for Waldenström's macroglobulinemia with productive in vivo engraftment in SCID-hu mice. *Experimental Hematology,* Vol. 35,. No. 9, (September, 2007), pp.1366-1375, ISSN 0301-472X

Scaglione, B.J., Salerno, E., Balan, M., Coffman, F., Landgraf, P., Abbasi, F., Kotenko, S., Marti, G.E. & Raveche, E.S. (2007). Murine models of chronic lymphocytic leukaemia: role of microRNA-16 in the New Zealand Black mouse model. *British Journal of Haematology,* Vol. 139, No. 5, (December, 2007), pp. 645–657, ISSN 0007-1048

Schmidtko, J., Wang, R., Wu CL, Mauiyyedi, S., Harris, N.L., Della, Pelle, P., Brousaides, N., Zagachin, L., Ferry, J.A., Wang, F., Kawai, T., Sachs, D.H., Cosimi, B.A. & Colvin, R.B. (2002). Posttransplant lymphoproliferative disorder associated with an Epstein-Barr-related virus in cynomolgus monkeys. *Transplantation.,* Vol. 73, No. 9, (May, 2002), pp. 1431-1439, ISSN 0041-1337

Seeman, E. (2008). Bone quality: the material and structural basis of bone strength. *Journal of Bone Mineral Metabolism,* Vol. 26, No. 1, (Epub January, 2008), pp. 1-8, ISSN 0914-8779

SEER Cancer Statisitcs Review, 1973-1995. (1998). National Cancer Institute. Available from: http://seer.cancer.gov/csr/1973_1995/overview.pdf

SEER (Surveillance Epidemiology and End Results); (2010), "SEER Cancer Statistics Review 1975–2007". Available from:
http://seer.cancer.gov/csr/1975 2007/results single/sect 28 table.09.pdf.

Shay, J.W., Werbin, H. & Wright, W.E. (1996). Telomeres and telomerase in human leukemias. *Leukemia,* Vol. 10, No. 8, (August, 1996), pp. 1255-1261, ISSN 0887-6924

Shipman, C.M., Rogers, M.J., Apperley, J.F., Russell, R.G. & Croucher, P.I. (1997). Bisphosphonates induce apoptosis in human myeloma cell lines: a novel anti-tumour activity. *Brtish Journal of Haematology,* Vol. 98, No. 3, (September, 1997), pp. 665-672, ISSN 0361-8609

Singhal, S., Mehta, J., Desikan, R., Ayers, D., Roberson, P., Eddlemon, P., Munshi, N., Anaissie, E., Wilson, C., Dhodapkar, M., Zeddis, J. & Barlogie, B. (1999). Antitumor activity of thalidomide in refractory multiple myeloma. *New England Journal of Medicine.,* Vol. 18, No. 341(21), (November, 1999), pp.1565-1571, ISSN 0028-4793

Sjak-Shie, N. N., Tsingotjidou, A. S., Zhang, K., Vescio, R. A., Said, J. W., Lieberman, J. R. & Berenson, J. R. (1999). Development of a SCID-hu animal model that more closely resembles human multiple myeloma. *Blood,* Vol. 94, No. 10, pp. 2447 Part 1 Supp., 1999, ISSN 0006-4971

Smith, A.C., Raimondi, A.R., Salthouse, C.D., Ignatius, M.S., Blackburn, J.S., Mizgirev, I.V., Storer, N.Y. de Jong, J.L., Chen, A.T., Zhou, Y., Revskoy, S., Zon, L.I., & Langenau, D.M. (2010). High-throughput cell transplantation establishes that tumor-initiating cells are abundant in zebrafish T-cell acute lymphoblastic leukemia. *Blood.,* Vol. 115, No. 16, (April, 2010), pp. 3296-3303, ISSN 0006-4971

Smith, M.A., Gloeckler Ries, L.A., Gurney, J.G. & Ross, J.A. (2010). "Leukemia. SEER Pediatric Monograph". Available from:
http://seer.cancer.gov/ publications/childhood/leukemia.pdf

Stehbens, J.A., Kaleita, T.A., Noll, R.B., MacLean, W.E. Jr, O'Brien, R.T., Waskerwitz, M.J. & Hammond, G.D. (1991). CNS prophylaxis of childhood leukemia: what are the long-term neurological, neuropsychological, and behavioral effects? *Neuropsychology Review,* Vol. 2, No. 2, (June, 1991), pp. 147-177, ISSN 1040-7308

Suljagic, M., Longo, P.G., Bennardo, S., Perlas, E., Leone, G., Laurenti, L. & Efremov, D.G. (2010). The Syk inhibitor fostamatinib disodium (R788) inhibits tumor growth in the Eµ- TCL1 transgenic mouse model of CLL by blocking antigen-dependent B-cell receptor signaling. *Blood.*, Vol. 116, No. 23, (December, 2010), pp. 4894-4905, ISSN 0006-4971

Swinnen, L.J. Costanzo-Nordin, M.R., Fisher, S.G., O'Sullivan, E.J., Johnson, M.R., Heroux, A.L., Dizikes, G.J., Pifarre, R. & Fisher, R.I. (1990). Increased incidence of lymphoproliferative disorder after immunosuppression with the monoclonal antibody OKT3 in cardiac-transplant recipients. *New England Journal of Medicine,* Vol. 323, No. 25, (December, 1990), pp. 1723-1728, ISSN 0028-4793

Szczepek, A.J., Seeberger, K., Wizniak, J., Mant, M.J., Belch, A.R. & Pilarski, L.M. (1998). A high frequency of circulating B cells share clonotypic Ig heavy-chain VDJ rearrangements with autologous bone marrow plasma cells in multiple myeloma, as measured by single-cell and in situ reverse transcriptasepolymerase chain reaction. *Blood.,* Vol. 92, No. 8, (October, 1998), pp. 2844-2855, ISSN 0006-4971

Tang, Y., He, R., Zhang, Y., Liu, F., Cheng, A., Wu, Y. & Gan, R. (2011). Human-derived IgG level as an indicator for EBV-associated lymphoma model in Hu-PBL/SCID chimeras. *Virology Journal,* Vol. 8, (May, 2011), pp. 213, ISSN 1743-422X

Tassone, P., Neri, P., Kutok, J.L., Tournilhac, O., Santos, D.D., Hatjiharissi, E., Munshi, V., Venuta, S., Anderson, K.C., Treon, S.P. & Munshi, N.C. (2005). A SCID-hu in vivo model of human Waldenström macroglobulinemia. *Blood.*, Vol. 106, No. 4, (August, 2005), pp. 1341-1345, ISSN 0006-4971

The Non-Hodgkin's Lymphoma Classification Project (1997). A clinical evaluation of the International Lymphoma Study Group classification of non-Hodgkin's lymphoma. *Blood*, Vol. 89, No. 11, (June, 1997), pp. 3909–3918, ISSN 0006-4971

Theofilopoulos, A.N. (1996). Genetics of systemic autoimmunity. *Journal of Autoimmunity,* Vol. 9, No. 2, (April, 1996), pp. 207–210, ISSN 0896-8411

Treon, S.P., Branagan, A.R., Hunter, Z., Santos, D., Tournhilac, O. & Anderson, K.C. (2004). Paradoxical increases in serum IgM and viscosity levels following rituximab in Waldenström's macroglobulinemia. *Annals in Oncology,* Vol. 15, No. 10, (October, 2004), pp. 1481-1483, ISSN 0923-7534

Treon, S.P., Gertz, M.A., Dimopoulos, M., Anagnostopoulos, A., Blade, J., Branagan, A.R., Garcia-Sanz, R., Johnson, S., Kimby, E., Leblond, V., Fermand, J.P., Maloney, D.G., Merlini, G., Morel, P., Morra, E., Nichols, G., Ocio, E.M., Owen, R. & Stone, M.J. (2006). Update on treatment recommendations from the Third International Workshop on Waldenström's Macroglobulinemia. *Blood,* Vol. 107, No. 9, (May, 2006), pp. 3442-3446, ISSN 0006-4971.

Tsingotjidou, A.S., Zotalis, G., Jackson, K.R., Sawyers, C., Puzas, J.E., Hicks, D.G., Reiter, R. & Lieberman, J.R. (2001). Development of an animal model for prostate cancer cell metastasis to adult human bone. *Anticancer Research,* Vol. 21, No. 2A, (March-April, 2001), pp. 971-978, ISSN 0250-7005

Tsingotjidou, A.S., Emmanouilides, C.E., Siotou, E., Poutahidis, T., Xagorari, A., Loukopoulos, P., Sotiropoulos, D., Bekiari, C., Doulberis, M., Givissis, P., Fassas, A. & Anagnostopoulos, A. (2009). Establishment of an animal model for Waldenström's macroglobulinemia. *Experimental Hematology,* Vol. 37, No.4, (April, 2009), pp. 469-476, ISSN 0301-472X

U.S. Cancer Statistics Working group. Statistics Working Group (2009). United States Cancer Statistics: 1999–2005 Incidence and Mortality Web-based Report. Atlanta: U.S.

Department of Health and Human Services, Centers for Disease Control and Prevention and National Cancer Institute. Available from: www.cdc.gov/uscs

van Esser, J.W., Niesters, H.G., van der Holt, B., Meijer, E., Osterhaus, A.D., Gratama, J.W., Verdonck, L.F., Löwenberg, B. & Cornelissen, J.J. (2002). Prevention of Epstein-Barr virus-lymphoproliferative disease by molecular monitoring and preemptive rituximab in high-risk patients after allogeneic stem cell transplantation. *Blood,* Vol. 99, No. 12, (June, 2002), pp. 4364-4369, ISSN 0006-4971

Vijay, A. & Gertz, M.A. (2007). Waldenström macroglobulinemia. *Blood,* Vol. 109, No. 12, (June, 2007), pp. 5096-5103, ISSN 0006-4971

Virgilio, L., Lazzeri, C., Bichi, R., Nibu, K., Narducci, M.G., Russo G., Rothstein, J.L. & Croce C. M. (1998). Deregulated expression of TCL1 causes T cell leukemia in mice. *Proceedings of the National Academy of Sciences* USA, Vol. 95, No. 7, (March, 1998), pp. 3885-3889, ISSN 0027-8424

Waldenström, J. (1944). Incipient myelomatosis or 'essential' hyperglobulinemia with fibrinogenopenia: a new syndrome? *Acta Medica Scandinavica,* Vol. 117, pp. 216-222, ISSN 0001-6101

Watson, L., Wyld, P. & Catovsky D. (2008). Disease burden of chronic lymphocytic leukaemia within the European Union. *European Journal of Haematology*, Vol. 81, No. 4, (December 2008), pp. 253-258, ISSN 0902-4441

World Health Organization (2010), "Disease and injury regional estimates for 2004". Available from: http://www.who.int/healthinfo/global_burden_disease/estimates_regional/en/index.html

Witherspoon, R.P., Fisher, L.D., Schoch, G., Martin, P., Sullivan, K.M., Sanders, J., Deeg, H.J., Doney, K., Thomas, D., Storb, R. & Thomas, E.D. (1989). Secondary cancers after bone marrow transplantation for leukemia or aplastic anemia. *New England Journal of Medicine*, Vol. 321, No. 12, (September, 1989), pp. 784-789, ISSN 0028-4793

Yaccoby, S., Barlogie, B. & Epstein, J. (1998). Primary myeloma cells growing in SCID-hu mice: a model for studying the biology and treatment of myeloma and its manifestations. *Blood,* Vol. 92, No. 8, (October, 1998), pp. 2908-2913, ISSN 0006-4971

Yaccoby, S. & Epstein, J. (1999). The proliferative potential of myeloma plasma cells manifest in the SCID-hu host. *Blood.,* Vol. 94, No. 10, (November, 1999), pp. 3576-3582, ISSN 0006-4971

Yaccoby, S, Pearse, R.N., Johnson, C.L., Barlogie, B., Choi, Y. & Epstein, J. (2002). Myeloma interacts with the bone marrow microenvironment to induce osteoclastogenesis and is dependent on osteoclast activity. *British Journal of Haematology,* Vol. 116, No. 2, (February, 2002), pp. 278-290, ISSN 0007-1048

Yaccoby, S., Wezeman, M.J., Zangari, M., Walker, R., Cottler-Fox, M., Gaddy, D., Ling, W., Saha, R., Barlogie, B., Tricot, G., & Epstein, J. (2006). Inhibitory effects of osteoblasts and increased bone formation on myeloma in novel culture systems and a myelomatous mouse model. *Haematologica, Vol.* 91, No. 2, (February, 2006), pp. 192-199, ISSN 0390-6078

Yaccoby, S, Ling, W., Zhan, F., Walker, R., Barlogie, B., Shaughnessy, J.D. Jr. (2007). Antibody-based inhibition of DKK1 suppresses tumor-induced bone resorption and multiple myeloma growth in vivo. *Blood.,* Vol. 109, No. 5, (March 2007), pp: 2106-2111, ISSN 0006-4971

Yata, K., & Yaccoby, S. (2004). The SCID-rab model: a novel in vivo system for primary human myeloma demonstrating growth of CD138-expressing malignant cells. *Leukemia,* Vol.18, No. 11, (November 2004), pp.1891–1897, ISSN 0887-6924.

Yonou, H., Yokose, T., Kamijo, T., Kanomata, N., Hasebe, T., Nagai, K., Hatano, T., Ogawa, Y. & Ochiai, A. (2001). Establishment of a novel species- and tissue-specific metastasis model of human prostate cancer in humanized non-obese diabetic/severe combined immunodeficient mice engrafted with human adult lung and bone. *Cancer Research,* Vol. 61, No. 5, (March, 2001), pp. 2177-2282, ISSN 0008-5472

Yu, B.H., Zhou, X.Y., Zhang, T.C., Zhang, T.M. & Shi, D.R. (2011). Establishment and characterization of a nude mice model of human diffuse large B-cell lymphoma. *Chinese Journal of Pathology* (*Zhonghua Bing Li Xue Za Zhi.),* Vol. 40, No. 4, (April, 2011), pp. 246-250, ISSN 0529-5807

Yun, J.P., Behan, J.W., Heisterkamp, N., Butturini, A., Klemm, L., Ji, L., Groffen, J., Müschen, M. & Mittelman S.D. (2010). Diet-induced obesity accelerates acute lymphoblastic leukemia progression in two murine models. *Cancer Prevention Research (Philadelphia, PA).,* Vol. 3, No. 10, (October, 2010), pp. 1259-1264, ISSN 1940-6215

Zhang, J., Xiao, Y., Guo, Y., Breslin, P., Zhang, S., Wei, W,, Zhang. Z. & Zhang, J. (2011). Differential requirements for c-Myc in chronic hematopoietic hyperplasia and acute hematopoietic malignancies in Pten-null mice. *Leukemia,* Sep. 16. doi: 10.1038/leu.2011.220, ISSN 0887-692

7

Epstein-Barr Virus-Encoded miRNAs in Epstein-Barr Virus-Related Malignancy

Jun Lu[1,*], Bidisha Chanda[2,*] and Ai Kotani[1,*]
[1]*Tokai University Institute of Innovative Science and Technology*
[2]*University of Tokyo Institute of Medical Science*
Japan

1. Introduction

In 1958, Denis Burkitt described B cell lymphomas in 2- to 14-year-old African children from malaria-endemic areas.[1] In 1964, Michael Anthony Epstein and Yvonne Barr found that immortalized B lymphocyte cell lines derived from these tumors spontaneously released a herpesvirus.[2] Thus, Epstein-Barr virus (EBV) was discovered by examining electron micrographs of cells cultured from Burkitt's lymphoma; its unusual geographic distribution indicated a viral etiology. It was Gertrud and Werner Henle who demonstrated that EBV is ubiquitous in the human population.[3] Far from having a restricted distribution, EBV, a member of the γ-herpesvirus family, was found to be widespread in all human populations and to persist in the vast majority of individuals as a lifelong, asymptomatic infection of B lymphocytes. Therefore, EBV is usually the cause of clinically inconspicuous infections, although it can cause infectious mononucleosis. The most severe, albeit rare, result of EBV infection is malignant transformation and the development of cancer in various forms, including Burkitt's lymphoma and nasopharyngeal carcinoma, the latter of which is one of the most common cancers in China.[4] The link between EBV and "endemic" Burkitt's lymphoma proved constant and became the first of an unexpectedly wide range of associations discovered between this virus and tumors.[5] As a ubiquitous human pathogen, EBV is responsible for several lymphoid malignancies, including a subset of Burkitt's lymphoma, acquired Immune deficiency syndrome (AIDS)-associated lymphoma, Hodgkin's lymphoma, post-transplant lymphoma, age-associated B cell lymphoma, and peripheral T and NK cell lymphomas.[6,7]

1.1 EBV infection

The primary site of EBV infection is the oropharyngeal cavity.[8] Children and teenagers are often infected after oral contact, hence the nickname "kissing disease". Like other herpesviruses, infection with EBV can exhibit two distinct patterns, or states, of gene expression. During acute (lytic) EBV infection, the virus sequentially expresses its entire repertoire of genes. In this lytic state, linear, double-stranded viral genomes are produced and packaged into virions that spread infection from cell to cell. Shortly after the initial

---

[*] These authors equally contributed to this work.

infection, EBV enters into a latent state, whereupon only select "latent" genes are expressed, thereby evading host immune surveillance mechanisms, and establishing a lifelong, persistent infection in the host.[9] During latency, only a few viral genes are transcribed, no viral progeny are produced, and infected cells are protected from apoptotic stimuli and, in some circumstances, driven to proliferate. Based on serology, about 95% of the world's adult population is infected with EBV, and following primary infection, hosts remain lifelong carriers of the virus.[10] In developed countries, exposure to EBV occurs relatively late; only 50–70% of adolescents and young adults are EBV seropositive. About 30% of seronegative individuals will later develop infectious mononucleosis as a result of primary EBV infection. This disease is characterized by fever, pharyngitis, generalized lymphadenopathy, splenomegaly, intense asthenia, hyper-lymphocytosis (>50%) with atypical lymphocytes, and elevated transaminase levels. In developing countries, EBV antibodies are acquired early in life and the disease is mostly asymptomatic.

1.2 EBV-related cancer

EBV has been etiologically linked to a variety of human cancers, such as Burkitt's lymphoma, nasopharyngeal carcinoma (NPC), Hodgkin's disease, and more recently with sporadic cases of gastric adenocarcinoma and invasive breast carcinoma.[11,12] Nearly 100% of NPC tumors, 90% of Burkitt's lymphoma tumors of African origin, and 40–60% of Hodgkin's and non-Hodgkin's lymphomas contain EBV episomes. Clonality of the EBV genome has been confirmed in these tumors, suggesting that the tumors arose from a single EBV-infected cell, and that EBV infection is a very early, if not causal, event. EBV is also commonly associated with lymphoproliferative diseases in patients with congenital or acquired immunodeficiencies. Examples include X-linked lymphoproliferative syndrome, human immunodeficiency virus (HIV)-related non-Hodgkin's lymphoma, and perhaps most importantly post-transplantation lymphoproliferative disease.[5]

Burkitt's lymphoma is a malignant tumor associated with EBV that is endemic to central parts of Africa and New Guinea with an annual incidence of 6–7 cases per 100,000 and a peak incidence in children of 6 or 7 years of age. The epidemiological involvement of EBV in Burkitt's lymphoma was first suspected due to the presence of the EBV viral genome in tumor cells and elevated antibody titers against EBV viral capsid antigen in cancer patients. The highest prevalence of Burkitt's lymphoma occurs in the "lymphoma belt," a region that extends from West Africa to East Africa, between the 10th degree north and 10th degree south of the equator, and continues south along the eastern coast of Africa. This area is characterized by high temperature and humidity, which is likely the reason why an association between malaria and Burkitt's lymphoma was once suspected. In African countries within the lymphoma belt, such as Uganda, the association of Burkitt's lymphoma with EBV is very strong (97%), whereas it is less so elsewhere (e.g., 85% in Algeria and 10–15% in France and the USA). (World Health Organization, WHO)

NPC incidence rates are less than 1 per 100,000 in most populations, except for those in southern China, where an annual incidence of more than 20 cases per 100,000 is reported.[4] Isolated northern populations, such as Eskimos and Greenlanders, also have high incidences. Moderate incidences occur in North Africa, Israel, Kuwait, the Sudan, and parts of Kenya and Uganda. Men are twice as likely to develop NPC as women. The rate of incidence generally increases at ages 20–50 years. In the USA, Chinese-Americans comprise the majority of NPC patients, along with workers exposed to fumes, smoke, and chemicals, implicating a role for chemical carcinogenesis. Studies assessing nutrition and diets have demonstrated an association between eating highly salted foods and NPC. Vitamin C deficiency at a young age may also be a contributing factor. Finally, a study of human leukocyte antigen (HLA) haplotypes revealed a genetically distinct subpopulation in southern China, with an increased frequency of haplotype A-2/B-Sin-2, which may account for the higher disease incidence in that area. (WHO)

1.3 Cytotoxic T lymphocyte therapy for EBV-related cancer

EBV, together with human herpesvirus (HHV)-8 (also known as Kaposi sarcoma-associated virus), belongs to the genus *Lymphocryptovirus* in the subfamily Gammaherpesvirinae of the family Herpesviridae. These are complex, enveloped, DNA viruses, which multiply in the nucleus of the host cell. EBV infects resting human B lymphocytes and epithelial cells, multiplies in the latter, and establishes latent infection in memory B lymphocytes. Thus, infected individuals may produce virions, carry virus-specific cytotoxic T lymphocytes (CTLs), produce EBV-specific antibodies, and yet harbor latently infected memory B cells. EBV-infected individuals maintain the latent EBV genome as an episome that expresses only part of its genetic information, including EBV nuclear antigens (EBNA)-1 (a latent DNA replication factor), EBNA-2 (a transcriptional activator), and EBNA-3A and -3C (involved in the establishment of latency). Also expressed are latent membrane protein (LMP)-1 and LMP-2, which play major roles in the maintenance of latency and escape from the host immune response. Latently infected cells do not express the B7 coactivator receptor and, therefore, are not targeted by CTLs. When peripheral blood from an infected individual is cultured, latently infected B cells replicate and become immortalized lymphoblasts that can be indefinitely propagated in the laboratory.[13]

In a previous study, CTL therapy was proven to be safe and effective as a treatment for patients with EBV-related cancers, and was found to enable the complete remission of patients who failed all previous standard treatments. The first clinical trials using EBV-specific CTLs tested their utility for both prophylaxis and treatment of post-transplant lymphoproliferative diseases arising in stem cell transplant or solid organ transplant recipients.[5]

Nucleoside analogs, such as acyclovir (ACV) and ganciclovir (GCV), are often used as antiviral drugs against acute EBV and other herpesvirus infections.[14] The virally encoded thymidine kinase enzyme converts these analogs into their phosphate forms, which, after conversion into their triphosphate form by host kinases, are then incorporated into newly synthesized DNA, leading to the premature termination of DNA synthesis and apoptosis of the infected cell. The EBV thymidine kinase, however, is only expressed during lytic replication of the virus. Because EBV maintains a latent state of replication in all EBV-associated malignancies, nucleoside analog drugs have very limited, or no, cytopathic effect on virus-infected cells. Novel therapeutic approaches to target EBV-infected tumor cells, which include inducing lytic replication of EBV followed by treatment with nucleoside analogs, have been proposed.

Arginine butyrate induces the expression of the viral thymidine kinase gene in EBV-positive, immunoblastic, non-Hodgkin's lymphoma cell lines and lymphoblastic cell lines (LCLs) and acts synergistically with GCV to inhibit cell proliferation and decrease cell viability.[15] Various other agents have also been used to induce lytic replication of the EBV genome. For example, treatment of EBV-positive lymphoblastoid cells, or primary central nervous system lymphoma, with γ-irradiation promotes GCV-susceptibility of target cells.[15] Other studies successfully used 5-azacytidine, gemcitabine, doxorubicin, or a combination of anti-CD20 monoclonal antibody (Rituximab) and dexamethasone to induce lytic-phase gene expression and sensitize EBV-infected tumor cells to GCV or other nucleoside analogs.[15]

Butyric acid, a short-chain fatty acid, and its derivatives have been experimentally employed in attempts to treat leukemias and other diseases. Butyrate induces the expression of certain EBV lytic proteins, including the thymidine kinase enzyme, from latent EBV-infected cells.[16] The inhibitory effect of butyrate on histone deacetylase (HDAC) is required for this effect. In previous clinical studies, systemic administration of arginine butyrate was used to induce expression of the latent EBV thymidine kinase in the tumors of patients with EBV-positive post-transplantation lymphoproliferative disease or non-Hodgkin's lymphomas, followed by treatment with GCV.[16,17]

Bortezomib, a proteasome inhibitor, also activates EBV lytic gene expression.[18] Bortezomib leads to increased levels of CCAAT/enhancer-binding protein β (C/EBPβ) in a variety of tumor cell lines.[18] C/EBPβ activates the promoter of the EBV lytic switch gene *ZTA* (BZLF1). Bortezomib treatment leads to increased binding of C/EBPβ to sites within the *ZTA* promoter. Knockdown of C/EBPβ inhibits bortezomib activation of EBV lytic gene expression.[18] Bortezomib also induces the unfolded protein response (UPR). Thapsigargin, an inducer of the UPR that does not interfere with proteasome function, also induces EBV lytic gene expression.[18,19] The effect of thapsigargin on EBV lytic gene expression is also inhibited upon C/EBPβ knock-down.[18] Therefore, C/EBPβ mediates the activation of EBV lytic gene expression associated with bortezomib and thapsigargin.[18]

Pretreatment of naturally infected EBV tumor cell lines (from Burkitt's lymphoma and gastric carcinoma) with bortezomib activates viral gene expression.[20] Marked changes in tumor growth are also achieved in naturally infected Kaposi's sarcoma herpesvirus tumors after pretreatment with bortezomib.[20] Bortezomib-induced, enzyme-targeted radiation therapy illustrates the potential of pharmacological modulation of tumor gene expression for targeted radiotherapy.

There is increasing interest in the pharmacologic activation of lytic viral gene expression in tumors. Several therapeutic strategies requiring activation of EBV lytic genes for tumor cell lysis have been described, but concerns have been raised about the possible adverse effects of viral gene activation patients treated with pharmacologic activators.

2. EBV-encoded miRNA

2.1 miRNA

Micro (mi)RNAs are small, non-coding, single-stranded RNAs of approximately 21 to 25 nucleotides (nt) in length. They post-transcriptionally regulate mRNA expression in animals and plants and are transcribed from the non-coding regions of genes in all multi-cellular organisms and certain viruses and are often phylogenetically conserved across species.[21,22] EBV was the first human virus found to encode miRNA.[23] EBV encodes 44 viral miRNAs and a small RNA. EBV-encoded miRNAs are located within the *BHRF1* and BamHI A rightward transcript (*BART*) loci of the EBV genome. The BHRF1 cluster of miRNAs includes BHRF1-1, BHRF1-2, BHRF1-3, and BHRF1-4.[22-24] The other EBV-encoded miRNAs are encoded by BART cluster 1 and BART cluster 2, except miR-BART2, which is expressed from a sight outside of the BART clusters.[22-25] miRNAs bind to the 3′ untranslated region (UTR) of mRNA and interfere with their translation, leading to downregulated protein expression levels. EBV-encoded miRNAs have been found in various EBV-associated carcinomas and lymphomas, such as NPC, gastric carcinoma, diffuse large B cell lymphoma, nasal NK/T cell lymphoma, and Hodgkin's lymphoma.[23,26] Viral miRNAs play vital roles in immunogenesis, host cell survival and proliferation, differentiation, lymphomagenesis, and regulation of viral infection and latency.[23,27-29]

2.2 EBV miRNA-mediated regulation of viral infection states

During lytic infection, EBV genomes are amplified into 1000 copies per cell with the help of replication proteins.[30] EBV expresses six replication proteins, the most important of which are BZLF1 and BALF5. BALF5 is a catalytic DNA polymerase encoded by the *balf5* gene during lytic infection;[30] it is not present in latent infection. This DNA polymerase is a single-stranded DNA binding protein, which functions within viral replication factories in the nucleus, likely generating replication forks on the replicating EBV genome. EBV-encoded miR-BART2 is expressed at low levels during latency, prevents aberrant expression of BALF5 mRNA, and prevents inadvertent viral replication.[31] The sequence of miR-BART2 is perfectly complementary to the 3′UTR of BALF5 mRNA. Therefore, miR-BART2 serves as an inhibitor of viral DNA replication through the degradation of BALF5 mRNA. The miRNA-guided cleavage of mRNA requires an association with Ago2,[32] which is a member of the Argonuate family of proteins and a part of the RNA-induced silencing complex (RISC). Upon its association with Ago2, miR-BART2 guides the sequence-specific cleavage of BALF5 mRNA. This miR-BART2-guided cleavage is substantially reduced after induction of the lytic cycle in EBV-infected cells.[31] The amount of miR-BART2 is reduced during lytic infection, and this causes a de-repression of BALF5 protein expression.[31] However, it is unclear whether the miR-BART2-mediated regulation of viral replication is fully controlled by BALF5 protein or not.

Another regulator of the shift from EBV latency to lytic infection is miR-BART6, which itself is regulated by RNA editing.[33] Editing of the wild-type primary (pri)-miR-BART6 sequence dramatically reduces the loading of miR-BART6-5p onto RISC, without affecting the processing of precursor (pre) or mature miRNAs.[33] Editing of pri-miRNA might affect the selection and loading of the guide strand onto RISC.[34] miR-BART6-5p silences Dicer through multiple target sites located in the 3′UTR of Dicer mRNA, but miR-BART6-3p is unable to perform this function.[33]

In EBV-infected human cells, Dicer protein levels are substantially reduced by miR-BART6-5p,[33] suggesting that miR-BART6-5p may indirectly regulate the biogenesis of all miRNAs. It may even affect the latency of EBV by modulating the expression of viral proteins, including EBNA2, LMP1, RTA, and ZTA. EBNA2 is required for the transition from the less immunologically confrontational type I or type II latency to the more immunity-stimulating type III latency, which occurs through the upregulation of all latent EBV genes and the transformation of infected B lymphocytes.[35,36] However, EBNA2 deficiency is observed in type I and type II latency.[35,36] Low-level expression of LMP1 is also observed in type II latency, but is absent in type I. LMP1 controls the NF-κB signaling pathway and the growth and apoptosis of host cells. RTA and ZTA proteins initiate lytic infection of EBV. Thus, it is clear that miR-BART6-5p regulates EBV infection and latency by suppressing RTA and ZTA protein expression. To modulate protein expression, miR-BART6-5p downregulates viral promoters, such as Cp and Wp, which are characteristic of type III latency, and reduces transcriptional activity via its silencing effect on Dicer. Mutation and adenosine-to-inosine (A-to-I) editing are adaptive mechanisms that antagonize miR-BART6 activities and affect the latent state of viral infection.[33] Therefore, we conclude that miR-BART6-5p, and its mutant or edited versions, are critical for the establishment and maintenance of latent EBV infection.

2.3 EBV miRNA-mediated host cell survival

The miR-BART5 miRNA promotes host cell survival by regulating the p53 upregulated modulator of apoptosis (PUMA) protein.[37] PUMA is an apoptotic protein belonging to the "BH3-only" group of the Bcl-2 family and is encoded by the *BBC3* gene.[38-40] PUMA is regulated by the tumor suppressor p53 and is involved in both p53-mediated and non-mediated apoptosis via independent signaling pathways. PUMA is an important downstream regulator of p53, both of which are master regulators of host cell growth and apoptosis. PUMA function is downregulated or absent in cancer cells, but the absence of PUMA activity alone is not sufficient for the spontaneous formation of malignancies.[41-45] PUMA has four isoforms (i.e., α, β, γ, and δ), which share the same 3′UTR.[39] Only PUMA-α and PUMA-β have pro-apoptotic activity. The PUMA 3′UTR sequence is perfectly complementary to miR-BART5. Thus, binding of miR-BART5 and the PUMA 3′UTR suppresses the expression of the pro-apoptotic protein. PUMA-β protein expression is also reduced by pre-miR-BART5.[37] Abundant expression of miR-BART5 in NPC cells is correlated with significant downregulation of PUMA in 60% of NPC tissues.[37] By this mechanism, miR-BART5 induces anti-apoptotic activity in NPC cells, EBV-infected gastric carcinoma cells, and EBV-infected epithelial cells.[37] Therefore, miR-BART5 may be a good target for anti-cancer therapy in EBV-infected cancer cells.

LMP1 is a viral protein expressed during the type III latency period of EBV infection.[35,36] LMP1 promotes cell growth, resistance to serum deprivation-induced apoptosis, and phenotypic changes in epithelial cells and B cell transformation. It activates the NF-κB, JNK, JAK/STAT, p38/MAP, and RAS/MAPK pathways and regulates host gene expression.[5] NF-κB transcription factors influence proliferation, apoptosis, oncogenesis, and inflammation.[46] Low levels of LMP1 activate NF-κB, but with increasing amounts of LMP1, NF-κB activation reaches a plateau, after which small increases in LMP1 reduces NF-κB activity.[47] Thus, a threshold level of LMP1 can maintain peak NF-κB activity. LMP1 regulates the level of NF-κB activity by modulating the UPR pathway and autophagy. *BARTI* cluster miRNAs negatively regulate LMP1 expression, limiting inappropriately high levels, thereby preventing apoptosis that would otherwise result from LMP1-mediated changes in the UPR. Such *BART1* cluster miRNAs include BART16, BART17-5p, and BART1-5p, which target sites within the 3′UTR of LMP1 mRNA.[47] These miRNAs regulate LMP1 expression at the post-transcriptional level, regulating NF-κB-mediated gene expression. Therefore, the negative regulation of LMP1 expression by *BART1* cluster miRNAs may affect EBV-associated cancer development by balancing the effect of LMP1 on cellular proliferation.

BHRF1 is a latent protein expressed in growth-transformed cells that contributes to virus-associated lymphomagenesis.[48] miR-BHRF1 downregulates this protein, modulates cell transformation,[49] and promotes B cell proliferation after EBV infection. EBV-infected B cells lacking miR-BHRF1 progress less efficiently into the cell cycle and eventually die by apoptosis.[49] miR-BHRF1 is constitutively expressed in LCLs.[49] Without miR-BHRF1, the proportion of G1/G0 cells increases while the numbers of S-phase cells decreases,[49] indicating a definite role of miR-BHRF1 in the control of proliferation of latently infected cells. miR-BHRF1 acts at a stage of the EBV life cycle when multiple EBV-encoded oncogenes become activated.

2.4 EBV-encoded miRNAs regulate immune evasion

Major histocompatibility complex (MHC) class I polypeptide-related sequence B (MICB) protein is a ligand for the NKG2D type II receptor, which is a stress-induced immune molecule.[50,51] B cells and endothelial cells, which are targets of EBV, both express this protein. Binding of MICB activates NK, $CD8^+$ $\alpha\beta$, and $\gamma\delta$ T cells.[52] MICB is upregulated at the cell surface due to various insults, such as viral infection, tumor transformation, heat shock, and DNA damage. Thus, it would be beneficial for a virus to downregulate the expression of this protein ligand to avoid immune detection. Previous studies have shown that downregulated MICB expression leads to reduced lysis of infected cells by NK cells.[53] EBV-expressed miR-BART2-5p has potential binding sites in the MICB mRNA 3′UTR.[54] EBV downregulates MICB via miR-BART2-5p, resulting in decreased NK cell-mediated lysis, to avoid detection by immune cells.

miR-BHLF1-1 is expressed from the 5′UTR, and miR-BHLF1-2 and miR-BHLF1-3 are expressed from the 3′UTR, of the *bhrf1* gene in EBV-infected cells.[28] miR-BHLF1-3 is markedly elevated in EBV-infected, type III latent cell lines[28] and is also detected in EBV-positive primary effusion lymphoma and AIDS-related diffuse large B cell lymphoma.[28] BHRF1 miRNA is characteristic of EBV type III latent infections.[55] EBV miR-BHRF1-3 regulates host immunity by downregulating the interferon (IFN)-inducible T cell attracting chemokine (I-TAC; also known as CXCL-11). CXCL-11/I-TAC belongs to the CXC family of chemokines, and both IFN-β and IFN-γ strongly induce its transcription.[56] CXCL-11/I-TAC promotes cell-mediated immunity by attracting activated T cells. The 3′UTR of CXCL-11/I-TAC mRNA is 100% complementary to the sequence of miR-BART1-3 and, therefore, serves as a target of miR-BART1-3. miR-BART1-3 inversely regulates the expression of CXCL-11/I-TAC; the anti-sense sequence of miR-BART1-3 has the reverse effect.[23] miR-BART1-3 significantly reduces the expression of CXCL-11/I-TAC at both the mRNA and protein levels.[28] Thus, as cellular chemokines can be targets of viral miRNA, EBV-mediated regulation of antigen processing and presentation, and the downregulation of CTL cytokine networks, may occur through such a mechanism.

2.5 Small nucleolar RNAs encoded by the EBV genome

A small nucleolar (sno)RNA, named v-snoRNA1, has been identified within the EBV genome in EBV-infected B lymphocytes.[57] snoRNAs, 60–300 nt in length, guide nucleotide modifications of ribosomal (r)RNAs, i.e., 2′O-ribose methylation or pseudouridylation, that are located in subnuclear compartments.[58,59] snoRNAs are subdivided into the C/D box and H/ACA box classes. The majority of snoRNAs located within introns of protein-encoding genes are processed by splicing, followed by endo- and exonucleolytic cleavage.[60-62] However, some of them are orphan snoRNAs that lack rRNA or small modulatory (sm)RNA targets. v-snoRNA is processed into 24 nt long miRNAs, which then target the 3'UTR of viral DNA polymerase mRNA.

The *v-snoRNA1* gene is located within the *BART* sense stand of the EBV genome.[57] Both v-snoRNA1 and miR-BART2 arise from the same intron. Although v-snoRNA1 is an integral part of the EBV latent transcription program, it is highly expressed during lytic infection. The 3'UTR of the BHLF5 mRNA is fully complementary to v-snoRNA1, so v-snoRNA1 binds and cleaves BALF5 mRNA, enabling its exonucleolytic degradation.[57] It is unclear whether v-snoRNA1 serves an important function during the viral life cycle.

3. Editing and mutation of EBV-encoded miRNAs

Recently widespread RNA-DNA differences in the human transcriptome were found. It also occurs to miRNAs including EBV-encoded miRNAs.[63]

3.1 RNA editing

RNA editing is carried out by enzymes that target mRNA post-transcriptionally, such as adenosine deaminases that act on RNA (ADARs, which convert adenosine to inosine, which is subsequently recognized by translation machinery as a guanosine, i.e., A-to-G mutation) and apolipoprotein B mRNA-editing enzyme catalytic polypeptide-like (APOBEC) proteins, which convert cytidine to uridine (i.e., C-to-U mutation). Editing of pri-miR-142, the primary transcript form of miR-142 that is expressed in hematopoietic tissues, results in suppression of its processing by Drosha.[64] The mutated pri-miR-142 is degraded by Tudor-SN, a component of RISC and also a ribonuclease that is specific to inosine-containing double-stranded (ds)RNAs. Mature miR-142 is substantially upregulated in ADAR1- or ADAR2-null mice,[64] demonstrating that RNA editing helps control miRNA biogenesis. Kawahara et al. found that primary transcripts of certain miRNA genes are subject to RNA editing that converts adenosine to inosine. By way of ADAR, tissue-specific A-to-I editing of miR-376 cluster transcripts lead to the predominant expression of edited miR-376 isoform RNAs. One highly edited site is located in the middle of the 5'-proximal "seed" region of miR-376 critical for its hybridization to its targets, providing evidence that the mutated miR-376 specifically targets a set of genes that is different than those targeted by wild-type miR-376.[65] Mutated miR-376 represses phosphoribosyl pyrophosphate synthetase 1, an enzyme involved in the uric-acid synthesis pathway.

Iizasa et al. reported that the primary transcripts of four EBV miRNAs, including miR-BART6, are subject to A-to-I editing. Moreover, it was demonstrated that editing of pri-miR-BART6, as well as mutations of miR-BART6, found in latently EBV-infected cells prevented its loading onto functionally active RISC.[33] As mentioned, miR-BART6 targets Dicer and affects the latent state of EBV viral infection. Therefore, regulation of miR-BART6 expression and function through A-to-I editing may be critical for the establishment or maintenance of latent EBV infection.

3.2 Mutation of the EBV genome affects encoded miRNAs

Sequence variation in the EBV genome has been extensively studied for a long time; in particular, *BLRF1* and other genes have been reported to have sequence variation in EBV-infected cancer patients.[66] Mechanistic analysis of this sequence variability has recently been reported by Suspène et al.[67] Human APOBEC3 cytidine deaminases target and edit single-stranded DNA, which can be of viral, mitochondrial, or nuclear origin. Retroviral genomes, such those of HIV, deficient in the *vif* gene, and hepatitis B virus, are particularly vulnerable.

The genomes of DNA viruses, such as herpesviruses, are also subject to editing. This is the case for herpes simplex virus type 1 (HSV-1), at least in tissue culture, where APOBEC3C (A3C) overexpression reduces viral titers and the particle/plaque forming unit (PFU) ratio by approximately 10-fold. A3A, A3G, and activation-induced cytidine deaminase (AICDA) can edit what is thought to be a small fraction of HSV genome in an experimental setting without seriously impacting viral titers. Hyper-editing was found to occur in HSV genomes recovered from four of eight uncultured buccal lesions, but the phenomenon was not restricted to HSV; hyper-mutated EBV genomes were readily recovered from four of five established cell lines, indicating that episomes are also vulnerable to editing [67]. These findings suggest that the widely expressed A3C cytidine deaminase can function as a restriction factor for some human herpesviruses.

Other studies reported sequence variation in BART miRNAs.[68] The significance of these mutations and their effect on miRNA processing, as well as the mechanism of mutation, whether it is mediated by A3C, members of other APOBEC families, or other mechanisms, have yet to be determined.

4. Regulation of EBV-encoded miRNA processing

4.1 Processing of miRNAs under normal versus cancerous conditions

The mechanism of miRNA biosynthesis involves sequential endonucleolytic cleavages mediated by two RNase III enzymes, Drosha and Dicer (Fig.1). Following transcription by RNA pol II, Drosha processes the primary miRNA transcript (pri-miRNA) into a 60–100 nt hairpin structure, termed the precursor miRNA (pre-miRNA), in the nucleus (Fig. 1). Following cleavage by Drosha, the pre-miRNA is transported out of the nucleus through an interaction with Exportin-5 and Ran-GTP. Then, the pre-miRNA undergoes further processing catalyzed by Dicer (Fig. 1). This cleavage event gives rise to an approximately 22 nt dsRNA product containing the mature miRNA guide strand and the miRNA* passenger strand (Fig. 1). Then, the mature miRNA guide strand is loaded onto the RISC, while the passenger strand is degraded (Fig. 1).

Although substantial progress has been made in understanding the basic mechanism of miRNA biogenesis, less is known about the mechanisms that regulate miRNA biogenesis and how these systems might be deregulated during oncogenesis. Several studies have reported that various regulatory mechanisms of miRNA biosynthesis are potentially involved in carcinogenesis.[69]

The tumor suppressor protein p53 was recently found to modulate miRNA processing through its association with p68 and Drosha.[70,71] Under conditions of DNA damage, several miRNAs, such as miR-143 and miR-16, are post-transcriptionally induced. This process requires p53, as p53-null HCT116 cells do not induce miRNAs in response to DNA damage.[72] Co-immunoprecipitation studies have indicated that p53 is present in a complex with both Drosha and p68, and the addition of p53 to *in vitro* pri-miRNA processing assays enhances the activity of Drosha. Interestingly, several p53 mutant-containing cells that are linked to oncogenesis have low post-transcriptional miRNA expression.[72]

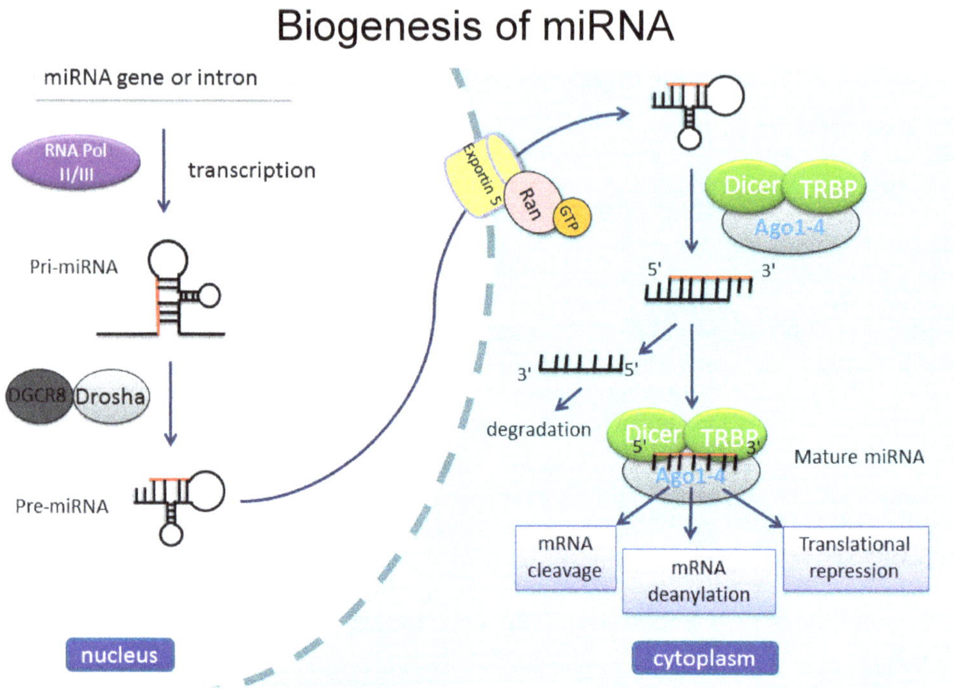

Fig. 1. Processing machinery of miRNA
miRNA genes are transcribed by RNA polymerase II or III into long primary (pri) miRNA transcripts, processed by the nuclear nuclease Drosha into ~60 bp hairpins termed precursor (pre) miRNAs, and further cleaved in the cytosol by the Dicer nuclease into mature miRNAs. Mature miRNAs are then incorporated into the multiprotein RNA-induced silencing complex (RISC), exerting post-transcriptional repression of target mRNAs, either by inducing mRNA cleavage, mRNA degradation or blocking mRNA translation.

4.2 Processing of EBV-encoded miRNAs

For EBV-encoded miRNAs, several regulatory processes have been reported[68]. Almost all of the EBV-encoded miRNAs originate from one of three sequence clusters. Two of the three clusters of miRNAs are made from the BARTs, a set of alternatively spliced transcripts that are highly abundant in NPC, but have not been shown to produce a detectable protein. Edwards et al. investigated the mechanism of BART-derived miRNA processing by comparing the processed miRNAs with the original BART transcript and residual transcripts after processing.[68] First, they showed that residual pieces of the intron sequence were detectable in the nucleus of cells that express the miRNAs. Characterization of these residual pieces indicated that the miRNAs were produced from one large initial transcript prior to splicing and that a specific spliced form of the transcript favored the production of miRNAs. Second, they found that miR-BART12 is not detected at all, even though the primary transcript is abundant. Third, pre-miR-BART5 could be detected in all cell lines and tumors tested, despite low or undetectable expression of the mature miR-BART5, indicating that the processing of pre-miR-BART5 was inhibited.

	function	target viral	Host target	
BLHF1-1	transformation	BFLF2	LILRB-5,E2F1,p53,CBFA2T2	BHRF1
BLHF1-2	transformation	BFLF2	PIK3R1	BHRF1
BLHF1-3	transformation	BFLF2	CXCL11,PRF1,TGIF,NSEP1	BHRF1
BART1-5p	Cancer development	LMP1	CXCL12	BART Cluster1
BART2-5p	viral replication	BALF5、LMP1	MIC B, Bim	
BART3		LMP1	IPO7, Bim	BART Cluster1
BART4		LMP1	Bim	BART Cluster1
BART5	Host cell survival	LMP1	PUMA, Bim	BART Cluster1
BART6	maintain viral latency	LMP1	Dicer, Bim	BART Cluster1
BART7		LMP1	Bim	BART Cluster2
BART8				BART Cluster2
BART9				BART Cluster2
BART10				BART Cluster2
BART11				BART Cluster2
BART12				BART Cluster2
BART13				BART Cluster2
BART14				BART Cluster2
BART15				BART Cluster1
BART16	Cancer development	LMP1	TOMM22	BART Cluster1
BART17	Cancer development	LMP1		BART Cluster1
BART18				BART Cluster2
BART19				BART Cluster2
BART20				BART Cluster2
BART21				BART Cluster2
BART22		LMP2		BART Cluster2

Table 1.

Amoroso et al. reported that the levels of the different BART miRNAs vary up to 50-fold within a given cell line.[73] However, this variation cannot be explained by differential miRNA turnover, as all EBV miRNAs appear to be remarkably stable, suggesting that miRNA maturation is a key step in regulating steady-state levels of EBV miRNAs. Future studies should further investigate the mechanism of miRNA transcript processing in EBV-infected cells, highlighting any differences between the three types of latent infections.

5. Secretory EBV-encoded miRNAs

5.1 Secretory miRNAs

Cellular and viral miRNAs control gene expression by repressing the translation of mRNAs into protein, a process that is tightly regulated in healthy cells, but is deregulated in cancerous and virus-infected cells. Curiously, miRNAs are not strictly intracellular, but are also secreted through the release of small vesicles called exosomes and, therefore, exist extracellularly in the peripheral blood and in cell culture media.[74] It has been suggested that exosome-associated miRNAs play a role in intercellular communication [74], although concrete evidence for this has been lacking. The dynamics of miRNA secretion via exosomes and the proposed transfer mechanisms remain poorly understood. In addition, it is unclear whether miRNAs are secreted in physiologically relevant amounts.

5.2 Existence of secretory EBV-encoded miRNAs

Pegtel et al. were the first to show that exosomes deliver viral miRNAs to non-infected cells.[75] They used EBV B95.8-immortalized LCLs and demonstrated that exosomes contained

BHRF1 miRNAs, which could target the *CXCL11/ITAC* gene in nearby uninfected cells. Furthermore, they showed that non-B cells in EBV-infected patients with elevated viral loads contained EBV miRNAs, demonstrating that exosomes apparently transfer miRNAs *in vivo* to uninfected cells. These findings were confirmed by two studies that demonstrated the release of exosomes from NPC cells. Gourzones et al. showed that EBV miR-BARTs present within exosomes can be detected in the serum of mice xenografted with human NPC cells and that the sera of NPC patients also contain BART miRNAs.[76]

6. Concluding remarks

EBV-related cancers are generally difficult to cure. Despite extensive studies based on well-known concepts and methods, the molecular basis by which EBV mediates tumorigenesis and eludes immunosurveillance remains unclear. Mouse models of EBV-mediated lymphoproliferative disease have recently revealed that EBV infection of B cells is necessary, but not sufficient, for tumorigenesis, as all peripheral mononuclear cells are needed to generate tumors in these mice.[77] Immune cells are also indispensable for EBV-mediated tumorigenesis . The relationship between these cells and EBV-infected cells with regard to tumorigenesis remains unclear. Moreover, the mechanism of drug resistance, which causes poor prognosis of EBV-related tumors, has not yet been elucidated. Therefore, it is important to study the tumor biology of EBV-related tumors from a fresh perspective, such as EBV-encoded miRNAs.

7. References

[1] Burkitt D. A sarcoma involving the jaws in African children. Br J Surg. 1958;46:218-223.

[2] Epstein MA, Achong BG, Barr YM. Virus Particles in Cultured Lymphoblasts from Burkitt's Lymphoma. Lancet. 1964;1:702-703.

[3] Henle G, Henle W. Immunofluorescence in cells derived from Burkitt's lymphoma. J Bacteriol. 1966;91:1248-1256.

[4] Fang W, Li X, Jiang Q, et al. Transcriptional patterns, biomarkers and pathways characterizing nasopharyngeal carcinoma of Southern China. J Transl Med. 2008;6:32.

[5] Young LS, Rickinson AB. Epstein-Barr virus: 40 years on. Nat Rev Cancer. 2004;4:757-768.

[6] Parkin DM, Bray F, Ferlay J, Pisani P. Global cancer statistics, 2002. CA Cancer J Clin. 2005;55:74-108.

[7] Parkin DM. The global health burden of infection-associated cancers in the year 2002. Int J Cancer. 2006;118:3030-3044.

[8] Borza CM, Hutt-Fletcher LM. Alternate replication in B cells and epithelial cells switches tropism of Epstein-Barr virus. Nat Med. 2002;8:594-599.

[9] Ghosh SK, Forman LW, Akinsheye I, Perrine SP, Faller DV. Short, discontinuous exposure to butyrate effectively sensitizes latently EBV-infected lymphoma cells to nucleoside analogue antiviral agents. Blood Cells Mol Dis. 2007;38:57-65.

[10] Thorley-Lawson DA. Epstein-Barr virus: exploiting the immune system. Nat Rev Immunol. 2001;1:75-82.

[11] Thorley-Lawson DA, Allday MJ. The curious case of the tumour virus: 50 years of Burkitt's lymphoma. Nat Rev Microbiol. 2008;6:913-924.

[12] Deyrup AT. Epstein-Barr virus-associated epithelial and mesenchymal neoplasms. Hum Pathol. 2008;39:473-483.
[13] Murray RJ, Kurilla MG, Brooks JM, et al. Identification of target antigens for the human cytotoxic T cell response to Epstein-Barr virus (EBV): implications for the immune control of EBV-positive malignancies. J Exp Med. 1992;176:157-168.
[14] Crumpacker CS. Ganciclovir. N Engl J Med. 1996;335:721-729.
[15] Jones K, Nourse J, Corbett G, Gandhi MK. Sodium valproate in combination with ganciclovir induces lysis of EBV-infected lymphoma cells without impairing EBV-specific T-cell immunity. Int J Lab Hematol;32:e169-174.
[16] He Y, Cai S, Zhang G, Li X, Pan L, Du J. Interfering with cellular signaling pathways enhances sensitization to combined sodium butyrate and GCV treatment in EBV-positive tumor cells. Virus Res. 2008;135:175-180.
[17] Westphal EM, Blackstock W, Feng W, Israel B, Kenney SC. Activation of lytic Epstein-Barr virus (EBV) infection by radiation and sodium butyrate in vitro and in vivo: a potential method for treating EBV-positive malignancies. Cancer Res. 2000;60:5781-5788.
[18] Shirley CM, Chen J, Shamay M, et al. Bortezomib induction of C/EBPbeta mediates Epstein-Barr virus lytic activation in Burkitt lymphoma. Blood. 2011;117:6297-6303.
[19] Taylor GM, Raghuwanshi SK, Rowe DT, Wadowsky R, Rosendorff A. ER-stress causes Epstein-Barr virus lytic replication. Blood. 2011.
[20] Fu DX, Tanhehco Y, Chen J, et al. Bortezomib-induced enzyme-targeted radiation therapy in herpesvirus-associated tumors. Nat Med. 2008;14:1118-1122.
[21] Wang X, Gu J, Zhang MQ, Li Y. Identification of phylogenetically conserved microRNA cis-regulatory elements across 12 Drosophila species. Bioinformatics. 2008;24:165-171.
[22] Chen K, Rajewsky N. The evolution of gene regulation by transcription factors and microRNAs. Nat Rev Genet. 2007;8:93-103.
[23] Pfeffer S, Zavolan M, Grasser FA, et al. Identification of virus-encoded microRNAs. Science. 2004;304:734-736.
[24] Grundhoff A, Sullivan CS, Ganem D. A combined computational and microarray-based approach identifies novel microRNAs encoded by human gamma-herpesviruses. RNA. 2006;12:733-750.
[25] Griffiths-Jones S, Grocock RJ, van Dongen S, Bateman A, Enright AJ. miRBase: microRNA sequences, targets and gene nomenclature. Nucleic Acids Res. 2006;34:D140-144.
[26] Kim do N, Chae HS, Oh ST, et al. Expression of viral microRNAs in Epstein-Barr virus-associated gastric carcinoma. J Virol. 2007;81:1033-1036.
[27] Rana TM. Illuminating the silence: understanding the structure and function of small RNAs. Nat Rev Mol Cell Biol. 2007;8:23-36.
[28] Xia T, O'Hara A, Araujo I, et al. EBV microRNAs in primary lymphomas and targeting of CXCL-11 by ebv-mir-BHRF1-3. Cancer Res. 2008;68:1436-1442.
[29] Barth S, Meister G, Grasser FA. EBV-encoded miRNAs. Biochim Biophys Acta. 2011.
[30] Tsurumi T, Daikoku T, Kurachi R, Nishiyama Y. Functional interaction between Epstein-Barr virus DNA polymerase catalytic subunit and its accessory subunit in vitro. J Virol. 1993;67:7648-7653.

[31] Barth S, Pfuhl T, Mamiani A, et al. Epstein-Barr virus-encoded microRNA miR-BART2 down-regulates the viral DNA polymerase BALF5. Nucleic Acids Res. 2008;36:666-675.
[32] Meister G, Landthaler M, Patkaniowska A, Dorsett Y, Teng G, Tuschl T. Human Argonaute2 mediates RNA cleavage targeted by miRNAs and siRNAs. Mol Cell. 2004;15:185-197.
[33] Iizasa H, Wulff BE, Alla NR, et al. Editing of Epstein-Barr virus-encoded BART6 microRNAs controls their dicer targeting and consequently affects viral latency. J Biol Chem. 2010;285:33358-33370.
[34] Khvorova A, Reynolds A, Jayasena SD. Functional siRNAs and miRNAs exhibit strand bias. Cell. 2003;115:209-216.
[35] Hislop AD, Taylor GS, Sauce D, Rickinson AB. Cellular responses to viral infection in humans: lessons from Epstein-Barr virus. Annu Rev Immunol. 2007;25:587-617.
[36] Pagano JS, Blaser M, Buendia MA, et al. Infectious agents and cancer: criteria for a causal relation. Semin Cancer Biol. 2004;14:453-471.
[37] Choy EY, Siu KL, Kok KH, et al. An Epstein-Barr virus-encoded microRNA targets PUMA to promote host cell survival. J Exp Med. 2008;205:2551-2560.
[38] Han J, Flemington C, Houghton AB, et al. Expression of bbc3, a pro-apoptotic BH3-only gene, is regulated by diverse cell death and survival signals. Proc Natl Acad Sci U S A. 2001;98:11318-11323.
[39] Nakano K, Vousden KH. PUMA, a novel proapoptotic gene, is induced by p53. Mol Cell. 2001;7:683-694.
[40] Yu J, Zhang L, Hwang PM, Kinzler KW, Vogelstein B. PUMA induces the rapid apoptosis of colorectal cancer cells. Mol Cell. 2001;7:673-682.
[41] Jeffers JR, Parganas E, Lee Y, et al. Puma is an essential mediator of p53-dependent and -independent apoptotic pathways. Cancer Cell. 2003;4:321-328.
[42] Villunger A, Michalak EM, Coultas L, et al. p53- and drug-induced apoptotic responses mediated by BH3-only proteins puma and noxa. Science. 2003;302:1036-1038.
[43] Hemann MT, Zilfou JT, Zhao Z, Burgess DJ, Hannon GJ, Lowe SW. Suppression of tumorigenesis by the p53 target PUMA. Proc Natl Acad Sci U S A. 2004;101:9333-9338.
[44] Erlacher M, Labi V, Manzl C, et al. Puma cooperates with Bim, the rate-limiting BH3-only protein in cell death during lymphocyte development, in apoptosis induction. J Exp Med. 2006;203:2939-2951.
[45] Nelson DA, Tan TT, Rabson AB, Anderson D, Degenhardt K, White E. Hypoxia and defective apoptosis drive genomic instability and tumorigenesis. Genes Dev. 2004;18:2095-2107.
[46] Rayet B, Gelinas C. Aberrant rel/nfkb genes and activity in human cancer. Oncogene. 1999;18:6938-6947.
[47] Lo AK, To KF, Lo KW, et al. Modulation of LMP1 protein expression by EBV-encoded microRNAs. Proc Natl Acad Sci U S A. 2007;104:16164-16169.
[48] Kelly GL, Long HM, Stylianou J, et al. An Epstein-Barr virus anti-apoptotic protein constitutively expressed in transformed cells and implicated in burkitt lymphomagenesis: the Wp/BHRF1 link. PLoS Pathog. 2009;5:e1000341.

[49] Seto E, Moosmann A, Gromminger S, Walz N, Grundhoff A, Hammerschmidt W. Micro RNAs of Epstein-Barr virus promote cell cycle progression and prevent apoptosis of primary human B cells. PLoS Pathog. 2010;6:e1001063.
[50] Bahram S, Bresnahan M, Geraghty DE, Spies T. A second lineage of mammalian major histocompatibility complex class I genes. Proc Natl Acad Sci U S A. 1994;91:6259-6263.
[51] Groh V, Bahram S, Bauer S, Herman A, Beauchamp M, Spies T. Cell stress-regulated human major histocompatibility complex class I gene expressed in gastrointestinal epithelium. Proc Natl Acad Sci U S A. 1996;93:12445-12450.
[52] Suarez-Alvarez B, Lopez-Vazquez A, Baltar JM, Ortega F, Lopez-Larrea C. Potential role of NKG2D and its ligands in organ transplantation: new target for immunointervention. Am J Transplant. 2009;9:251-257.
[53] Stern-Ginossar N, Elefant N, Zimmermann A, et al. Host immune system gene targeting by a viral miRNA. Science. 2007;317:376-381.
[54] Nachmani D, Stern-Ginossar N, Sarid R, Mandelboim O. Diverse herpesvirus microRNAs target the stress-induced immune ligand MICB to escape recognition by natural killer cells. Cell Host Microbe. 2009;5:376-385.
[55] Xing L, Kieff E. Epstein-Barr virus BHRF1 micro- and stable RNAs during latency III and after induction of replication. J Virol. 2007;81:9967-9975.
[56] Rani MR, Foster GR, Leung S, Leaman D, Stark GR, Ransohoff RM. Characterization of beta-R1, a gene that is selectively induced by interferon beta (IFN-beta) compared with IFN-alpha. J Biol Chem. 1996;271:22878-22884.
[57] Hutzinger R, Feederle R, Mrazek J, et al. Expression and processing of a small nucleolar RNA from the Epstein-Barr virus genome. PLoS Pathog. 2009;5:e1000547.
[58] Samarsky DA, Fournier MJ, Singer RH, Bertrand E. The snoRNA box C/D motif directs nucleolar targeting and also couples snoRNA synthesis and localization. EMBO J. 1998;17:3747-3757.
[59] Matera AG, Terns RM, Terns MP. Non-coding RNAs: lessons from the small nuclear and small nucleolar RNAs. Nat Rev Mol Cell Biol. 2007;8:209-220.
[60] Huttenhofer A, Brosius J, Bachellerie JP. RNomics: identification and function of small, non-messenger RNAs. Curr Opin Chem Biol. 2002;6:835-843.
[61] Huttenhofer A, Schattner P, Polacek N. Non-coding RNAs: hope or hype? Trends Genet. 2005;21:289-297.
[62] Huttenhofer A, Schattner P. The principles of guiding by RNA: chimeric RNA-protein enzymes. Nat Rev Genet. 2006;7:475-482.
[63] Li JB, Levanon EY, Yoon JK, et al. Genome-wide identification of human RNA editing sites by parallel DNA capturing and sequencing. Science. 2009;324:1210-1213.
[64] Yang W, Chendrimada TP, Wang Q, et al. Modulation of microRNA processing and expression through RNA editing by ADAR deaminases. Nat Struct Mol Biol. 2006;13:13-21.
[65] Kawahara Y, Zinshteyn B, Sethupathy P, Iizasa H, Hatzigeorgiou AG, Nishikura K. Redirection of silencing targets by adenosine-to-inosine editing of miRNAs. Science. 2007;315:1137-1140.
[66] Jia Y, Wang Y, Chao Y, Jing Y, Sun Z, Luo B. Sequence analysis of the Epstein-Barr virus (EBV) BRLF1 gene in nasopharyngeal and gastric carcinomas. Virol J. 2010;7:341.

[67] Suspene R, Aynaud MM, Koch S, et al. Genetic editing of herpes simplex virus 1 and Epstein-Barr herpesvirus genomes by human APOBEC3 cytidine deaminases in culture and in vivo. J Virol. 2011;85:7594-7602.

[68] Edwards RH, Marquitz AR, Raab-Traub N. Epstein-Barr virus BART microRNAs are produced from a large intron prior to splicing. J Virol. 2008;82:9094-9106.

[69] Davis BN, Hata A. microRNA in Cancer---The involvement of aberrant microRNA biogenesis regulatory pathways. Genes Cancer. 2010;1:1100-1114.

[70] Denli AM, Tops BB, Plasterk RH, Ketting RF, Hannon GJ. Processing of primary microRNAs by the Microprocessor complex. Nature. 2004;432:231-235.

[71] Shiohama A, Sasaki T, Noda S, Minoshima S, Shimizu N. Nucleolar localization of DGCR8 and identification of eleven DGCR8-associated proteins. Exp Cell Res. 2007;313:4196-4207.

[72] Suzuki HI, Yamagata K, Sugimoto K, Iwamoto T, Kato S, Miyazono K. Modulation of microRNA processing by p53. Nature. 2009;460:529-533.

[73] Amoroso R, Fitzsimmons L, Thomas WA, Kelly GL, Rowe M, Bell AI. Quantitative studies of Epstein-Barr virus-encoded microRNAs provide novel insights into their regulation. J Virol. 2010;85:996-1010.

[74] Kosaka N, Iguchi H, Ochiya T. Circulating microRNA in body fluid: a new potential biomarker for cancer diagnosis and prognosis. Cancer Sci. 2010;101:2087-2092.

[75] Pegtel DM, Cosmopoulos K, Thorley-Lawson DA, et al. Functional delivery of viral miRNAs via exosomes. Proc Natl Acad Sci U S A. 2010;107:6328-6333.

[76] Gourzones C, Gelin A, Bombik I, et al. Extra-cellular release and blood diffusion of BART viral micro-RNAs produced by EBV-infected nasopharyngeal carcinoma cells. Virol J. 2010;7:271.

[77] Kuppers R. Molecular biology of Hodgkin lymphoma. Hematology Am Soc Hematol Educ Program. 2009:491-496.

8

Systemic Mastocytosis: An Intriguing Disorder

Antonia Rotolo[1], Ubaldo Familiari[2], Paolo Nicoli[1], Daniela Cilloni[1], Giuseppe Saglio[1] and Angelo Guerrasio[1]
[1]M.D., Division of Hematology and Internal Medicine,
[2]M.D., Pathology Department,
Department of Clinical and Biological Sciences,
San Luigi Gonzaga Hospital, University of Turin, Turin,
Italy

1. Introduction

Systemic Mastocytosis (SM) is a mast cell (MC) neoplasm of the haematopoietic tissue. It is a rare disorder, but perhaps its prevalence is underestimated, as MC infiltrates may often be undetected. The aim of this chapter is to emphasize the importance of an active and careful work-up through multimodality approaches in order to achieve the diagnosis of SM. This might increase the incidence of SM. Moreover, it must be considered that SM is frequently associated with a second and, in rare cases, a third clonal blood disorder that isn't mast cell derived. Similar cases may be important for the correct initial evaluation and classification, as well as for a better risk stratification and management of patients with haematopoietic malignancies. Therapy could also improve, being personalized and tailored for each single SM patient.

2. Disease overview

Mastocytosis is a disorder characterised by clonal mast cells (MC) proliferation and accumulation. It has been described for the first time in 1869 by Nettleship and Tay as a form of urticaria resulting in a "brownish discoloration". Some years later Ehrlich used "mastzellen" to designate MC (Ehrlich, 1877). The term is derived from the German mästung, that means "to overfeed". In fact, the MCs have metachromatic properties that have been originally attributed to an excessive intake of aniline dye. In 1949 Ellis reported the first observation of MCs infiltrating visceral organs. Hence, several reports allowed standardizing the definition and classification of Mastocytosis.

According to the latest WHO classification Mastocytosis is a myeloproliferative neoplasm (MPN) (Vardiman, 2009). Clonal MCs proliferate, infiltrate and accumulate in skin and/or other organ systems. In Cutaneous Mastocytosis (CM) only skin is involved. In Systemic Mastocytosis (SM) at least one extracutaneous organ is infiltrated. This leads to a heterogeneous clinical presentation.

2.1 Epidemiology

Mastocytosis is a rare disorder. Several studies reported an incidence of 5-10 cases/10^6 people/year. However, there's a risk of underestimation due to the difficulty in getting a diagnosis. Recently Nowak et al. have published results of a monocentric retrospective study, reporting that in most patients mastocytosis was correctly diagnosed over a period of 2 years (up to 11 years in some cases), and often required consultation of three or more clinicians (Nowak, 2011). This was consistent with experiences reported by other authors. There are several possible explanations for such diagnostic delays. First, initial symptoms and signs are usually unspecific and overlap with many other diseases. For instance, at presentation some patients show neurological, psychological and psychiatric symptoms, leading to a misdiagnosis of somatoform disorder instead of mast cell syndrome (Amon, 2010). Second, morphological detection of pathological MCs is not obvious, mainly if they exhibit atypical features, such as hypogranulation or abnormal nuclear morphology (Pardanani, 2011). Moreover, as the second most frequent MC disorder is SM associated with haematological non mast cell disorder (SM-AHNMD), extensive bone marrow involvement by a second haematological neoplasm may obscure or distort MC aggregates (Horny, 2004), delaying or obviating at all the correct diagnosis. Taken together, these observations suggest that clinicians should become more confident with MC syndrome and MC disorders, as clinical suspicion should stimulate further appropriate immunochemical and molecular analysis. According to this, Horny proposed a novel routine approach, using antibodies against neoplastic MC markers in all bone marrow trephines presenting Myelodisplastic Syndrome, Acute Myeloid Leukemia and Chronic Myelomonocytic Leukemia (Horny, 2004).

Mastocytosis is more frequent in children, as CM. Adults represent one third of all cases and they are almost all affected by SM. There are no gender differences in incidence rate and clinical presentation. It can onset at any age, with an incidence peak in the first 2 years of life (Pardanani, 2011). Familiar cases have been occasionally observed. Survival is shorter in SM compared to the general population. However, patients classified according to the WHO 2008 system classification show great differences in demographical and clinical features, prognosis and survival (Lim, 2009). Nevertheless, quality of life is generally poor irrespective to subgroups.

3. Mast cells

Typical MCs are round or oval cells. Their size is small to medium, with a low nucleus/cytoplasm ratio. The nucleus is round or oval, in a central position, with condensed chromatin. The cytoplasm is large with plenty of metachromatic granules. However granules may also be few or lack at all, resulting in hypo-/de-granulated mast cells. Atypical MCs may present an oval nucleus and a hypogranulated cytoplasm. Generally they are spindle-shaped or with prominent projections on membrane surface and their nucleus is eccentric, sometimes with two or more lobes. Cells may appear more immature, with a large size, a high nucleus/cytoplasm ratio and a dispersed chromatin with nucleoli. The grade of immatureness may allow to the diagnosis of mast lineage blasts, characterized by the virtual absence of cytoplasm, with or without metachromatic granules, and fine chromatin with nucleoli.

3.1 Mast cell physiology

Mastocyte is a cell of the immune system. It derives from the haematopoietic stem cell. It is preferentially localized in the skin, respiratory and gastrointestinal mucosa.

MC growth, differentiation, proliferation, survival and activation are mediated by several factors The most important is SCF, that interacts with the tyrosine kinase receptor KIT (CD117 antigen). KIT is a key protein, either in normal or in clonal MCs, and its detection is essential in order to identify MCs and achieve the diagnosis of mastocytosis. Therefore, a multimodality approach should be routinely performed, including flow cytometry, immunochemistry and PCR (see below).

MCs play a main role in type I hypersensitivity reactions. Antigen-IgE complexes bind to the $Fc_{\varepsilon}RI$ on MC membrane and induce MC degranulation. Secretory granules contain histamine, tryptase, proteoglycans, TNF-α and other proteases. Tryptase is the most important mediator: it is virtually present in all MCs, therefore its expression on membrane surface identifies MCs, and serum levels may represent a useful marker of disease (see below).

After MC activation and degranulation, new phospholipid derived mediators are generated (e.g. leukotrienes, prostaglandins and PAF). The clinical manifestations are therefore heterogeneous and depend on the site of reaction. Atopic responses may vary in severeness between transient urticarial eruption and life-threatening anaphylactic shock. Several dermal inflammatory diseases are MC mediated, e.g. atopic dermatitis, bullous pemphigoid and psoriasis. However, MCs have also important physiological fuctions, as they are involved in antimicrobial defense, wound healing, angiogenesis, tumor surveillance and graft tollerance.

4. Pathogenesis

In more than 90% of affected adults a recurrent somatic mutation of *kit* can be detected (Garcia-Montero et al, 2006), suggesting that KIT plays a central role in autonomous proliferation of MC clone as well as in normal mastocytes (Orfao et al., 2007). Usually mutation occurs on exon 17 and results in a substitution of aspartic acid at codon 816 with valine. This mutation affects the tyrosine kinase TK2 domain and activates the receptor independently on ligand binding and dimerisation. According to its high occurrence, WHO diagnostic criteria for SM include *kit*D816V screening. Thus, it should be always investigated in bone marrow or blood or other organs when mastocytosis is suspected. Moreover, *kit*D816V represents an important prognostic factor and should be considered for planning and personalizing the therapeutic strategy.

The same mutation is less frequent in children, with an incidence of 42%. However, also most of the affected children share somatic *kit* point mutations that often involve exon 8 or 9, resulting in changes of the extracellular part of receptor (Bodemer, 2009).

Other mutations have been reported: they usually cluster at exon 11 or 17 affecting the juxtamembrane regulatory domain or TK2 enzymatic domain. Sometimes they've been reported at exons 2, 8, 9, 13 or 14 involving extracellular or TK1 domains. Interestingly, it has been observed a significant correlation between mutation type and disorder class. In fact, these specific genetic alterations have not been detected in different *kit* related neoplasms (e.g. GIST) and seem to be strictly associated with MC disorders (Orfao et al., 2007).

As *kit* is mutated in most patients without subgroup differences, the heterogeneous behaviour of each variant suggests that perhaps several different pathways may be involved in the pathogenesis and progression of the disease. Some authors have demonstrated that NF-κB and cyclin D3 may play a role. (Tanaka A, 2005). In addition, since a second haematological neoplasm is often associated with SM, the pathogenic mechanisms can be more difficult to understand.

Several studies suggests that mastocytosis is a haematopoietic stem cell disease (Horny, 2008). It can be hypothesized that *kit* mutation occurs at the level of leukaemia stem cell, the original clone that is responsible of leukaemia relapse. The occurrence of *kit* mutation confers either proliferative or mast cell lineage differentiative potential. Additional aberrations can then occur in the leukaemia stem cell, leading to the development of the associated myeloid neoplasm. Another possibility is the acquisition of *kit* mutation and transformation of a more mature leukaemia progenitor, resulting in the development of a synchronous mast cell malignancy (Pullarkat, 2003). Even less mature progenitors may be involved as also intra- and peri-lesional B and T cells have been demonstrated to carry the *kit*D816V point mutation. However, in SM patients without any associated clonal lymphoid disease most of the lymphocytes are reactive oligoclonal cells.

5. Clinical findings

Clinical features and course are variable, depending on the site and degree of infiltration and WHO subvariant.

Skin is often involved. Pruritus, erithema and orticarioid lesions usually occurs after mechanic irritation (Darier's sign). Hypercromic and infiltrated lesions affect body trunk, upper and lower limbs in 80% of adults, and head in all children. A frequent symptom is hypotension, often with headache and flushing, sometimes of high grade, resulting in syncope and shock. Diarrhoea is very common, with abdominal pain. Sometimes malabsorption cause a severe worseness of general conditions and must be considered clinically equivalent to organ damage. Bone is always involved: usually patients complain of bone pain, with signs of osteopenia, osteoporosis or atypical atraumatic fracture. Bone marrow infiltration may result in pancytopenia. Organomegaly, in particular enlargement of the lymph nodes, spleen and liver, may be present and causes organ damage (hepatic failure, low levels of albumin, etc.). Neuropsychiatric symptoms could be prevalent at diagnosis and they can be related to disfigurement in appearance: depression, suicide ideation, social and professional inefficiency have been reported (Amon, 2010). Risk of anaphylaxis is increased compared with health population, especially after a trigger exposition (physical exercise, psychic stress, alcohol, NSAID, infections and pregnancy) wich can result in MC activation. Based on this, it is recommended to perform a complete work-up after a first case of a severe anaphylactic reaction, especially in the absence of an evident trigger. Finally, there is a high risk of peptic ulcer. Patients must be closed monitored for all these symptoms in order to prevent complications and improve quality of life with anti-mediator drugs. Moreover, recording symptoms is a key part of staging, as established by WHO, and should drive the correct treatment choice and timing (WHO 2008).

Practically, two groups of clinical findings have been defined, the B and the C group. (Table 1). B stands for "burden of disease" and refers to symptoms that reflect the extension of disease. C stands for "cytoreduction requiring" and refers to signs of organ impairment indicating the need of therapy with cytostatic drugs.

C-findings are due to extensive MC infiltration, with direct organ damage and tissue destruction. The presence of at least one C-finding denotes a high grade disorder, referred as advanced systemic mastocytosis. After excluding any other causes of organ failure, cytoreduction must be considered. Symptoms due to MC infiltrates may be difficult to distinguish from indirect symptoms due to massive mediator release. When relationship between MC infiltration and organ impairment is not clear, patients must be closed monitored with serial dosages of serum tryptase level. An increase trend confirms the progression of the disease and the need of cytoreduction. CD30 expression may also be of help, since a strong positivity in most MCs denotes more likely ASM and MCL, while a weak positivity suggests a diagnosis of ISM. According to this, CD30 may perhaps become a useful tool in grading SM (Valent, 2010).

B-findings related to MC mediators	C-findings due to direct MC infiltration	Organ failure
1. **High MC burden**	**Organopathy**	
Marrow MCs > 30%		
Serum tryptase >200ng/ml		
2. **Dysmyelopoiesis**		
Hypercellular marrow with signs of myelodisplasia or myeloproliferation	Dysmyelopoiesis, with one or more peripheral cytopenias	Severe progressive pancytopenia
3. **Palpable Organomegaly**		
Hepatomegaly	Hepatomegaly with - ascites - abnormal liver function tests - portal hypertension	Progression to liver failure
Splenomegaly	Splenomegaly, with hypersplenism	
Lymph node enlargement	Bone lesions, with - osteolysis - osteoporosis and pathologic fractures	
	Malabsorption, with - hypoalbuminemia - weight loss.	

Table 1. Clinical findings (adapted from Valent *et al.*, 2001).

6. Diagnosis

Mastocytosis must be suspected.

WHO updated diagnostic criteria in 2008. The demonstration of neoplastic MC infiltrates in skin or extracutaneous organ is the *condition sine qua non*. The presence of typical MCs in dermal multifocal aggregates or diffusely infiltrating the skin allows the diagnosis of CM. The involvement of at least one visceral organ denotes SM. However, other criteria must be satisfied, i.e. clinical or biochemical, morphologic, immunophenotypic, molecular (Table 2). This is important to distinguish between any reactive MC proliferation and true clonal MC proliferation, that means Mast Cell Activation Syndrome (MCAS) from Mastocytosis.

Cutaneous mastocytosis (CM) usually presents as maculopapular infiltrates or diffuse erythrodermic rash, with thick skin or multiple nodules. Skin lesions must be biopsied to demonstrate the co-existence of pathological MCs.

The suspicion of mast cell syndrome without any cutaneous signs exclude the diagnosis of CM and requires bone marrow analysis to investigate the possible diagnosis of systemic mastocytosis (SM). Bone marrow biopsy and aspiration should always be performed in such cases as SM involves bone marrow in almost all affected patients. Other specimens may be obtained from other involved organs.

Pathological MCs infiltrates result as aggregates of at least 15 tryptase positive MCs. This is the first major criterion. The following diagnostic steps are BM smear evaluation, flow cytometry characterization and KIT mutational analysis. Finally serum tryptase levels must be dosed.

Cutaneous Mastocytosis	**Typical skin lesions**
• Clinical signs	- Maculopapular cutaneous mastocytosis - Diffuse cutaneous mastocytosis - Mastocytoma
• Microscopic findings	Multifocal or diffuse MC infiltrates
Systemic Mastocytosis	**SM criteria = 1 major + 1 minor or 3 minor criteria**
• Major criterion	Infiltrates of >15 aggregated MCs identified through tryptase immune-histochemistry or other stains in sections obtained from bone marrow or other extracutaneous organs
• Minor criteria	More than 25% spindle shaped MCs in histological sections or more than 25% atypical MCs in BM smear
	Detection of *kit* 816 mutation in BM or blood or any extracutaneous organ
	MC coexpression of CD25 and/or CD2 with CD117
	Serum tryptase levels > 20 ng/ml

Table 2. Proposed criteria to diagnose Mastocytosis (adapted from Valent *et al.*, 2001).

6.1 Histology

The typical histological mast cell lesion consists in focal typical and atypical MC aggregates infiltrating tissues. Giemsa or toluidine blue stains can reveal metachromatic granules, allowing discriminating between spindle mastocytes and fibroblasts.

Skin lesions are characterized by perivascular and periadnexal MC accumulation in upper dermis (Amon, 2010). In bone marrow compact infiltrates are perivascular, sharply demarcated from normal tissue, sometimes intermingled with macrophages and eosinophils. Spindle shaped MCs are often more than 25% of the total MCs. Rarely, infiltration is diffuse, with scattered cells that are difficult to recognize. In particular, in SM-AHNMD it is not unusual for the SM component to be unrecognized due to the extensive infiltration of bone marrow by the AHNMD component. This is commonly seen, for example, in SM-acute leukemia and SM with intense eosinophilic infiltration. Monotonous sheets of blasts may help to detect isolated clonal MCs (Horny, 2004). On the contrary, infiltration due to either reactive benign-looking lymphocytes or low grade lymphomatous cells is usually well defined and spindle mast cells cluster in different nodular lesions (Du, 2010). In some cases reactive well-differentiated lymphocytes have been reported to surround central aggregates of clonal mast cells or to be enclosed within malignant mast cells lesions (Kim, 2010). It must be clearly realized that MCs largely infiltrating malignant cells in haematopoietic disorders are clonal in most synchronous myeloid neoplasia, while they are reactive in all described lymphoid associated disorders so far reported. However, our group observed a case that may perhaps represent the first reported exception to this rule (see below).

Immunochemistry is important to recognize clonal MCs and get the right diagnosis. Spindle-shaped instead of round mast cells are more likely pathological and immunochemical reactions demonstrating co-expression of KIT, tryptase and CD25 enhance the probability of the clonal nature of the MCs (Pardanani et al., 2011).

6.2 Immunophenotyping

Flow cytometry represents the gold standard to identify, enumerate and characterise human MCs. The co-expression of CD2 and/or CD25 with CD117 is a minor WHO criterion to diagnose SM (Valent et al, 2010).

6.3 Molecular studies

Routine diagnostics should include the screening for *kit*D816V. Highly sensitive techniques (e.g. PCR) are recommended as the detection of this specific somatic mutation has been recognized as a valid minor diagnostic criterion by WHO system. *kit*D816V may be found also in myeloid and, less frequently, in lymphoid cells associated within the focal MC lesions, particularly in ASM and MCL. On the contrary, the same finding is rare in SM-AHNMD and depends on the concomitant disorder. In fact, the occurrence of *kit*D816V decreases through CMML, MPN, AML and lymphoproliferative disorders respectively.

Identification of different genetic abnormalities is not requested, since it does not have clinical relevance either for diagnosis or for therapy. However, in case of blood eosinophilia clinicians must consider screening for FIP1L1-PDGFRA fusion protein, since it predicts a great response to imatinib. Other rearrangements involving PDGFRB may be appropriately investigated through conventional cytogenetic analysis, allowing to the diagnosis of the entity defined by WHO as myeloid or lymphoid neoplasms with eosinophilia and abnormalities of PDGFRA, PDGFRB or FGFR1 (WHO 2008).

6.4 Biochemistry

Serum tryptase dosage and levels monitoring are a useful tools for diagnosis (WHO 2008) and follow-up, as they correlate with MC load and activation and disease progression (Pardanani, 2011). Elevated levels of serum tryptase (>20ng/ml) are consistent with the diagnosis, representing the fourth validated minor criterion to be evaluated according WHO system. Very high levels (>200ng/ml) correlate with more aggressive subvariants, severe course and poor prognosis. Anyway, serum tryptase levels are not clinically significant in case of a concomitant myeloid disorder as a proportion of patients affected by AML, CML and MDS usually show high levels of tryptase without any detectable MC disorder.

Serial dosages are recommended after anaphylactic or anaphylactoid episodes to distinguish between a transient elevation and an abnormal persistent increase. In addition, stable levels during follow up are consistent with stable disease (Quintas-Cardama et al., Cancer 2006).

6.5 Further considerations

SM diagnosis requires the presence of the major criterion together with one minor criterion or three isolated minor criteria (Table 2). Subvariants may be classified depending on the percentage of MCs in BM and PB smears and the clinical presentation. More than 20% MCs in BM smear denotes MCL, in the leukemic or aleukemic (more or less than 10% MC in PB smear) subvariants. Less than 20% MCs in BM smear connotes ISM in asymptomatic patients, SSM or ASM in patients suffering from B- or C-findings respectively.

A cytomorphological grading system has been also proposed (Valent et al., 2001). At BM smear analysis MCs may be typical or atypical. Atypical MCs are classified either type I or type II according to the nuclear feature, oval or bi-/polylobed respectively. The proportion of atypical MCs together with metachromatic blasts define the grade of the disorder: high grade > 20%, low grade < 10%, intermediate grade 10-20% MCs (Valent et al., 2001).

There are some peculiar conditions to be considered. First, sometimes a focal MC infiltrate is found without any MC related symptom or sign and coexists with normal skin and bone marrow, denoting a finding of MC tumour. If the growth pattern is destructive and the cytopathologycal grade is high, the diagnosis is of MC sarcoma. Otherwise, a low grade morphology and a respected tissue architecture denotes benign mastocytomas.

Second, MC aggregates may be scattered. This finding is often consistent with reactive MC hyperplasia and occasionally may be observed during the diagnostic approach for non MC haematologic diseases. A WHO entity is SM-AHNMD, where a myelo-/lymphoproliferative disorder coexists with a clonal MC growth. Myeloid neoplasms usually share the peculiar pattern of diffuse cells proliferation admixed with malignant mast cells, on the contrary lymphoid clones are clearly distinct, with a well-cut separation between the two clonal components, and generally the demonstration of SM in the bone marrow is an occasional histological finding in patients with a previous diagnosis of LNH in a lymph node (Schipper et al, 2011). Thus, a diffuse MC infiltration in the fields of LNH always suggests a reactive MC hyperplasia (Valent, 2001).

Also AHNMD is recommended to be investigated for biomolecular markers, in order to get a complete characterization and evaluate the event of therapeutic targets.

With regard to MCL, histology must refer to bone marrow areas away from spicules and the proportion of blasts must be cytomorphologically evaluated on the bone marrow smear. Thus histological detection of even more than 20% of blasts is not enough to make a diagnosis of MCL (Valent, 2010).

7. Classification and prognosis

MC disorders are classified in two groups: cutaneous and systemic. The former seems to have a good prognosis (Koga et al., 2011), the latter shows a poor prognosis. More precisely, in case of systemic involvement the observed survival is shorter than general population. The median overall survival is about 5 years (Pardanani et al., 2009), with excess deaths occurring between the third and the fifth year after diagnosis (Pardanani et al., 2011). However, prognosis is heterogeneous among SM subgroups and correlates with the WHO system. In fact, stratifying by the WHO classes, the Kaplan-Meier analysis allows distinguishing between an indolent and a rapidly progressive course. In the first case there is not a significant difference between affected patients and matched controls. By contrast, in the so-called aggressive forms median survival ranges between 2 and 41 months, depending on the variant (Pardanani et al. 2009).

7.1 CM

Cutaneous mastocytosis (CM) is a disorder characterized by accumulation of clonal mast cells isolated in the skin. Dermatologists are used to differentiate some clinical variants based on macroscopic presentation. Maculopapular Cutaneous Mastocytosis denotes the most frequent form, often described as urticaria pigmentosa (UP). It is the typical manifestation of CM, with disseminated small plaques. Sometimes lesions limits appear undefined and skin may be extensively involved, leading to the clinical condition referred as Diffuse Cutaneous Mastocytosis. Children rather than adults may carry a single blistering lesion known as solitary Mastocytoma, that generally goes to spontaneous regression with time. Other rare variants occur almost exclusively during childhood, with aspects of infiltration (bullae, plaques or nodules) or hyperpigmentation (Telangiectasia Macularis Eruptiva Perstans or TMEP) with or without erythema (Amon et al., 2010).

7.2 SM

Systemic mastocytosis (SM) is a disorder classified among Myeloproliferative Neoplasms by WHO in 2008. Unlike CM, clinical SM variants have been universally accepted and included in the international classification system since 2001. In addition, in 2010 Pardanani et al. published results of an observational study on 342 patients, leading to a formal validation of the WHO classification. Thus, SM subgroups are clinical evidence-based entities, with clear definition, characteristic features, definite prognosis and tailored management indications, beyond the clinical usage.

7.2.1 ISM

Indolent systemic mastocytosis (ISM) is the most frequent variant in adults (46%). Patients are young (median age 49) and usually show urticarioid skin lesions, gastrointestinal symptoms and MC mediator related syndrome. Almost all affected patients show bone marrow involvement, but no B- nor C- findings. Prognosis is very good, life expectancy is similar to general population, but quality of life is definitely poor. No progression risk has been observed, thus no cytoreduction has to be considered and only management of symptoms is needed (Valent et al., 2010).

7.2.2 SSM

Smoldering systemic mastocytosis is a recent subvariant of ISM. B-findings are always present, C-findings never. It is defined by high burden of MC (tryptase levels more than 200 ng/mL), enlarged spleen and/or lymph nodes, multilineage myelodysplasia or myeloid proliferation in the absence of diagnostic criteria for MDS, MPD, LMMC or AML. c-kit D816V should be detected in at least one non MC lineage. 14% of the patients with ISM are SSM affected individuals. They are older than typical ISM variant. Constitutional symptoms are almost constant. 23% patients are affected by a subvariant defined by isolated bone marrow involvement (BMM, Bone Marrow Mastocytosis), often associated with severe MC mediators related syndrome, including anaphylaxis. Prognosis is good, expected survival is even more than ten years, so symptomatic treatment may be enough. However, it must be stated that median survival is significantly inferior in SSM than in ISM (120 *versus* 301 months respectively). Moreover, there is an up to 18% risk of progression to aggressive subvariants as ASM, MCL and SM-AHNMD. Thus, patients must be strictly monitored, in order to switch to a cytoreductive therapeutic program if required. Cytoreduction is indicated even in absence of aggressive SM variants, if tryptase reach levels greater than 1000 ng/mL or symptoms show a worsening trend. Also, recurrent anaphylaxis unresponsive to immunotherapy or without specific IgE suggests that splenectomy or cytoreduction are needed for a better control of MC burden. This is in order to prevent a severe adverse event, as well as in myeloproliferative disorders hydroxyurea is administered to prevent deep venous thrombosis/pulmonary embolism (Valent et al., 2010).

7.2.3 ASM

Aggressive systemic mastocytosis is less frequent (12%) and occurs generally in adults. It is defined by the presence of at least one C-finding, associated with constitutional symptoms and visceromegaly, particularly of liver, spleen and lymph nodes. Prognosis is poor, with an overall median survival of 41 months. Leukemic transformation occurs in 5% of the patients. Affected patients must be always treated. Treatment depends on clinical course. According to time to progression, patients should be stratified in slowly and rapidly progressing. In the first case the natural history is similar to SSM. In the second case the disease is difficult to control and its behavior is similar to MCL: early blasts may increase, satisfying diagnostic criteria for leukemia. In addition, in some *kit*D816V patients the same mutation may become undetectable with progression. This is somewhat similar to disease progression in acute myeloid leukemia. In slowly progressing ASM milder therapeutic options may be considered, while rapidly progressing ASM always requires heavy chemotherapeutic approaches, according to the rapid multiorgan failure occurring in such patients. Tryptase levels usually increase every day, reflecting the poor clinical course (Valent et al., 2010).

7.2.4 MCL

Mast cell leukemia is the most rare variant, virtually limited to adulthood. In Pardanani's analysis it occurred in 1% of the patients. Median survival is 2 months. Usually MC blasts infiltrate extensively BM, with a range of 60-90%. High intensity chemiotherapy has to be administered, but patients generally result refractory (Valent et al., 2010).

7.2.5 SM-AHNMD

Systemic mastocytosis with an associated non-mast cell lineage disease (SM-AHNMD) is an heterogeneous and intriguing group of haematological malignancies, in which clonal proliferation of mast cells is associated with a second and, in rare cases, a third (Kim, 2010) clonal blood disorder that is not mast cell derived (Horny, 2008; Pardanani, 2010).

SM-AHNMD accounts for 40% of all cases of SM. About 89% of the patients show concomitant myeloid neoplasms: MPN (45%), CMML (29%) and MDS (23%). Among MPN, there is a high prevalence FIP1L1-PDGFRA related HES. In the remaining cases (21%) SM is associated with lymphoma, myeloma, CLL or amyloidosis. Prognosis is poor, with a median overall survival of 31 months in patients with MPN compared to 15, 13 and 11 months in patients with CMML, MDS and AML respectively. Transformation in MC leukemia occurs more frequently in SM-MDS (29%) (Pardanani, 2010).

WHO diagnostic criteria for SM remain valid, except for elevated serum tryptase levels, as they could be very high also in patients affected by AML, MDS and MPS without MC disorders.

The pathogenesis is not clear: in SM associated with myeloid malignancies mast cells and myeloid cells seem to originate from the same clone (Pardanani, 2009; Garcia-Montero 2006); according to this, in SM-LMMC *kit*D816V has been shown in both components. However, in SM-AML the leukemic counterpart generally lacks of *kit* mutation, suggesting a different origin for the two clones. At the opposite, in SM associated with lymphoid proliferative disease a distinct clonal origin has been demonstrated at least in some cases (Kim, 2007). Moreover, it has been hypothesized that malignant mast cells may support and promote the growth of the associated lymphoid disorder (Merluzzi, 2010).

Lymphoid proliferation as AHNMD component has been rarely observed. More precisely, B cell lymphomas associated with SM usually are low grade. To the best of our knowledge, the occurrence of SM and synchronous high grade lymphoma has been reported so far only by Schipper *et al.*, which described a case of SM associated with diffuse large B cell lymphoma (SM-DLBCL) (Schipper, 2011). Interestingly, we observed another patient, which is unlike to represent an accidental case. In our patient the diagnosis of mast cell disease was made concurrently with that of lymphoma, but we cannot state whether both the malignancies were synchronous or occurred at different time. In addition, the morphological evaluation of the bone marrow revealed a peculiar pattern of diffuse large B-cells proliferation admixed with malignant mast cells (fig. 1). Compared to what we observed, in Schipper *et al.* reported a sharp separation between the two clonal components, with the histological demonstration of SM in the bone marrow and DLBCL in a lymph node at different time. According to typical morphological findings, mastocytes appeared either solitary or clustered in a separate contest from malignant B cell. By contrast, our case of SM with concurrent large cell lymphoma seems to be unusual because of the great overlap between the two clonal populations of large B lymphocytes and mastocytes. Indeed, in our case, the lymphoid component resulted histologically atypical and new, as diffusely infiltrating within the malignant proliferating mast cells.

As expected, our case was positive for the D816V mutation in exon 17 like the vast majority of SM. Unfortunately, we do not know whether this mutation occurred also in clonal B cells, since they were not sorted from bone marrow specimen for DNA extraction. Therefore it is not possible to rule out any hypothesis about the pathogenesis of such an association.

On the therapeutical side, in SM-AHNMD it is recommended to treat SM as pure SM and AHNMD as pure AHNMD (Valent, 2003; Valent 2010). Accordingly, it is important a complete molecular characterization of both the disorders (Valent et al., 2010).

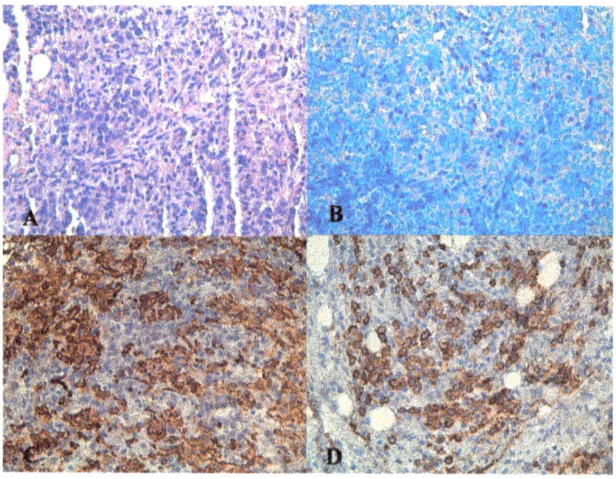

Fig. 1. **A-B** Bone marrow sections stained with haematoxylin and eosin (A) and Giemsa (B), 40x. **C-D** Immunohistochemistry on bone marrow sections with antibodies against tryptase to detect mast cells (C) and antibodies against CD79a to detect B lymphocytes (D), 40x. A great overlap between lymphocytes and mast cells lesions is observed, resulting in a diffuse proliferation of B-cells admixed with mast cells.

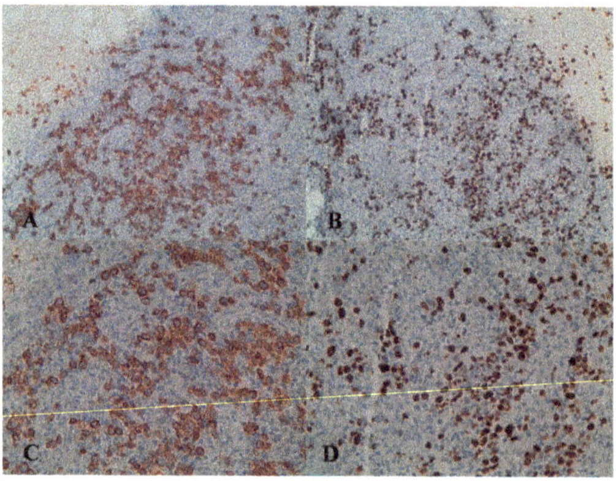

Fig. 2. Immunoperoxidase staining detecting large B lymphocytes, positive for CD79a (A, 20x; C, 40x) and exhibiting nuclear Ki-67 reactivity (B, 20x; D, 40x).

8. Treatment

To date Mastocytosis is incurable, thus clinicians should personalize treatment for each patients in order to reduce symptoms and complications (Molderings et al., 2011).

Exposition to triggers (animal venoms, extreme temperatures, mechanical irritation, alcohol, medications, etc.) should be avoided, but often no clear trigger may be identified, therefore active therapy must be considered (Valent et al., 2010).

Treatment in Mastocytosis may be symptomatic or cytoreductive. Symptoms could be managed with both non specific and tailored drugs. Cytoreduction should be considered if symptoms are refractory to basic therapy, rapidly worsening or life-threatening, or in the presence of complications (C-finding).

In summary, in CM and ISM therapeutic approach may be just symptomatic. In advanced forms of SM schedules must be personalized, depending on progression risk. In SSM and slowly progressing ASM IFNα and 2CdA may be appropriated. In rapidly progressing ASM, MCL and SM-AHNMD high intensity chemotherapy and allogeneic bone marrow transplantation represent the current therapeutic approach.

8.1 Symptomatic treatment

The so-called basic therapy consists in antihistaminic medications and MC membrane stabilizers. Usually relief occurs many days or weeks after the introduction of a new drug, therefore the persistence of symptoms does not justify an earlier shift to others therapeutic schedules. As each new drug can trigger a hypersensitive reaction, one drug at a time should be introduced (Quintas-Cardama et al., 2006).

When first line fails, immunomodulating agents may be considered, such as prednisone, cyclosporine, methotrexate, and azathioprine (Quintas-Cardama et al., 2006). IFNα might be combined with prednisone, but it generally represents the first line agent for cytoreduction in ASM.

Omalizumab, a humanized murine antibody targeted to IgE, is now available as an experimental option (Quintas-Cardama et al., 2006). It seems to control MC activation syndrome also in patients resistant to conventional fist line therapy. Recently, Molderings *et al.*, reporting their experience in four patients, showed its good risk-benefit profile. Two patients benefit a rapid remission, the third had a progressive improvement, only the fourth suffered from a worsening in MC-mediators syndrome (Molderings et al., 2011). Such isolated experience suggests that omalizumab could represent a new promising option.

Epinephrine on demand remains the gold standard during life-threatening anaphylactic or anaphylactoid episodes.

8.2 Cytoreductive treatment

Cytoreduction consists in single (IFNα and 2CdA) or multidrug (Fludarabine, Cytarabine, Mitoxantrone) approaches.

Usually IFNα represents the first line of treatment in slowly progressing variants. Cladribine is the second line, sometimes associated with novel agents (e.g. Imatinib).

In rapidly progressing variants Mito FLAG must be considered, with or without a previous treatment with 2CdA, in order to perform HSCT as soon as possible. In these cases BMT represents the only effective strategy to cure mastocytosis. If patient is ineligible, experimental trials remain the next option. Palliation is the last choice.

8.3 Novel agents

8.3.1 Tyrosine kinase inhibitors

Tyrosine kinase inhibitors have been under investigation since several years, particularly imatinib, dasatinib and midostaurin. Some clinical trials have been performed and many reports have been described. Target therapy has been observed to reduce both MC proliferation and infiltration, and sometimes to normalize BM histology. However, mediators related syndrome improved or got complete remission just in isolated reports.

8.3.1.1 Imatinib

Among the TK inhibitors, Imatinib is the most studied molecule. Low doses of Imatinib can inhibit wild type KIT. However, since D816V alters the kinase domain conformation, inhibiting steric interaction between the drug and the TK domain, efficacy of imatinib on *kit*D816V SM is still controversial. A phase II study conducted by Vega-Ruiz *et al.*, showed that imatinib has no significant clinical activity in patients carrying the D816V mutation. By contrast, in a different phase II trial Droogendij *et al.* observed an apparent remission in 11 *kit*D816V positive SMs (Droogendij et al., 2006). Some authors underline that concomitant use of prednisone may perhaps justify their results (Vega-Ruiz et al., 2009). Nevertheless, in some of these patients the observed reduction of symptoms was only transient. The case of SM with wild type kit or other sporadic mutations is different, since the conformational structure of the TK domain does not seem to be impaired. Moreover, these patients usually show an objective response, consisting in reduction of seric tryptase levels and bone marrow MC percentage (Vega-Ruiz, 2009). In summary, on one hand available data seem to suggest that imatinib is active against sporadic *kit* mutations, on the other hand the activity on *kit*D816V is not well established yet. Accordingly, in 2006 FDA approved the use of imatinib in adults with ASM without the D816V mutation.

Imatinib is also a potent competitive inhibitor of PDGFR and has been demonstrated to be either active or effective in FIP1L1/PDGFRA related HES. Consequently, SM patients with blood eosinophilia are recommended to be screened for this fusion protein. However, cardiogenic shock has been reported in patients with HES after the start of therapy with imatinib. Such an adverse event could be easily avoided by concomitant administration of corticosteroids during the first one or two weeks of treatment, mostly in case of echocardiographic abnormalities or high serum troponin levels at baseline.

Nilotinib is another TK inhibitor that has shown an in vitro activity against *kit* similar to imatinib, but no clinical experiences have been reported yet (Quintas-Cardama et al., Cancer 2006).

8.3.1.2 Dasatinib

Dasatinib is a dual SRC/ABL kinase inhibitor that is more potent than imatinib also against KIT. Preliminary data from either preclinical or clinical studies seemed to suggest a key role in SM, independently on mutational state of *kit* (Shah et al., 2006). However, data are too limited to draw any conclusion and the efficacy of dasatinib still remains controversial. Some authors described long lasting histological responses (Verstovsek et al, 2007) and both groups of patients with wild type and *kit*D816V improved in symptoms and quality of life. Wild type kit and *kit*D816V improved in symptoms and quality of life. It has been proposed a weekly dose escalation from 20 mg QD up to 100 mg QD during the first month of therapy (Rondoni et al., 2007). The proportion of responses may increase administering a dose of 120 mg QD in case of suboptimal or no response after three months of therapy. Based on this, the GIMEMA group is conducting an Italian multicenter phase II study in which subjects with SM are treating with a continuous regimen of dasatinib at a starting dose of 20 mg once daily. The primary endpoint is the evaluation of clinical response in terms of proportion of subjects experiencing a regression in B/C findings and mediator-related symptoms. The secondary endpoints include duration of response, progression free survival and time to response (GIMEMA, 2008).

8.3.1.3 Midostaurin

Midostaurin is a multi-kinase inhibitor with a demonstrated *in vitro* activity against KIT, but there are only sporadic observations of effectiveness *in vivo*. Gotlib *et al.* reported a case of MCL associated with MDS/MPD who received a transient benefit from administration of midostaurin (Gotlib et al., 2005). More interestingly, midostaurin seems to exhibit a synergic activity with nilotinib (Quintas-Cardama et al., 2006), suggesting a more attracting role of these small molecules, as useful tools to combine in multidrug strategies in order to avoid the resistance to single agent approaches.

8.3.1.4 Other TK inhibitors

Several more small molecules have been identified as potential agents against MC diseases: e.g. ATP analogs (OSI-930, MLN518, PD180970, PD180970, PD173955, AP23464 and AP23848), indolinone-based products (SU11652, SU11654 and SU11655) or quinoxaline derivatives (AGL2043). To date there are no data on clinical tolerability and efficacy yet (Quintas-Cardama et al., 2006).

8.3.2 Monoclonal antibodies

Monoclonal antibodies might play a crucial role in the future. The antiCD25 antibody conjugated with the pseudomonas exotoxin-A generates a potent immunotoxin with proapoptotic activity, associated with a significant reduction in the number of MCs (Valent et al., 2004). The effect is similar to that reported by other authors after in vitro exposure to Ontak, also known as denileukin diftitox, consisting in recombination of CD25 ligand and diphtheria toxin. Based on data on Ontak preclinical activity as well as clinical effectiveness in cutaneous T-cell lymphoma, there are ongoing phase II trials to test Ontak also in SM patients.

Other monoclonal antibodies are under investigation in Mastocytosis: the antiCD25 Daclizumab and Basiliximab, the antiCD33 Gemtuzumab with the toxic compound calicheamicin and the antiCD87 and antiCD45 antibodies, conjugated to $_{131}$I radioisotope or diphtheria toxin (Quintas-Cardama et al., Cancer 2006).

8.3.3 mTor inhibitors

mTor inhibitors have been tested since it has been demonstrated, both *in vitro* and *in vivo,* that the mTor pathway is active in SM and contributes to MC survival, growing and proliferation (Kim et al, 2008). Preclinical observations suggest that mTor inhibitors act against clonal MCs. Particularly, rapamycin inhibits selectively the mTor pathway, either in fresh MCs collected from KITD816V patients or in KITD816 cell lines. Hence, everolimus was tested in a clinical trial, but it did not show any apparent significant effectiveness. Perhaps some more experiences must be collected to determine whether mTor inhibitors may play any role in SM (Quintas-Cardama et al., 2006).

8.3.4 Future perspectives in SM therapy

Apoptosis still remains an attractive way to be investigated. Several drugs have shown some activity on Bcl-2 family members, as bortezomib, obatoclax and geldanamycin. The first one acts promoting Bim expression, the second one is known as BH3-mimetic (Aichberger et al., 2009), the last one inhibits the hsp90-bcl2 complex (Quintas-Cardama et al., 2006).

9. Conclusion

SM is a rare disorder, but its prevalence might be underestimated. Afar from drafting a complete and exhaustive review on mastocytosis, the aim of this chapter was to remark the relevance of SM. Clinical suspicion is really important and multimodality approaches must be considered to get the right diagnosis. Then, treatment must be personalized for each patient, accordingly with a careful and complete characterization of the disease.

Prospectively, two major challenges still have to be faced in SM research: first, the molecular and cellular pathogenesis; second, the definition of new strategies of treatment. About the former goal, we do believe that reporting new cases may be of great usefulness and is needed to better understand the nature of the disorder. In order to this, the case we described may perhaps represent a paradigmatic example. Referring to treatment, several novel agents are under investigation. However, preliminary clinical data seem to suggest that the use of a single drug may be insufficient. That means that a multidrug strategy is needed within a multitarget approach.

10. References

Aichberger, KJ.; Gleixner, KV.; Mirkina, I.; Cerny-Reiterer, S.; Peter, B.; Ferenc, V.; Kneidinger, M.; Baumgartner, C.; Mayerhofer, M.; Gruze, A.; Pickl, W F.; Sillaber, C. & Valent, P. (2009) Identification of proapoptotic Bim as a tumor suppressor in neoplastic mast cells: role of KIT D816V and effects of various targeted drugs, *Blood*, vol.114, no.26, pp.5342-5351, doi: 10.1182/blood-2008-08-175190

Amon, U.; Hartmann, K.; Horny, HP. & Nowak, A. (2010) Mastocytosis – an update *JDDG*; Vol.8, pp.695–712, DOI: 10.1111/j.1610-0387.2010.07482.x

Bodemer, C.; Hermine, O.; Palmérini, F.; Yang, Y.; Grandpeix-Guyodo, C.; Leventhal, PS.; Hadj-Rabia, S.; Nasca, L.; Georgin-Lavialle, S.; Cohen-Akenine, A.; Launay, JM.; Barete, S.; Feger, F.; Arock, M.; Catteau, B.; Sans, B.; Stalder, JF.; Skowron, F.; Thomas, L.; Lorette, G.; Plantin, P.; Bordigoni, P.; Lortholary, O.; de Prost, Y.;

Moussy, A.; Sobol, H.& Dubreuil, P. (2010) Pediatric mastocytosis is a clonal disease associated with D816V and other activating c-KIT mutations. *J Invest Dermatol*, Vol.130, pp.804–15.

González de Olano D, Alvarez-Twose I, Esteban-López MI, Sánchez-Muñoz L, de Durana MD, Vega A, García-Montero A, González-Mancebo E, Belver T, Herrero-Gil MD, Fernández-Rivas M, Orfao A, de la Hoz B & Castells MC, Escribano L. (2008) Safety and effectiveness of immunotherapy in patients with indolent systemic mastocytosis presenting with Hymenoptera venom anaphylaxis. *J Allergy Clin Immunol.* Vol.121(2), pp.519-526

Droogendijk. HJ.; Kluin-Nelemans, HJC.; van Doormaal, JJ.; Oranje, AR.; van de Loosdrecht, AA. & van Daele PLA (2006) Imatinib mesylate in the treatment of systemic mastocytosis - A phase II trial. *Cancer*, Vol.107, pp.345-351.

Du, S.; Rashidi, HH.; Le, DT.; Kipps, TJ.; Broome, HE. & Wang, HY. (2010) Systemic Mastocytosis in association with chronic lymphocytic leukaemia and plasma cell myeloma. *Int J Clin Exp Pathol*, Vol.3, No.4, pp.448-457.

Ehrlich P. (1877) Berträge zur Kenntnis der anilifarbungen und ihrer Verwendung in der microscopischem Technik. *Arch. Mikros. Anat.* Vol.13, pp.163-77.

Ellis, JM. (1949) Urticaria pigmentosa: a report of a case with autopsy. *AMA Arch Pathol,* Vol.48(5) , pp. 426–435.

Garcia-Montero, AC.; Jara-Acevedo, M.; Teodosio, C.; Sanchez, ML.; Nunez, MR.; Prados, A., Aldanondo, I.; Sanchez, L.; Dominguez, M.; Botana, LM.; Sanchez-Jimenez, F.; Sotlar, K.; Almeida, J.; Escribano, L. & Orfao, A. (2006) KIT mutation in mast cells and other bone marrow hematopoietic cell lineages in systemic mast cell disorders: a prospective study of the Spanish Network on Mastocytosis (REMA) in a series of 113 patients, *Blood,* Vol.108, pp.2366-2372, DOI 10.1182/blood-2006-04-015545

Gotlib, J.; Berube, C.; Growney, JD.; Chen, CC.; George, TI.; Williams, C.; Kajiguchi, T.; Ruan, J.; Lilleberg, SL.; Durocher, JA.; Lichy, JH.; Wang, Y.; Cohen, PS.; Arber, DA.; Heinrich, MC.; Neckers, L.; Galli, SJ.; Gilliland, DG. & Coutre SE. (2005) Activity of the tyrosine kinase inhibitor PKC412 in a patient with mast cell leukemia with the D816V KIT mutation. *Blood*. Vol.106, pp.2865–2870.

Gotlib J, George TI, Corless C, Linder A, Ruddell A, Akin C, DeAngelo DJ, Kepten I, Lanza C, Heinemann H, Yin O, Gallagher N, Graubert T (2008) The Kit tyrosine kinase inhibitor midostaurine (PKC412) exhibits a high response rate in aggressive systemic mastocytosis (ASM): interim results of a phase II trial. *Blood,* Vol.110, No. 11, pp.3536, ISSN 0006-4971.

Hissard, R.; Moncourier, L. & Jacquet, J. (1951) Study of a case of mastocytosis, *Ann Med Interne (Paris),* Vol.52, No.6, pp. 583-607.

Horny, HP.; Sotlar, K.; Sperr, WR. & Valent, P. (2004) Systemic mastocytosis with associated clonal haematological non-mast cell lineage, diseases: a histopathological challenge. *J Clin Pathol,* Vol.57, pp.604–608.

Horny, HP.; Sotlar, K. & Valent P. (2007) Mastocytosis: state of the art. *Pathobiology*, Vol.74, pp.121–32.

Horny, HP.; Sotlar, K.; Valent, P. & Hartmann, K. (2008) Mastocytosis. A disease of the Hematopoietic Stem Cell. *Dtsch Arztebl Int.*, Vol.105, No.40, pp.686–692. doi:10.3238/arztebl2008.0686

Kim Y, Weiss L, Chen Y & Pullarkat V (2007) Distinct clonal origins of systemic mastocytosis and associated B-cell lymphoma *Leukemia* Research Vol.31, No.12, pp.1749-1754.

Kim, MK.; Kuehn, HS.; Metcalfe, DD. & Gilfillan, AM. (2008) Activation and Function of the mTORC1 Pathway in Mast Cells *J Immunol*, Vol.180, pp.4586-4595.

Koga, H.; Kokubo, T.; Akaishi, M.; Iida, K. and Korematsu, S. (2011) Neonatal Onset Diffuse Cutaneous Mastocytosis: A Case Report and Review of the Literature *Pediatric Dermatology* Vol.28,No.5, pp.542–54

Metcalfe, DD. (2008) Mast cells and mastocytosis. *Blood,* Vol.112, pp.946–56

Merluzzi, S.; Frossi, B.; Gri, G.; Parusso, S.; Tripodo, C.; & Pucillo, C. (2010), Mast cells enhance proliferation of B lymphocytes and drive their differentiation toward IgA-secreting plasma cells *Blood;* Vol.115, No.14, pp.2810-2817.

Middelkamp Hup, MA.; Heide, R.; Tank, B.; Mulder, PGH. & Oranje, AP. (2002) Comparison of mastocytosis with onset in children and adults *Journal of the European Academy of Dermatology and Venereology,* Vol.16, No.2, pp.115–120. doi:10.1046/j.1468-3083.2002.00370.x

Molderings, GJ.; Brettner, S.; Homann, J.; Afrin, LB. (2011) Mast cell activation disease: a concise practical guide for diagnostic workup and therapeutic options. *Journal of Hematology & Oncology,*4:10, available from http://www.jhoonline.org/content/4/1/10

Molderings, GJ.; Raithel, M.; Kratz, F.; Azemar, M.; Haenisch, B.; Harzer. S. & Homann, J. (2011) Omalizumab treatment of systemic mast cell activation disease: experiences from four cases. *Intern Med.* Vol.50, No.6, pp.611-5

Nettleship, E. &Tay, W.(1869) Rare forms of urticaria. *Br Med J,* Vol.2, pp.323-330.

Nowak, A.; Gibbs, BF. & Ulrich Amon, U. (2011) Pre-inpatient evaluation on quality and impact of care in systemic mastocytosis and the influence of hospital stay periods from the perspective of patients: a pilot study JDDG. *Journal der Deutschen Dermatologischen Gesellschaft* Vol.9, No.7, pp.525–532. doi: 10.1111/j.1610-0387.2011.07638.x

Orfao, A., Garcia-Montero, AC.; Sanchez, L. & Escribano, L for the Spanish Network on Mastocytosis (REMA) (2007) Recent advances in the understanding of mastocytosis: the role of KIT mutations, *British Journal of Haematology,* Vol.138, pp.12–30, doi:10.1111/j.1365-2141.2007.06619.x

Pardanani, A.; Kim, KH.; Lasho, TL.; Finke, C.; McClure, RF.; Li, CY. & Teffery, A. (2009) Prognostically relevant breakdown of 123 patients with systemic mastocytosis associated with other myeloid malignancies. *Blood,* Vol.114, pp.3769-3772.

Pardanani A, Tefferi A. Proposal for a revised classification of systemic mastocytosis (2010) *Blood* Vol.115, No.13, pp.2720-1.

Pardanani, A (2011) Systemic mastocytosis in adults: 2011. update on Diagnosis, Risk-stratification and Management, *American Journal of Hematology,* Vol.86, No.4, pp.362–371

Parikh, SA.; Kantarjian, HM.; Richie, MA.; Cortes, JE.& Verstovsek, S (2010) Experience with everolimus (RAD001), an oral mammalian target of rapamycin inhibitor, in patients with systemic mastocytosis. *Leuk Lymph,* Vol.51,pp.269-274.

Quintas-Cardama, A.; Aribi, A.; Cortes, J.; Giles, F.J.; Kantarjian, H. & Verstovsek, S. (2006) Novel Approaches in the Treatment of Systemic Mastocytosis, *Cancer,* Vol.107, No.7, pp. 1429-39 doi: 10.1002/cncr.22187

Rondoni, M.; Paolini, S.; Colarossi, S.; Piccaluga, PP.; Papayannidis, C.; Palandri, F.; Laterza, C.; De Rosa F.; Pregno, P.; Gatto, S.; Ottaviani, E.; Saglio, G.; Cilloni, D.; Pane, F.; Triggiani, M.; Soverini, S., Zaccaria, A.; Baccarani, M & Martinelli G. (2007) Response to Dasatinib in Patients with Aggressive Systemic Mastocytosis with D816V Kit Mutation. *ASH Annual Meeting Abstracts* 2007 110: 3562.

Schipper, EM.; Posthuma, W.; Snieders, I.; & Brouwer, R.E. (2011). Mastocytosis and diffuse large B-cell lymphoma, an unlikely combination, *Neth J Med.* Vol.69, No.3, pp.132-4.

Shah, NP.; Lee, FY.; Luo, R.; Yibin, J.; Donker, M. & Akin, C. (2006) Dasatinib (BMS-354825) inhibits KITD816V, an imatinib-resistant activating mutation that triggers neoplastic growth in most patients with systemic mastocytosis. *Blood,* Vol.108, pp.286-291.

Sotlar, K.; Fridrich, C.; Mall, A.; Jaussi, R.; Bültmann, B.; Valent, P.& Horny, HP. (2002) Detection of c-kit point mutation Asp-816→Val in microdissected pooled single mast cells and leukemic cells in a patient with systemic mastocytosis and concomitant chronic myelomonocytic leukemia. *Leuk Res,* Vol.26, pp.979–984.

Tanaka, A.; Konno, M.; Muto, S.; Kambe, N.; Morii, E.; Nakahata, T.; Itai, A. & Matsuda, H. (2005) A novel NF-kB inhibitor, IMD-0354, suppresses neoplastic proliferation of human mast cells with constitutively activated c-kit receptors. *Blood.* Vol.2005, No.105, pp.2324–23

Taylor, ML.; Sehgal, D.; Raffeld, M.; Obiakor, H.; Akin, C.; Mage; RG. & Metcalfe, DD. (2004) Demonstration that mast cells, T cells, and B cells bearing the activating kit mutation D816V occur in clusters within the marrow of patients with mastocytosis. *Journal of Molecular Diagnostics,* Vol.6, No.4, pp.335-42. PMID:15507672, doi:10.1186/1756-8722-4-10

Travis, WD.; Li, CY.; Yam, LT.; Bergstralh, EJ.& Swee, RG (1988) Significance of systemic mast cell disease with associated hematologic disorders. *Cancer,* Vol.62, pp.965–972.

Triggiani, M.; Multicenter, Open-Label, Single Arm Phase II Clinical Trial of Dasatinib in the Treatment of Systemic Mastocytosis Writing Committee: Martinelli, G.; Merante, S.; Rondoni, M.; Zanotti, R.; Pagano, L.; Musto, P.; Cilloni, D.; Pulsoni, A.; Colarossi, S.; Venditti, A.; Amadori, S.; Beghini, A.; Cairoli, S.; Morra, E.; Pane, F.; Saglio, G. & Baccarani, M. Available from *ClinicalTrials.gov*

Valent, P.; Horny, HP.; Escribano, L.; Longley; BJ.; Li, CY.; Schwartz, LB.; Marone, G.; Nun˜ez, R.; Akin, C.; Sotlar, K.; Sperr, WR.; Wolff, K.; Brunning, RD.; Parwaresch RM.; Austen, KF.; Lennert, K.; Metcalfe, DD.; Vardiman, JW.; Bennett, JM.; (2001), Diagnostic criteria and classification of mastocytosis: a consensus proposal, *Leukemia Research,* Vol.25, pp.603–625

Valent, P.; Akin, C.; Sperr, WR.; Horny, HP.; Arock, M.; Lechner, K.; Vardiman, JW. & Metcalfe, DD.; Diagnosis and treatment of systemic mastocytosis: state of the art. (2003) *Br J Haematol* Vol.122,No.5, pp.695–717.

Valent, P.; Ghannadan, M.; Akin, C.; Krauth, MT.; Selzer, E.; Mayerhofer, M.; Sperr, WR.; Arock, M.; Samorapoompichit. P.; Horny, HP. & Metcalfe, DD. (2004) On the way to targeted therapy of mast cell neoplasms: identification of molecular targets in neoplastic mast cells and evaluation of arising treatment concepts. *Eur J Clin Invest.* Vol.34, No.2, pp.41–52.

Valent, P.; Sperr, WR. & Akin, C. (2010) How I treat patients with advanced systemic mastocytosis, *Blood,* Vol.116, pp.5812-5817

Valent, P.; Cerny-Reiterer, S.; Herrmann, H.; Mirkina, I.; George, TI.; Sotlar, K.; Sperr, WR. & Horny, HP. (2010) Phenotypic heterogeneity, novel diagnostic markers, and target expression profiles in normal and neoplastic human mast cells *Best Practice & Research Clinical Haematology* Vol.23, pp.369–378, doi: 10.1016 / j.beha.2010.07.003

Vardiman, JW.; Thiele, J.; Arber, DA.; Brunning, RD.; Borowitz, MJ.; Porwit, A.; Harris, NL.; Le Beau, MM.; Hellström-Lindberg, E.; Tefferi, A. & Bloomfield, CD. (2009) The 2008 Revision of the WHO Classification of Myeloid Neoplasms and Acute Leukemia: Rationale and Important Changes, *Blood,* available from bloodjournal.hematologylibrary.org, doi:10.1182/blood-2009-03-209262 ISSN 1528-0020

Vega-Ruiz A, Cortes JE, Sever M, Manshouri T, Quintás-Cardama A, Luthra R, Kantarjian HM, Verstovsek S (2009) Phase II study of imatinib mesylate as therapy for patients with systemic mastocytosis. *Leuk Res*, Vol.33, pp.1481-1484.

Verstovsek, S.; Tefferi, A.; Cortes, J.; Susan O'Brien, S.; Garcia-Manero, G.; Pardanani, A.; Akin, C.; Faderl, S.; Ma n s h o u r i , T.; Thomas, D. & Kantarjian, H. (2007) Phase II Study of Dasatinib in Philadelphia Chromosome-Negative Acute and Chronic Myeloid Diseases, Including Systemic Mastocytosis. *Clin Cancer Res* Vol.2008; No.14, pp.3906-3915, doi:10.1158/1078-0432.CCR-08-036

Part 2

Hematology in the Clinic

9

Heparin-Induced Thrombocytopenia

Kazuo Nakamura
Nihon Pharmaceutical University
Japan

1. Intoduction

Heparin is an effective anti-coagulant for the prevention of venous thromboembolism and for the treatment of venous thrombosis and pulmonary embolism (Girolami et al., 2003; Hirsh et al., 2004; Shantsila et al., 2009). It is often used for patients with unstable angina and acute myocardial infarction, and for patients who have undergone vascular surgery (Battistelli et al., 2010). The administration of heparin frequently induces a reduction in platelet counts. This phenomenon is called heparin-induced thrombocytopenia (HIT) and be classified as either type I or II. To avoid confusion between the syndromes, "HIT type I" has been changed to "non-immune heparin associated thrombocytopenia", and "HIT type II" is simply called "HIT".

The origin of non-immune heparin associated thrombocytopenia is not yet completely understood, though it is thought to be caused by heparin-induced platelet clumping (Fabris et al., 1983; Chong & Ismail, 1989). Thrombocytopenia of this type is mild (platelet count, >100 x 10^9 cells/L), not progressive, nor associated with bleeding or thrombosis (Salzman et al., 1980), and is independent of any immune reaction (Chong et al., 1993a; Burgess & Chong, 1997; Shantsila et al., 2009). It is characterized by a transitory, slight and asymptomatic reduction in platelet count, occurring during the first 1-2 days of heparin administration. This phenomenon gradually resolves without interruption of heparin administration, and platelet counts gradually rises to pre-treatment levels within a few days without special treatment. Non-immune heparin associated thrombocytopenia may be related to the direct binding of heparin to platelet membranes (Salzman et al., 1980; Fabris et al., 1983; Chong & Ismail, 1989).

In this view, the term HIT refers only to HIT type II. HIT is associated with a heparin-related immune reaction. It is a prothrombotic disease initiated by administration of heparin, and is related to antibody-mediated platelet activation causing thrombin generation and thrombotic complications. Thrombocytopenia is common in hospitalized patients, occurring in up to 58% of critically ill individuals, and can be caused by a variety of factors (Strauss et al., 2002). HIT, which is associated with significant morbidity and mortality if unrecognized, can be regarded as a very severe side effect of a drug, (Chong, 1992; Aster, 1995; Chong, 2003). Unfortunately, HIT often remains unrecognized, undiagnosed, and untreated, a problem that can be rectified with increased awareness and a high degree of suspicion for HIT. Current treatment recommendations are based on recent advances in research on the pathophysiology and the natural history of HIT (Jang & Hursting, 2005). HIT should be considered a clinicopathologic syndrome (Warkentin et al., 1998; Warkentin, 2002, 2003) since its diagnosis is based on both clinical criteria, such as thrombocytopenia and thrombosis, and laboratory data, such as platelet count dynamics and the detection of HIT antibodies (Shantsila et al., 2009).

However, HIT is often difficult to diagnose because of the following phenomena: 1) nonimmune heparin-associated thrombocytopenia occurs in 10-30% of patients receiving heparin (Blank et al., 2002); 2) HIT antibody seroconversion is observed in the absence of thrombocytopenia or other clinical sequelae; and 3) enzyme-linked immunosorbent assay (ELISA) detects both clinically irrelevant (non-pathogenic) and clinically relevant (pathogenic) antibodies (Shantsila et al., 2009). Seroconversion of anti-HIT antibody without thrombocytopenia or other clinical sequela is not considered HIT, whereas a diagnosis of HIT can be made when anti-HIT antibody formation is accompanied by an otherwise unexplained platelet count fall, or by skin lesions at heparin injection sites or acute systemic reactions after intravenous injection of heparin (Bartholomew et al., 2005). Furthermore, HIT formation may also be related to the occurrence of venous limb gangrene occurring in HIT patients treated with oral anticoagulants (Warkentin, 1996a). A mnemonic device, the "4 Ts" of HIT, has been developed to remember the salient clinical features of HIT, thus facilitating patient assessment and HIT diagnosis (Warkentin & Heddle, 2003): the degree of *T*hrombocytopenia, the *T*iming of the platelet fall, the presence of *T*hrombosis or other sequelae, and o*T*her potential causes of thrombocytopenia (Lillo-Le Louët et al., 2004; Denys et al., 2008; Gruel et al., 2008).

Despite the utility of this memory device, severe morbidity and mortality in HIT patients persists because of lack of awareness accompanied by a delayed diagnosis. Thus, we have developed the following chapter to provide an overview of HIT, focusing particularly on the epidemiology, pathophysiology, diagnosis, laboratory evaluation, and treatment.

2. Overview of HIT

HIT type II, namely, HIT, is immune-mediated and associated with a risk of thrombosis. It develops in approximately 5-10% of patients treated with heparin and is characterized by a significant reduction in platelets (levels fall by 30% or more), generally after the fifth day of therapy (Warkentin et al., 1998; Warkentin, 2002). Although, this phenomenon is usually resolved by therapy within 5-15 days, some cases may require months of treatment (Chong, 1992; Warkentin et al., 1998; Warkentin, 2002).

Platelet count monitoring is recommended for heparin-treated patients in whom the risk of HIT is high (e.g., postoperative patients) or intermediate (e.g., medical or obstetric patients receiving a prophylactic dose of heparin or postoperative patients receiving antithrombotic prophylaxis) (Chong et al., 1993a; Jang & Hursting, 2005). Shantsila et al. (2009) have recommended measurement of platelet counts before, and 24 h after, initiation of heparin therapy in patients who have received heparin within the past 100 days. Platelet counts should also be performed every 2-3 days in intermediate-risk patients, every other day in high-risk patients, and immediately in patients with systemic, cardiorespiratory, or neurologic symptoms that occur within 30 min after an intravenous injection of heparin.

HIT should be suspected when thrombocytopenia (<15-20×10^9 cells/L, or a >50% decrease in platelet count) occurs during heparin administration, typically 5-14 days after initiation of heparin administration (Warkentin & Kelton, 2001a); however, very severe thrombocytopenia (platelet count <15-20 × 10^9 cells/L) is generally not due to HIT. Routine platelet count monitoring for HIT may be appropriate in a least some clinical situations, and it may be reasonable to stratify the intensity of need for platelet count monitoring in relation to the risk of HIT.

Although it is difficult to predict which heparin-exposed patients will develop HIT, one consistent factor is a property of heparin preparation. HIT antibodies occur at higher levels in patients given bovine unfractionated heparin (UFH) than in those treated with porcine UFH or low molecular weigh heparin (LMWH) (Green et al., 1984; Bailey et al., 1986; Monreal et al., 1989; Rao et al., 1989; Warkentin et al., 1995; Warkentin et al., 2003a; Lee & Warkentin, 2004; Denys et al., 2008; Gruel et al., 2008).

HIT antibody formation is also influenced by the medical circumstances in which heparin is administered. For example, approximately 20% of heparin-exposed patients develop HIT antibodies after orthopedic surgery, while as many as 70% develop antibodies after receiving a cardiopulmonary bypass (CPB) (Amiral et al., 1996a). However, it can be difficult to compare results across studies because of differences in duration and route of anticoagulant administration, as well as patient group composition (Lee et al., 2004).

3. Epidemiology

There is a need for studies on HIT incidence. The work that has been done is sufficient, and they have so many differences that it is difficult to compare results across studies in order to uncover broader trends. Most HIT studies are retrospective, and differ with respect to patient characteristics, type of heparin preparation, duration of therapy, definition of thrombocytopenia, and laboratory tests used for confirm thrombocytopenia diagnosis (Schmitt & Adelman, 1993; Magnani, 1993; Chong, 2003). Despite these problems, it is possible to draw some general conclusions about HIT epidemiology.

There are 3 characteristic profiles in the timing of the onset of thrombocytopenia. Approximately 70% of HIT patients are classified as "typical-onset HIT". In these patients, platelet counts begin to decrease (serocnversion and initial platelet count fall) within 5-10 days after beginning heparin treatment (Warkentin & Kelton, 2001a). Approximately 25-30% of HIT patients are classified as having "Rapid-onset HIT", which occurs when platelet counts fall abruptly within 24 h of starting heparin therapy (Warkentin & Kelton, 2001a; Lubenow et al., 2002). "Rapid-onset HIT" is strongly associated with recent heparin exposure, usually within the preceding 100 days (Warkentin & Kelton, 2001a; Lubenow et al., 2002). Because of the previous exposure, patients already have circulating HIT antibodies, which cause platelet counts to fall quickly once heparin is re-administered. The last category of HIT, affecting approximately 3-5% of HIT patients, is "delayed-onset HIT" in which the onset of thrombocytopenia begins several days after completion of heparin treatment (Warkentin & Kelton, 2001b; Rice et al., 2002; Warkentin & Bernstein, 2003; Warkentin, 2004a). This type of syndrome is often clinically severe, as it is associated with high-titer, platelet-activating HIT antibodies that do not require ongoing heparin administration to exert their pathogenic effect (Rice et al., 2002). Furthermore, this type may occur in patients exposed to minimal amounts of heparin, although it has also been observed in patients exposed to large amounts of heparin during coronary artery bypass grafting (Rice et al., 2002; Jackson et al., 2006). Rarely, patients who received intravenous heparin develop acute inflammatory or cardiorespiratory symptoms and signs within 30 min (Warkentin, 2007).

HIT severity is mainly determined by the extent of thrombotic complications (Girolami et al, 2003). Many HIT patients develop thrombosis after receiving as an antithrombotic prophylaxis (Warkentin, 1996a; Wallis et al., 1999). The thrombotic event is frequently a worsening of pre-existing thrombosis in heparin-treated HIT patients, and this worsening of thrombosis may cause a new thromboembolic complication (Magnani, 1993; Warkentin & Kelton, 1990, 1996; Nands et al., 1997); this has been observed in approximately 20% of cases (Wakentin, 2004a). Development of a new thrombus or extension of an existing thrombus during treatment with prophylactic or therapeutic UFH or LMWH should always raise a suspicion of HIT (Shantsila et al., 2009). The first event to be associated with HIT was arterial thrombosis, which seems to be more frequent in patients with cardiovascular disease (Nands et al., 1997); venous complications may be common in patients undergoing post-surgical prophylaxis (Rhodes et al., 1973; Magnani, 1993; Warkentin & Kelton, 1996;). In most cases, arterial complications manifest as thromboses of the large vessels, leading to gangrene and limb amputation, stroke, myocardial infarction, and cardiac thrombosis (Warkentin & Kelton, 1990; Boshkov et al., 1993; Fondu, 1995; Chong, 1995).

Approximately 10-20% of patients who develop HIT while receiving subcutaneous injections of heparin experience skin lesions, ranging from painful erythematous plaques to skin necrosis, at the injection sites (Warkentin, 2004a; Chong, 1995). Skin lesions have been observed in patients without thrombocytopenia but with circulating HIT antibodies (Warkentin, 1996b). Occasionally, HIT associated with intravenous heparin injection also manifests as an acute systemic reaction developing within 5-30 min after heprin administration (Ansell et al., 1986; Popov et al., 1997; Warkentin, 2004a).

Estimates of HIT prevalence among heparin-treated patients differ depending on heparin type. Fabris et al. (2000) found that laboratory-confirmed HIT occurs in approximately 2% of patients receiving UFH. Among patients given therapeutic doses of bovine UFH, HIT has been observed in approximately 5% of patients. This is a much higher rate than that observed in patients given procine UFH (1%). Prophylactic doses of porcine heparin have been reported to cause HIT in <1% of patients (Warkentin & Kelton, 1990). However, risk of HIT is relatively low in medical and obstetric patients receiving LMWH (Fabris et al., 2000). For instance, Warkentin (2004a) reorted that HIT was observed in 2.7% of patients treated with subcutaneous UFH injection, but in no patients receiving LMWH; further, thrombotic complications were more frequent in the former group (88.9%) than in the latter (17.8%). Both the bovine/procine UFH and the LMWH data were collected from medical patients receiving LMWH or UFH as "flushes", *e.g.*, oncology patients with indwelling catheters (Mayo et al., 1990; Kadidal et al., 1999). A randomized controlled trial that compared use of porcine UFH with LMWH after hip replacement surgery found that HIT was significantly less common among patients who received the latter treatment (Lee & Warkentin, 2004; Warkentin, 2004a).

4. Pathophysiology

Francis and colleagues have reported that HIT antibody formation in cardiac surgery patients who received procine UFH was significantly lower than those with bovine UFH (Francis et al., 2003). The IgG fraction of HIT patients serum has been found to cause *in vitro* platelet aggregation in the presence of therapeutic amounts of heparin (Rhodes et al., 1973), indicating that HIT has an immunologic etiology (Amiral et al., 1998; Warkentin et al., 2000).

Green *et al.* (1978) reported that immunoglobulin-heparin complexes form only in the presence of platelets (Green et al., 1978), and several platelet proteins have been proposed as the receptors of heparin-dependent antibodies (Lynch & Howe, 1985). Multiple studies have found that the pro-aggregating effect of heparin depends on the degree of sulfation and the molecular weight of the heparin (Geinacher et al., 1992; Geinacher et al., 1993; Kelton et al., 1994) and is mediated by the release of platelet alpha-granules (Gruel et al., 1993), which contain platelet factor 4 (PF4), a small, positively charged molecule produced by megakaryocytes. Although its biological function is unknown, it has been identified as the main co-factor of heparin (Amiral et al., 1992, Gentilini et al., 1999); it also binds to endothelial-surface glycosaminoglycans, *e.g.*, heparin sulfate (Visentin et al., 1994; Cines et al., 2007). Normal blood levels of PF4 are very low, as it is only released into circulation following weak platelet activation. However, PF4 levels may be high in specific clinical circumstances, such as prosthetic hip or cardiac surgery, which are associated with platelet activation (Greinacher et al., 1994a). When heparin binds with PF4, it undergoes a conformational change and becomes immunogenic, leading to the generation of anti-heparin/PF4 antibodies, namely, HIT antibodies (Suh et al., 1998; Ziporen et al., 1998). The PF4/heparin ratio is important for the constitution of the multimolecular antigenic complex, and the optimal PF4/heparin ratio has been reported to range from 4-6:1 (Kelton et al., 1994; Visentin et al., 1994; Amiral et al., 1995; Cines et al., 2007). The immunogenicity of heparin-PF4 conjugates may form the biological basis for differences in immunogenicity between bovine and porcine sources of heparin: Bovine lung heparin has longer polysaccharide chains and a higher degree of sulfation, which could increase reactivity with PF4 (Boshkov et al., 1993).

HIT antibodies activate platelets and stimulate an immunomedited endothelial lesion, followed by the appearance of thrombocytopenia and/or thrombosis (Fondu, 1995; Greinacher, 1995; Warkentin et al., 1998; Cines et al., 2007). Platelet activation is primarily caused by binding between the immunocomplex and FcγRIIa (CD32) receptors (Adelman et al., 1989; Anderson et al., 1995; Baglin, 2001), leading to degranulation and the release of pro-coagulant substances (*e.g.*, serotonin, histamine, and adenosine diphosphate), thromboxane biosynthesis, an influx of Ca^{2+}, and the generation of highly pro-thrombotic phospholipid microparticles (Chong et al., 1981; Chong et al., 1989a; Warkentin & Kelton, 2001a). The immunocomplex can bind to Fc receptors on the surfaces of monocytes, neutrophils, and endothelial cells, and the binding of the immunocomplex to so many types of cells can contribute to the profound thrombin generation seen in patients with HIT. Thrombin generation can be enhanced by HIT activation of monocytes and endothelial cell tissue factor on the surface of monocytes and endothelial cells (Visentin et al., 1994; Warkentin, 1999; Newman & Chong, 2000; Pouplard et al., 2001; Arepally & Mayer, 2001). These thrombotic processes may lead to a hypercoagulable state, thus increasing the risk of severe and extensive thromboembolic complications in many patients. Additional activation of platelets by thrombin and other released agonists results in a further increase in the numbers of FcγRIIa receptors on the platelet surface, facilitating even more platelet activation (Chong et al., 1993b; Anderson et al., 1995). However, some reports have indicated that platelet activation can be blocked by the FcγRIIa receptor-specific monoclonal antibody (IV.3) (Kelton et al., 1988; Visentin et al, 1994).

While IgG-class HIT antibody can be detected in most HIT patients, IgA and IgM HIT antibodies can be found in only a small portion of patients (Suh et al., 1997; Amiral et al.,

1996b). Given that IgA and IgM antibodies do not activate platelets in the presence of heparin *in vitro,* and that they are unable to bind FcγRIIa, their presence in HIT patients could simply be coincidental, though IgM and IgA are not able to bind to FcγRIIa (Amiral et al., 1996a; Amiral et al., 1996b; Amiral et al., 1996c; Blank et al., 1997). These data suggest that platelet activation occurs independently of the IgG FcγRIIa receptor. After heparin administration is interrupted, the HIT antibody gradually disappears; laboratory tests for HIT antibodies are usually "negative" or "weakly positive" at 100 days (Shantsila et al., 2009). For HIT to develop at this point, the HIT antibody would need to form again (Lubenow et al., 2002; Rice et al., 2002). Harris et al. (2008) have reported an association between the PLA2 polymorphism of glycoprotein IIIa and the risk of thrombosis in patients with HIT antibodies.

5. Diagnosis of HIT

The diagnosis of HIT should be based both on clinical criteria, such as the presence of thrombocytopenia and thrombosis, and laboratory data, such as platelet count dynamics and detection of HIT antibodies. However, it may be difficult to establish a general diagnostic protocol, given the lack of a readily accessible standard laboratory test and the frequent detection of elevated anti-HIT antibody levels in heparin-treated patients that display no clinical features of the disease (Arepally & Ortel, 2006).

In the majority of patients with HIT, thrombocytopenia is defined as an otherwise unexplained >50% drop in the platelet count (Warkentin et al., 2008a); thrombocytopenia is generally of moderate severity, and median platelet count is approximately 50-60 x 10^9 platelets/L (Jackson et al., 2006). In HIT patients, platelet counts are generally < 20 x 10^9 platelets/L. Clinical presentation of HIT in patients with profound thrombocytopenia can be rapidly progressive and include the development of disseminated intravascular coagulation and microvascular thrombotic complications (Ortel, 2009). Patients are likely to suffer from HIT when their platelet counts drop to less than 50% of normal levels and when they present with thrombosis or skin lesions at heparin injection sites (Jackson et al., 2006). Generally, platelet count decreases and/or thrombotic events begin 5–10 days after the initiation of heparin therapy in heparin-hypersensitive individuals, and platelet count in thrombocytopenic patients may not return to initiation levels until several days later (Warkentin & Kelton, 2001a). In patients who have undergone operation, the expected pattern would show a return of normal platelet count immediately after surgery, followed by an unexpected drop (Warkentin, 2003). Persistent thrombocytopenia following cardiac bypass surgery is usually not a result of HIT, but instead may stem from other causes, such as postoperative complications. However, postoperative thrombocytopenia lasting for >5 days without an apparent alternative cause may be the result of HIT (Lillo-Le et al., 2004).

Several diagnostic algorithms have been developed to provide a more systematic approach to the diagnosis of HIT. Patients can be assigned an HIT score using the "**4 Ts,**" an assessment protocol and memory device focused on the salient clinical features of HIT: degree of Thrombocytopenia (maximum points for a platelet count fall of >50% or a nadir of 20–100 × 10^9/L), the Timing of the fall in platelet count (maximum points for an onset of 5–10 days after initiation of heparin treatment or within 1 day if there has been recent heparin exposure), the presence of Thrombosis or other sequelae (maximum points for new thrombosis, skin lesions, or acute systemic reactions), and oTher causes of thrombocytopenia excluded (maximum points for no other cause event) (Warkentin, 2003, Warkentin et al., 2003b, Bryant et al., 2008). The "4 Ts" is useful for following the recommendation of Warkentin and Heddle, who suggest the employment of a clinical decision-making model to establish a pretest probability for HIT in patients who receive UFH or LMWH (Warkentin & Heddle, 2003). A diagnostic score for HIT after cardiopulmonary bypass surgery has also been proposed (Lillo-Le et al., 2004). Other studies have demonstrated the usefulness of combining the 4Ts score with laboratory testing when diagnosing HIT (Lillo-Le et al., 2004; Denys et al., 2008; Gruel et al., 2008); laboratory tests can also be used independently for confirming a clinical diagnosis.

5.1 Laboratory testing

Laboratory testing is necessary to confirm the diagnosis of HIT, and is most helpful in these patients clinically assessed to be at intermediate high clinical risk of HIT (Arepally & Ortel, 2006). Patients who have undergone cardiopulmonary bypass surgery frequently have elevated antiheparin/PF4 antibody levels; among these individuals, testing should not be used to "screen" patients for HIT or evaluate patients assessed to have a low pre-test probability for HIT (Warkentin et al., 2008a). Although a lot of laboratory tests are available for detection of heparin-PF4 antibody, these tests have several advantages and disadvantages. Blood sampling for the detection of HIT antibodies was performed in patients with clinically suspected HIT on days 5 to 14 following the initiation of heparin therapy (Warkentin et al., 2008a). Although HIT antibodies are detectable in the blood for several weeks after heparin administration, discontinuation of heparin administration, samples should be collected as soon as possible because antibody levels can decrease quite rapidly.

The first test developed for diagnosing HIT was the platelet aggregation test, which uses citrated platelet-rich plasma (PRP) and standard platelet aggregometry (Warkentin, 2004b). The platelet aggregation test is able to provide results quickly (Kelton et al, 1988), although results of this test is more influenced by heparin concentrations and donor platelet variability compared to those of ^{14}C-serotonin release assay (SRA) (Warkenin & Kelton, 1990; Chong, 1992, 1995). Accordingly, to increase sensitivity and specificity, test conditions need to be optimized- instance, by washed platelets (Chong et al., 1993a; Greinacher et al., 1994a; Pouplard et al., 1999a). Washed platelet activation assays, such as the platelet SRA, (Sheridan et al., 1986; Warkentin et al., 1992; Warkentin, 2001; Price E et al., 2007), and the heparin-induced platelet activation test (Greinacher et al., 1991; Greinacher et al,. 1994a) are used by a few reference laboratories. In these assays, it is necessary to use of apyrase in a wash step for maintenance of platelet reactivity to HIT antibodies, and to resuspend in a calcium- and magnesium-containing buffer (Polgár et al., 1998; Warkentin, 2001). The major limitation of this method is its technically demanding nature (Warkentin, 2000), which limits its use to a few reference laboratories. In most clinical laboratories, immunological tests such as ELISA are used because they are easy to perform, have a rapid turnaround time, and are highly sensitive (Price et al., 2007). There are 2 PF4-dependent antigen assays that are commercially available for detecting HIT antibodies (Amiral et al., 1992; Collins et al., 1997; Warkentin, 2000; Warkentin et al., 2001): the Asserachrom (Stago, Asnières, France), which detects antibodies that react with PF4-heparin complexes, and the GTI-PF4 (GTI, Brookfield, WI, USA), which detects antibodies that react with PF4 bound to polyvinyl sulfonate.

Prospective studies have shown that, among HIT antibody classes, only HIT-IgG antibodies have very high sensitivity for diagnosing clinical HIT (Warkentin et al., 2000; Lindhoff-Last et al., 2001). Detection of PF4-heparin antibodies is performed as followed. Unbound material is removed, and a chromogen is added to label the bound conjugate, producing a yellow color, read at 405 nm. The amount of yellow produced at the end point, as indicated by the optical density (OD), is proportional to the amount of antibody present. A positive result is reported if OD reading is 0.400 or more. Higher ELISA OD results have been shown to significant correlation of the serotonin release assay results and an increased risk for thrombosis in patients with HIT (Warkentin et al., 2008b). Furthermore, the ELISA results are most useful when combined with a clinical scoring system (Janatpour et al., 2007). Zwicker et al (2004) have reported that higher ELISA OD measurements correlated significantly with thrombosis, and patients with isolated HIT (HIT in the absence of thrombosis) and an OD level of 1.0 or more had a 6-fold increased risk of thrombosis compared with patients who had OD levels between 0.4 and 0.99 (Zwicker et al, 2004). The sensitivity of the ELISA for PF4-heparin antibodies is greater than functional assays (Greinacher et al., 1994b; Amiral et al., 1995; Pouplard et al., 1999b), though a "positive" result may not denote the same magnitude of thrombotic risk.

5.2 Laboratory data from 2 potential HIT patients

We examined 2 patients who experienced thrombocytopenia after being given UFH during percutaneous transluminal coronary angioplasty (PTCA) and cardiac surgery. For both individuals, we tested for HIT by measuring platelet aggregability and quantifying levels of both anti-heparin-PF4 complex antibody (anti-HIT antibody) and thrombin-antithrombin III complex (TAT). Platelet aggregation in response to 0.2 µg/mL collagen was measured using Born's turbidimetric methods (Born GVR, 1962), and quantified by light transmission, as previously reported (Toyohira et al., 1995; Kariyazono et al., 1997; Nakamura et al., 1999); platelet aggregation activity was evaluated as percent maximum aggregation (MA). First samples were prepared by incubating the PRP of suspected HIT patients with UFH (0.2 IU/mL), and second samples were prepared by separately adding plasma from the 2 patients to the PRP of healthy volunteers at a ratio of 1:1, then adding UFH (0.2 IU/mL). We then used a commercial ELISA kit (GTI Diagnostics, Waukesha, WI, NJ, USA) to measure anti-heparin antibodies in these samples.

As shown in Figure 1, platelet aggregation was much higher in the first set of sample than in the first control sample (without UFH); in other words, heparin had a strong positive effect on aggregation. As a result, MA of second sample was 68% (Figure 2), and showed strong aggregation. The ELISA results indicated significantly higher OD values for the 2 potential HIT patients than in the healthy volunteers. Furthermore, remarkably high levels of circulating TAT and TNF-alpha were found in the plasma of the suspected HIT patients. Our laboratory data indicate the likelihood that anti-HIT antibodies were present in the plasma of both patients. Furthermore, these data demonstrate the marked acceleration of blood coagulation in these patients, suggesting an increased risk of thrombosis.

These findings support previous reports that many HIT patients are hypercoagulable and have greatly elevated levels of TAT (Warkentin et al., 1997; Greinacher et al., 2000); furthermore, this helps explain the strong relationship between HIT and venous or arterial thrombosis (Warkentin & Kelton, 2001a).

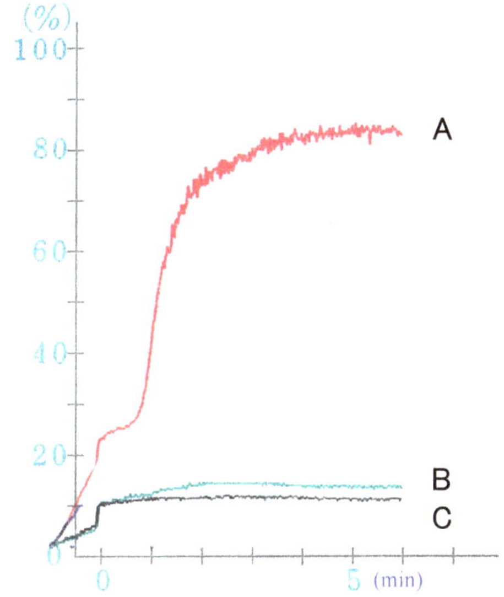

Fig. 1. Platelet aggregation was stimulated by 0.2 μg/mL collagen. In case A's PRP incubated without UFH (first control sample) (C). In healthy volunteer's PRP incubated with UFH (second control sample) (B). In case A's PRP incubated with UFH (A).

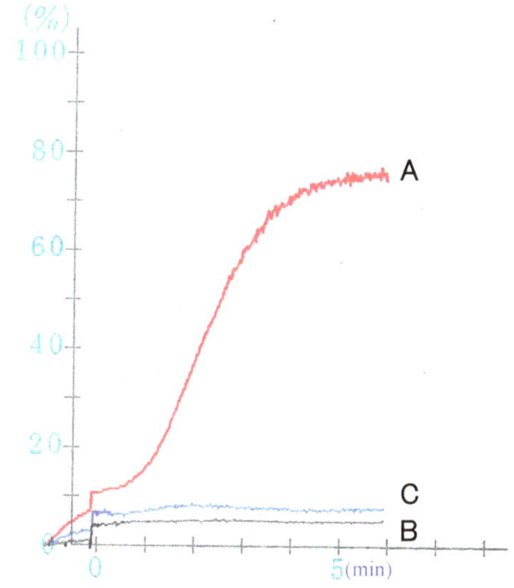

Fig. 2. Anti-heparin antibody was detected by turbidimetric method. Collagen (0.2 μg/mL) was used as agonist. In case A's PRP incubated without UFH (first control sample) (C). In healthy volunteer's PRP was mixed with case A's plasma following incubation without UFH (third control sample) (B). In healthy volunteer's PRP was mixed with case A's plasma following incubation with UFH (A).

Given these findings, we propose a model for the pathophysiological mechanism of HIT (Figures 3 and 4). This model helps explain observations that the hypercoagulable state, coupled with endothelial cell dysfunction due to injury from heparin antibody, activated platelets, leukocytes, platelet microparticles, atherosclerosis or medical intervention, can lead to arterial thrombosis (Walenga et al., 2000). Furthermore, the model is supported by the report that anti-HIT antibodies bind to and directly activate microvascular endothelial cells, whereas binding to and activating macrovascular endothelial cells requires pre-activation by platelets or TNF-alpha (Walenga et al., 2004).

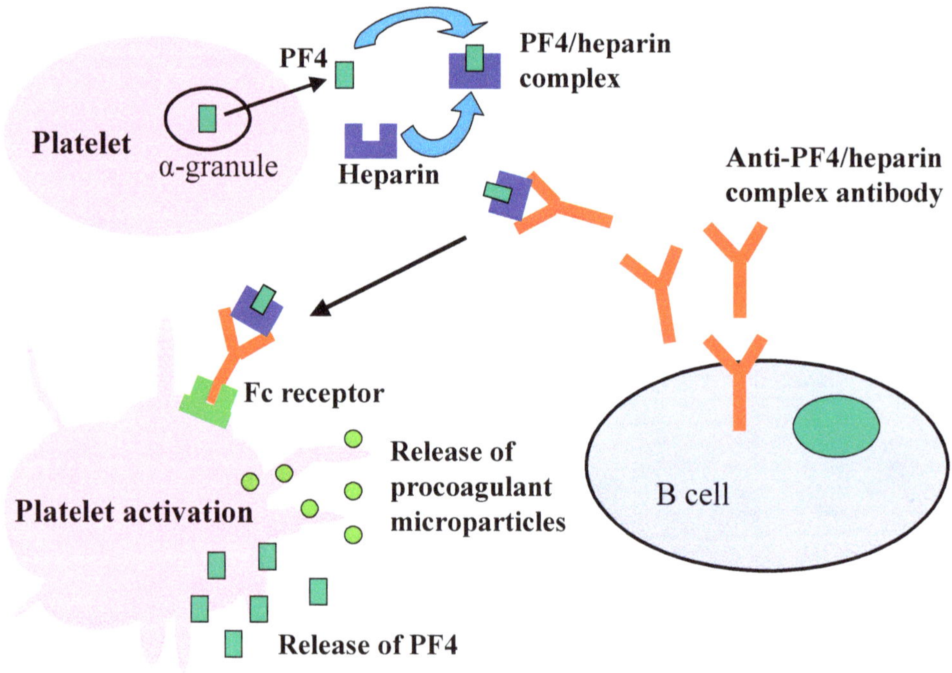

Fig. 3. Pathophysiological mechanism of HIT (1). Stage 1; binding of heparin to PF4 induces the formation of a neoepitope. Stage 2; an immune response against the PF4/heparin complex induces antibody formation. Stage 3; the complex of PF4/heparin and specific antibody associates with platelets via binding of the antibody Fc part to the platelet immunoglobulin receptor FcγRIIa (CD32), representing the major stage in platelet activation in HIT. Stage 4; activated platelets shed procoagulant microparticles which enhance thrombin generation.

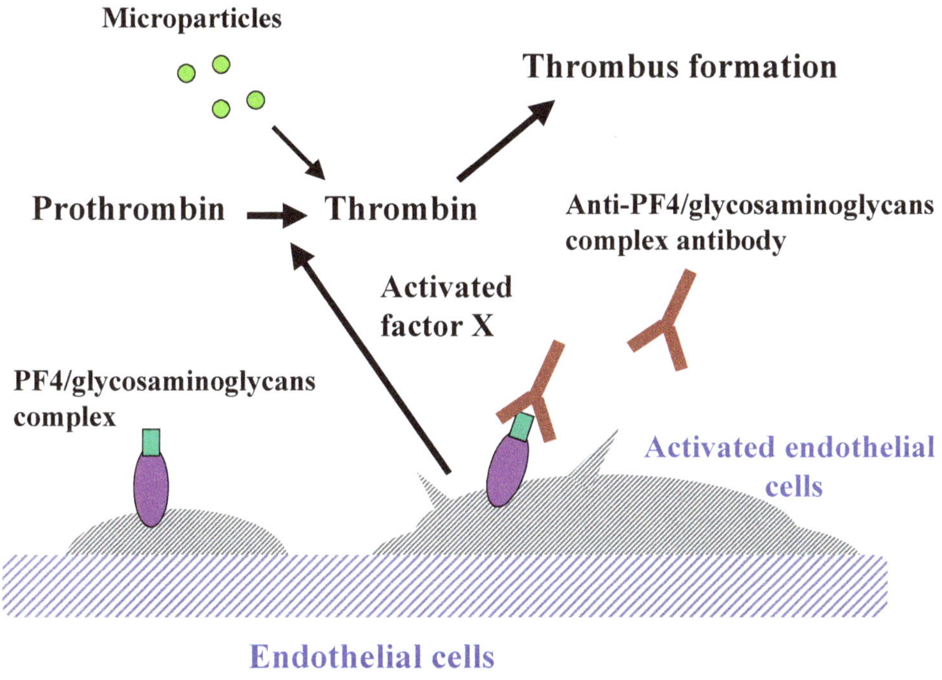

Fig. 4. Pathophysiological mechanism of HIT (2). Stage 5; binding of released PF4 to heparan sulfate of endothelial cell induces the formation of PF4/glycosaminoglycans complex on the surface of endothelial cell. Stage 6; PF4/glycosaminoglycans complex antibody binds to PF4/glycosaminoglycans complex on the surface of endothelial cell, and activates endothelial cell. Stage 7; activation of endothelial cells lead to the release of activated factor X. Stage 8; thrombin generation induces thrombus formation.

6. Management of HIT

All heparins must be avoided when treating patients suspected to have HIT; even exposure to very low amounts of heparin through heparin-coated catheters and heparin flushes used to maintain intravenous lines may trigger HIT (Laster et al., 1989). Likewise, preparations of LMWH can induce severe HIT, though they do so less frequently than UFH (Warkentin et al., 2003a; Warkentin & Greinacher, 2003; Walenga et al., 2004). Further, the cross-reactivity rate between heparin and LMWH is so high that LMWH is not recommended for the treatment of HIT patients (Chong, 2003; Warkentin et al., 2008a). Alternative anticoagulant therapy must be initiated immediately, both for HIT patients diagnosed with thrombocytopenia alone or with thromboembolism (Warkentin & Greinacher, 2004). In patients in whom treatment was delayed until an HIT diagnosis could be confirmed by laboratory tests, the incidence of new thrombosis was approximately 10-fold higher than in individuals treated promptly with a direct thrombin inhibitor (Greinacher et al., 2000).

Marked decreases of platelet counts in HIT patients require anticoagulation with an effective antithrombotic drug that does not cross-react *in vivo* with the circulating anti-heparin/PF4 antibodies. There are currently 3 thrombin inhibitors available for patients with HIT: lepirudin, argatroban, and bivalirudin, all of which directly bind and inactivate thrombin. Prospective cohort studies have been performed to investigate the efficacy and major bleeding endpoints for lepirudin (Greinacher et al., 1999a; Greinacher et al., 1999b; Lubenow et al., 2004; Lubenow et al., 2005) and argatroban (Lewis et al., 2001; Lewis et al., 2003) in patients with HIT complicated by thrombosis. When respective historical control data were taken into consideration, composite end point risk rates and new thrombosis risk rates were 0.48 and 0.28 for lepirudin, respectively, and 0.75 and 0.45 for argatroban, respectively. The corresponding absolute event rates were 19.2% (lepirudin) and 42.3% (argatroban) for the composite end point, and 7.0% (lepirudin) and 15.5% (argatroban) for new thrombosis. Patients who received lepirudin were less likely to require amputation than those who were given argatroban. Fatal bleeding after treatment with lepirudin has been found to range from 1.2% of patients (in a prospective study) to 3.9% of patients (in a retrospective observational study) (Lubenow et al., 2005; Tardy et al., 2006). Danaparoid and fondaparinux may also be used to manage HIT (Warkentin et al., 2008a). When abrupt decreases in platelet count (to $<10 \times 10^9$ clls/L) are observed in patients who underwent angioplasty and were treated with a combination of heparin and glycoprotein IIb/IIIa antagonist, the recommended antagonist is always glycoprotein IIb/IIIa (Shantsila et al., 2009)

6.1 Lepirudin

Lepirudin, a recombinant form of hirudin, is a direct, specific, and irreversible inhibitor of thrombin that is administered via intravenous injection (Greinacher & Lubenow, 2001). The Biggest drawback of Lepirudin is that it must be accompanied by the strict laboratory monitoring: activated partial thromboplastin time (aPTT) monitoring should be performed at 4-h intervals until it is clear that patients have reached a steady state within the normal range of values (Warkentin et al., 2008b). Moreover, patients should be informed that they have received lepirudin, since fatal anaphylactic reactions have been reported in patients re-exposed to lepirudin during a second round of intravenous treatment (Greinacher et al., 2003). Although similar bleeding rates have been observed in lepirudin-treated patients and historical control subjects, this drug has been found to significantly reduce the combined end point of death, limb amputation, and new thromboembolic complications in patients with HIT associated thrombosis (Greinacher et al., 1999a; Greinacher et al., 1999b).

6.2 Argatroban

Argatroban is a synthetic L-arginine-derived direct thrombin inhibitor that reversibly binds to the thrombin active site. Argatroban is administered by intravenous injection, with dose adjustment to maintain aPTT at 1.5-3.0 times the baseline value (Gosselin et al., 2004). It has been reported that, in HIT patients without thrombosis, treatment with argatroban produces a significant reduction in the composite end point, such as all-cause death, all-cause limb amputation, and new thrombosis at 37 days (Lewis et al., 2001; Lewis et al., 2003). In HIT patients who underwent lower extremity revascularization, the composite end point of deaths, urgent revascularization, and limb amputations developed in 25% of patients treated with argatroban, and 6% of patients had major bleeding episodes (Baron et al., 2008). Restoration of platelet counts is universally observed within 6–7 days of the initiation of argatroban therapy (Bartholomew et al., 2007). Some precautions are required when argatroban infusion is overlapped by warfarin anticoagulant therapy, although argatroban causes a further substantial increase in the international normalized ratio (INR). In addition, careful thought should be given to the participation of direct thrombin inhibitor to the patient's INR.

6.3 Danaparoid

Danaparoid is approved as an alternative anticoagulant for HIT in many countries. Danaparoid, a heparinoid with predominantly anti-Xa activity and some anti-IIa activity, is a mixture of three glycosaminoglycans such as heparin sulfate, dermatan sulfate, and chondroitin sulfate. Danaparoid presents its anticoagulant effect by catalyzing the inactivation of factor Xa in the presence of antithrombin, and has a unique property of specific suppression of HIT antibody-induced platelet activation that is not observed with other drugs used for HIT treatment (Chong et al., 1989b). Tardy-Poncet et al. reported that major bleeding episodes in those patients treated with danaparoid were significantly fewer compared with those treated with lepirudin (Tardy-Poncet et al., 1999). Among the drugs used for the treatment of HIT, danaparoid is the only drug whose efficacy and safety have been confirmed by a prospective randomized controlled study (Chong et al., 2001).

6.4 Bivalirudin

Bivalirudin, which is not approved as an HIT treatment, is a 20-amino acid polypeptide with sequence homology to hirudin. Campbell et al. (2000) reported 94% procedural success in a series of 17 percutaneous coronary intervention patients who were given bivalirudin as a treatment for HIT (Campbell et al., 2000). In the Anticoagulant Therapy with Bivalirudin to Assist in the Performance of Percutaneous Coronary Intervention in Patients with HIT (or ATBAT) multicenter open-label trial (Mahaffey et al., 2003), clinical percutaneous coronary intervention success, defined as the absence of death, emergency bypass surgery, or Q-wave infarction, was achieved in 96% of patients treated with bivalirudin; further, patients displayed a low rate of bleeding. Cumulatively, these results indicate that bivalirudin therapy is safe and effective during percutaneous coronary intervention.

6.5 Fondaparinux

Fondaparinux, a synthetic pentasaccharide with potent indirect anti-Xa inhibitor properties, is used only a limited number of patients with HIT. The generation of HIT-related antigen depends on the polysaccharide chain length (Amiral et al., 1995). Because patients have a very low risk of developing HIT while receiving fondaparinux (Warkentin et al., 2005), platelet count monitoring is not needed during administration of this drug. Despite these advantages, fondaparinux cannot be recommended for in the treatment of HIT until there are more data demonstrating its efficacy and safety (Rota et al., 2008; Lobo et al., 2008).

7. Conclusion

Heparin is one of the most widely used and valuable anticoagulants for the treatment and prophylaxis of thrombotic complications. However, HIT is not only a common but also a serious complication of heparin therapy with a high rate of morbidity and mortality. Its prompt clinical and laboratory recognition is necessary to stop heparin administration immediately and start an alternative anticoagulant. HIT antibody test results must be interpreted in the appropriate context of the available clinical information. Furthermore, additional diagnostic information is available as a result of considering the magnitude of a given positive test result. The diagnosis of HIT should be clearly recorded in the patient's notes and marked as a serious allergy.

8. References

Adelman B, Sobel M, Fujimura Y, Ruggeri ZM, & Zimmerman TS. (1989). Heparin-associated thrombocytopenia: observations on the mechanism of platelet aggregation. *J Lab Clin Med*, 113, 2, (Feb 1989), pp.204-210.

Amiral J, Bridey F, Dreyfus M, Vissoc AM, Fressinaud E, et al. (1992). Platelet factor 4 complexed to heparin is the target for antibodies generated in heparin-induced thrombocytopenia. *Thromb Haemost*, 68, 1, (Jun 1992), pp.95-96.

Amiral J, Bridey F, Wolf M, Boyer-Neumann C, Fressinaud E, et al. (1995). Antibodies to macromolecular platelet factor 4-heparin complexes in heparin-induced thrombocytopenia: a study of 44 cases. *Thromb Haemost*, 73,11, (Jan 1995), pp.21-28.

Amiral J, Marfaing-Koka A, Poncz M, & Meyer D. (1998). The biological basis of immune heparin-induced thrombocytopenia. *Platelets*, 9, 2, (1998), pp.77-91.

Amiral J, Marfaing-Koka A, Wolf M, Alessi MC, et al. (1996c). Presence of autoantibodies to interleukin-8 or neutrophil-activating peptide-2 in patients with heparin-associated thrombocytopenia. *Blood*, 88, 2, (Jul 1996), pp.410–416.

Amiral J, Peynaud-Debayle E, Wolf M, Bridey F, Vissac AM, et al. (1996a). Generation of antibodies to heparin-PF4 complexes without thrombocytopenia in patients treated with unfractionated or low-molecular-weight heparin. *Am J Hematol*, 52, 2, (Jun 1996), pp.90-95.

Amiral J, Wolf M, Fischer A, Boyer-Neumann C, Vissac A, et al. (1996b). Pathogenicity of IgA and/or IgM antibodies to heparin-PF4 complexes in patients with heparin-induced thrombocytopenia. *Br J Haematol*, 92,4, (Mar 1996), pp.954–959.

Anderson CL, Chacko GW, Osborne JM, & Brandt JT. (1995). The Fc receptor for immunoglobulin G (Fc gamma RII) on human platelets. *Semin Thromb Hemost*, 21, 1, (1995), pp.1-9.

Ansell JE, Clark WP Jr, Compton CC. (1986). Fatal reactions associated with intravenous heparin. *Drug Intell Clin Pharm*, 20, 1, (Jun 1986), pp.74-75.

Arepally GM, & Mayer IM. (2001). Antibodies from patients with heparin-induced thrombocytopenia stimulate monocytic cells to express tissue factor and secrete interleukin-8. *Blood*. 98, 4, (Aug 2001), pp.1252-1254.

Arepally GM, & Ortel TL. (2006). Clinical practice. Heparin-induced thrombocytopenia. *N Engl J Med*, 355, 8, (Aug 2006), pp.809-817.

Aster RH. (1995). Heparin-induced thrombocytopenia and thrombosis. *N Engl J Med*, 332, 20, (May 1995), pp. 1374–1376.

Baglin TP. (2001). Heparin induced thrombocytopenia thrombosis (HIT/T) syndrome: diagnosis and treatment. *J Clin Pathol*, 54, 4, (Apr 2001), pp.272-274.

Bailey RT Jr, Ursick JA, Heim KL, Hilleman DE, & Reich JW. (1986). Heparin-associated thrombocytopenia: a prospective comparison of bovine lung heparin, manufactured by a new process, and porcine intestinal heparin. *Drug Intell Clin Pharm*, 20, 5, (May 1986), pp.374-378.

Baron SJ, Yeh RW, Cruz-Gonzalez I, Healy JL, Pomerantsev E, et al. (2008). Efficacy and safety of argatroban in patients with heparin induced thrombocytopenia undergoing endovascular intervention for peripheral arterial disease. *Catheter Cardiovasc Interv*, 72, 1, (Jul 2008), pp.116–120.

Bartholomew JR, Begelman SM, & Almahameed A. (2005). Heparin-induced thrombocytopenia: principles for early recognition and management. *Cleve Clin J Med*, 72, (Suppl 1), (Apr 2005), pp.S31-S36.

Bartholomew JR, Pietrangeli CE, & Hursting MJ. (2007). Argatroban anticoagulation for heparin-induced thrombocytopenia in elderly patients. *Drugs Aging*, 24, 6, (Jun 2007), pp.489–499.

Battistelli S, Genovese A, & Gori T. (2010). Heparin-induced thrombocytopenia in surgical patients. *Am J Surg*, 199, 1, (Jan 2010), pp.43-51.

Blank M, Cines DB, Arepally G, Eldor A, Afek A, et al. (1997). Pathogenicity of human anti-platelet factor 4 (PF4)/heparin in vivo: generation of mouse anti- PF4/heparin and induction of thrombocytopenia by heparin. *Clin Exp Immunol*, 108, 2, (May 1997), pp.333-339.

Blank M, Shoenfeld Y, Tavor S, Praprotnik S, Boffa MC, et al. (2002). Anti-platelet factor 4/heparin antibodies from patients with heparin-induced thrombocytopenia provoke direct activation of microvascular endothelial cells. *Int Immunol*, 14, 2, (Feb 2002), pp.121-129.

Born GVR. (1962). Aggregation of blood platelets by adenosine diphosphate and its reversal. *Nature*, 194, (Jun 1962), pp.927-929.

Boshkov LK, Warkentin TE, Hayward CP, Andrew M, & Kelton JG. (1993). Heparin-induced thrombocytopenia and thrombosis: clinical and laboratory studies. *Br J Haematol*. 84, 2, (Jun 1993), pp.322-328.

Bryant A, Low J, Austin S, & Joseph J. (2008). Timely diagnosis and management of heparin-induced thrombocytopenia in a frequent request, low incidence single centre using clinical 4T's score and particle gel immunoassay. *Br J Haematol*, 143, 5, (Dec 2008), pp.721-726.

Burgess JK, & Chong BH. (1997). The platelet proaggregating and potentiating effects of unfractionated heparin, low molecular weight heparin and heparinoid in intensive care patients and healthy controls. *Eur J Haematol*, 58, 4, (Apr 1997), pp.279-285.

Campbell KR, Mahaffey KW, Lewis BE, Weitz JI, Berkowitz SD, et al. (2000). Bivalirudin in patients with heparin-induced thrombocytopenia undergoing percutaneous coronary intervention [abstract]. *J Invasive Cardiol*, 12, (Suppl F), (Dec 2000), pp.14F–19F.

Chong BH, & Ismail F. (1989). The mechanism of heparin-induced platelet aggregation. *Eur J Haematol*, 43, 3, (Sep 1989), pp.245-251.

Chong BH, Burgess J, & Ismail F. (1993a). The clinical usefulness of the platelet aggregation test for the diagnosis of heparin-induced thrombocytopenia. *Thromb Haemost*, 69, 4, (Apr 1993), pp.344-350.

Chong BH, Grace CS, & Rozenberg MC. (1981). Heparin-induced thrombocytopenia: effect of heparin platelet antibody on platelets. *Br J Haematol*, 49, 4, (Dec 1981), pp.531-540.

Chong BH, Ismail F, Cade J, Gallus AS, Gordon S, Chesterman CN. (1989a). Heparin-induced thrombocytopenia: studies with a new low molecular weight heparinoid, Org 10172. Blood, 73, 6, (May 1989), pp.1592-1596.

Chong BH, Ismail F, Cade J, Gallus AS, Gordon S, et al. (1989b). Heparin-induced thrombocytopenia: studies with a new low molecular weight heparinoid, Org 10-172. *Blood*, 73, 6, (May 1989), pp.1592–1596.

Chong BH, Pilgrim RL, Cooley MA, & Chesterman CN. (1993b). Increased expression of platelet IgG Fc receptors in heparin induced thrombocytopenia. *Blood*, 81, 4, (Feb 1993), pp.988–993.

Chong BH. (1995). Heparin-induced thrombocytopenia. *Br J Haematol*, 89, 3, (1995), pp.431-439.

Chong BH. (2003). Heparin-induced thrombocytopenia. *J Thromb Haemost*, 1, 7, (Jul 2003), pp.1471–1478.

Chong BH. Heparin-induced thrombocytopenia. (1992). *Aust N Z J Med*, 22, 2, (Apr 1992), pp.145-152.

Cines DB, Rauova L, Arepally G, Reilly MP, McKenzie SE, et al. (2007). Heparin-induced thrombocytopenia: an autoimmune disorder regulated through daynamic outoantigen assembly/disassembly. *J Clin Apheresis*, 22, 1, (Feb 2007), pp.31-36.

Collins JL, Aster RH, Moghaddam M, Piotrowski MA, Strauss TR, et al. (1997). Diagnostic testing for heparin-induced thrombocytopenia (HIT): an enhanced platelet factor 4 complex enzyme linked immunosorbent assay (PF4ELISA). *Blood*, 90, (suppl), p.461a.

Denys B, Stove V, Philippé J, & Devreese K. (2008). A clinical-laboratory approach contributing to a rapid and reliable diagnosis of heparin-induced thrombocytopenia. *Thromb Res*, 123, 1, (Jan 2008), pp.137-145.

Fabris F, Fussi F, Casonato A, Visentin L, Randi M, et al. (1983). Smith MR, Girolami A. Normal and low molecular weight heparins: interaction with human platelets. *Eur J Clin Invest*, 13, 2, (Apr 1983), pp.135-139.

Fabris F, Luzzatto G, Stefani PM, Girolami B, Cella G, et al. (2000). Heparin-induced thrombocytopenia. *Haematologica*, 85, 1, (Jun 2000), pp.72-81.

Fondu P. (1995). Heparin-associated thrombocytopenia: an update. *Acta Clin Belg*, 50, 6, (1995), pp.343-357.

Francis JL, Palmer GJ 3rd, Moroose R, & Drexler A. (2003). Comparison of bovine and porcine heparin in heparin antibody formation after cardiac surgery. Ann Thorac Surg, 75, 1, (Jun 2003), pp.17-22.

Gentilini G, Kirschbaum NE, Augustine JA, Aster RH, & Visentin GP. (1999). Inhibition of human umbilical vein endothelial cell proliferation by the CXC chemokine, platelet factor 4 (PF4), is associated with impaired downregulation of p21(Cip1/WAF1). *Blood*, 93, 1, (Jun 1999), pp.25-33.

Girolami B, Prandoni P, Stefani PM, Tanduo C, Sabbion P, et al. (2003). The incidence of heparin-induced thrombocytopenia in hospitalized medical patients treated with subcutaneous unfractionated heparin: a prospective cohort study. *Blood*, 101, 8, (April 2003), pp.2955-2959.

Gosselin RC, Dager WE, King JH, Janatpour K, Mahackian K, et al. (2004). Effect of direct thrombin inhibitors, bivalirudin, lepirudin, and argatroban, on prothrombin time and INR values. *Am J Clin Pathol*, 121, 4, (Apr 2004), pp.593–599.

Green D, Harris K, Reynolds N, Roberts M, & Patterson R. (1978). Heparin immune thrombocytopenia: evidence for a heparin-platelet complex as the antigenic determinant. *J Lab Clin Med*, 91, 1, (Jun 1978), pp.167-175.

Green D, Martin GJ, Shoichet SH, DeBacker N, Bomalaski JS, et al. (1984). Thrombocytopenia in a prospective, randomized, double-blind trial of bovine and porcine heparin. *Am J Med Sci*, 288, 2, (Sep 1984), pp.60-64.

Greinacher A, & Lubenow N. (2001). Recombinant hirudin in clinical practice: focus on lepirudin. *Circulation*, 103, 10, (Mar 2001), pp.1479–1484.

Greinacher A, Amiral J, Dummel V, Vissac A, Kiefel V, et al. (1994b). Laboratory diagnosis of heparin-associated thrombocytopenia and comparison of platelet aggregation test, heparin-induced platelet activation test, and platelet factor 4/heparin enzyme-linked immunosorbent assay. *Transfusion*, 34, 5, (May 1994), pp.381-385.

Greinacher A, Eichler P, Lubenow N, Kwasny H, & Luz M. (2000). Heparin-induced thrombocytopenia with thromboembolic complications: meta-analysis of 2 prospective trials to assess the value of parenteral treatment with lepirudin and its therapeutic aPTT range. *Blood*, 96, 3, (Aug 2000), pp.846-851.

Greinacher A, Janssens U, Berg G, Böck M, Kwasny H, et al. (1999a). Lepirudin (recombinant hirudin) for parenteral anticoagulation in patients with heparin-induced thrombocytopenia: Heparin-Associated Thrombocytopenia Study (HAT) investigators. *Circulation*, 100, 6, (Aug 1999), pp.587–593.

Greinacher A, Lubenow N, & Eichler P. (2003). Anaphylactic and anaphylactoid reactions associated with lepirudin in patients with heparin-induced thrombocytopenia. *Circulation*, 108, 17, (Oct 2003), pp.2062–2065.

Greinacher A, Michels I, & Mueller-Eckhardt C. (1992). Heparin-associated thrombocytopenia: the antibody is not heparin specific. *Thromb Haemost*, 67, 5, (May 1992), pp.545-549.

Greinacher A, Michels I, Kiefel V, Mueller-Eckhardt C. (1991). A rapid and sensitive test for diagnosing heparin-associated thrombocytopenia. *Thromb Haemost*, 66, 6, (Dec 1991), pp.734-736.

Greinacher A, Michels I, Liebenhoff U, Presek P, & Mueller-Eckhardt C. (1993). Heparin-associated thrombocytopenia: immune complexes are attached to the platelet membrane by the negative charge of highly sulphated oligosaccharides. *Br J Haematol*, 84, 4, (Aug 1993), pp.711-716.

Greinacher A, Pötzsch B, Amiral J, Dummel V, Eichner A, et al. (1994a). Heparin-associated thrombocytopenia: isolation of the antibody and characterization of a multimolecular PF4-heparin complex as the major antigen. *Thromb Haemost*, 71, 2, (Feb 1994), pp.247-251.

Greinacher A, Völpel H, Janssens U, Hach-Wunderle V, Kemkes-Matthes B, Eichler P, et al. (1999b). Lepirudin provides safe and effective anticoagulation in patients with heparin-induced thrombocytopenia: a prospective study. *Circulation*, 99, 1, (Jan 1999), pp.73–80.

Greinacher A. (1995). Antigen generation in heparin-associated thrombocytopenia: the nonimmunologic type and the immunologic type are closely linked in their pathogenesis. *Semin Thromb Hemost*, 21, 1, (1995), pp.106-116.

Gruel Y, Boizard-Boval B, & Wautier JL. (1993). Further evidence that alpha-granule components such as platelet factor 4 are involved in platelet-IgG-heparin interactions during heparin-associated thrombocytopenia. *Thromb Haemost*, 70, 2, (Aug 1993), pp.374-375.

Gruel Y, Régina S, & Pouplard C. (2008). Usefulness of pretest clinical score (4Ts) combined with immunoassay for the diagnosis of heparin-induced thrombocytopenia. Curr Opin Pulm Med, 14,5, (Sep 2008), pp.397-402.

Harris K, Nguyen P, & Van Cott EM. (2008). Platelet PLA2 polymorphism and the risk for thrombosis in heparin-induced thrombocytopenia. *Am J Clin Pathol*, 129, 2, (Feb 2008), pp.282-286.

Hirsh J, Heddle N, & Kelton JG. (2004). Treatment of heparin-induced thrombocytopenia: a critical review. *Arch Intern Med*, 164, 4, (Feb 2004), pp.361-369.

Jackson MR, Neilson WJ, Lary M, Baay P, Web K, & ET AL. (2006). Delayed-onset heparin-induced thrombocytopenia and thrombosis after intraoperative heparin anticoagulation: four case reports. *Vasc Endovasc Surgery*, 40, 11, (Jun-Feb 2006), pp.67-70.

Janatpour KA, Gosselin RC, Dager WE, Lee A, Owings JT, et al. (2007). Usefulness of optical density values from heparin-platelet factor 4 antibody testing and probability scoring models to diagnose heparin-induced thrombocytopenia. *Am J Clin Pathol*, 127, 3, (Mar 2007), pp.429-433.

Jang IK, & Hursting MJ. (2005). When heparins promote thrombosis: review of heparin-induced thrombocytopenia. *Circulation*, 111, 20, (May 2005), pp.2671-2683.

Kadidal VV, Mayo DJ, & Horne MK. (1999). Heparin-induced thrombocytopenia (HIT) due to heparin flushes: a report of three cases. *J Intern Med*. 246, 3, (Sep 1999), pp.325-329.

Kariyazono H, Nakamura K, Shinkawa T, Moriyama Y, Toyohira H, et al. (1997). Inhibitory effects of antibiotics on platelet aggregation in vitro. *Hum Exp Toxicol*, 16, 11, (Nov 1997), pp.662-666.

Kelton JG, Sheridan D, Santos A, Smith J, Steeves K, et al. (1988). Heparin-induced thrombocytopenia: laboratory studies. *Blood*, 72, 3, (Sep 1988), pp.925-930.

Kelton JG, Smith JW, Warkentin TE, Hayward CP, Denomme GA, & Horsewood P. (1994). Immunoglobulin G from patients with heparin-induced thrombocytopenia binds to a complex of heparin and platelet factor 4. Blood, 83, 11, (Jun 1994), pp.3232-3239.

Laster JL, Nichols WK, & Silver D. (1989). Thrombocytopenia associated with heparin-coated catheters inpatients with heparin-associated antiplatelet antibodies. *Arch Intern Med*, 149, 10, (Oct 1989), pp.2285–2287.

Lee DH, & Warkentin TE. (2004). Frequency of heparin-induced thrombocytopenia. In: Warkentin TE. Greinacher A. eds. Heparin-induced thrombocytopenia. 3rd ed. New York, NY: Marcel Dekker, pp.107-148

Lewis BE, Wallis DE, Berkowitz SD, Matthai WH, Fareed J, et al. (2001). Argatroban anticoagulant therapy in patients with heparin-induced thrombocytopenia. *Circulation*, 103, 14, (Apr 2001), pp.1833–1843.

Lewis BE, Wallis DE, Leya F, Hursting MJ, & Kelton JG; Argatroban-915 Investigators. (2003). Argatroban anticoagulation in patients with heparin-induced thrombocytopenia. *Arch Intern Med*, 163, 15, (Aug 1003), pp.1849–1856.

Lillo-Le Louët A, Boutouyrie P, Alhenc-Gelas M, Le Beller C, Gautier I, et al. (2004). Diagnostic score for heparin-induced thrombocytopenia after cardiopulmonary bypass. *J Thromb Haemost*, 2, 11, (Nov 2004), pp.1882-1888.

Lindhoff-Last E, Gerdsen F, Ackermann H, & Bauersachs R. (2001). Determination of heparin–platelet 4–IgG antibodies improves diagnosis of heparin-induced thrombocytopenia. *Br J Haematol*, 113, 4, (Jun 2001), pp.886–890.

Lobo B, Finch C, Howard A, & Minhas S. (2008). Fondaparinux for the treatment of patients with acute heparin-induced thrombocytopenia. *Thromb Haemost*, 99, 1, (Jan 2008), pp.208–214.

Lubenow N, Eichler P, Lietz T, & Greinacher A; Hit Investigators Group. (2005). Lepirudin in patients with heparin-induced thrombocytopenia: results of the third prospective study (HAT-3) and a combined analysis of HIT-1, HAT-2, and HAT-3. *J Thromb Haemost*, 3, 11, (Nov 2005), pp.2428–2436.

Lubenow N, Eichler P, Lietz T, Farner B, Greinacher A. (2004). Lepirudin for prophylaxis of thrombosis in patients with acute isolated heparin-induced thrombocytopenia: an analysis of 3 prospective studies. *Blood*, 104, 10, (Nov 2004), pp.3072-7.

Lubenow N, Kempf R, Eichner A, Eichler P, Carlsson LE, et al. (2002). Heparin-induced thrombocytopenia: temporal pattern of thrombocytopenia in relation to initial use or reexposure to heparin. *Chest*, 122, 1, (Jul 2002), pp.37-42.

Lynch DM, & Howe SE. (1985). Heparin-associated thrombocytopenia: antibody binding specificity to platelet antigen. *Blood*, 66, 5, (Nov 1985), pp.1176-1181.

Magnani HN. (1993). Heparin-induced thrombocytopenia (HIT): an overview of 230 patients treated with orgaran (Org 10172). *Thromb Haemost*, 70, 4, (Oct 1993), pp.554-561.

Mahaffey KW, Lewis BE, Wildermann NM, Berkowitz SD, Oliverio RM, et al. (2003). The anticoagulant therapy with bivalirudin to assist in the performance of percutaneous coronary intervention in patients with heparin-induced thrombocytopenia (ATBAT) study. *J Invasive Cardiol*, 15, 11, (Nov 2003), pp.611–616.

Mayo DJ, Cullinane AM, Merryman PK, & Horne MK 3rd. (1990). Serologic evidence of heparin sensitization in cancer patients receiving heparin flushes of venous access devices. *Support Care Cancer*, 7, 6, (Nov 1990), pp.425-427.

Monreal M, Lafoz E, Salvador R, Roncales J, & Navarro A. (1989). Adverse effects of three different forms of heparin therapy: thrombocytopenia, increased transaminases, and hyperkalaemia. *Eur J Clin Pharmacol,* 37, 4, (1989), pp.415-418.

Nakamura K, Kariyazono H, Moriyama Y, Toyohira H, Kubo H, et al. (1999). Effects of sarpogrelate hydrochloride on platelet aggregation, and its relation to the release of serotonin and P-selectin. *Blood Coagul Fibrinolysis*, 10, 8, (Dec 1999), pp.513-519.

Nand S, Wong W, Yuen B, Yetter A, Schmulbach E, et al. (1997). Heparin-induced thrombocytopenia with thrombosis: incidence, analysis of risk factors, and clinical outcomes in 108 consecutive patients treated at a single institution. *Am J Hematol*, 56, 1, (Sep 1997), pp.12-16.

Newman PM, & Chong BH. (2000). Heparin-induced thrombocytopenia: new evidence for the dynamic binding of purified anti-PF4-heparin antibodies to platelets and the resultant platelet activation. *Blood*, 96, 1, (Jul 2000), pp.182-187.

Ortel TL. (2009). Heparin-induced thrombocytopenia: when a low platelet count is a mandate for anticoagulation. *Hematology (Am Soc Heamatol Educ Prog)*, pp.225-232.

Polgár J, Eichler P, Greinacher A, Clemetson KJ. (1998). Adenosine diphosphate (ADP) and ADP receptor play a major role in platelet activation/aggregation induced by sera from heparin-induced thrombocytopenia patients. *Blood*, 91, 2, (Jun 1998), pp.549-554.

Popov D, Zarrabi MH, Foda H, & Graber M. (1997). Pseudopulmonary embolism: acute respiratory distress in the syndrome of heparin-induced thrombocytopenia. *Am J Kidney Dis*, 29, 3, (Mar 1997), pp.449-452.

Pouplard C, Amiral J, Borg JY, Laporte-Simitsidis S, Delahousse B, et al. (1999b). Decision analysis for use of platelet aggregation test, carbon 14-serotonin release assay, and heparin-platelet factor 4 enzyme-linked immunosorbent assay for diagnosis of heparin-induced thrombocytopenia. *Am J Clin Pathol*, 111, 5, (May 1999), pp.700-706.

Pouplard C, Iochmann S, Renard B, Herault O, Colombat P, et al. (2001). Induction of monocyte tissue factor expression by antibodies to heparin-platelet factor 4 complexes developed in heparin-induced thrombocytopenia. *Blood*, 97, 10, (May 2001), pp.3300-3302.

Pouplard C, May MA, Iochmann S, Amiral J, Vissac AM, et al. (1999a). Antibodies to platelet factor 4-heparin after cardiopulmonary bypass in patients anticoagulated with unfractionated heparin or a low-molecular-weight heparin : clinical implications for heparin-induced thrombocytopenia. *Circulation*, 99, 19, (May 1999), pp.2530-2536.

Price E, Hayward C, Moffat K, Moore J, Warkentin T, et al. (2007). Laboratory testing for heparin-induced thrombocytopenia is inconsistent in North America: a survey of North American specialized coagulation laboratories. *Thromb Haemost*, 98, 6, (Dec 2007), pp.1357-1361.

Rao AK, White GC, Sherman L, Colman R, Lan G, et al. (1989). Low incidence of thrombocytopenia with porcine mucosal heparin. A prospective multicenter study. *Arch Intern Med*, 6, (Jun 1989), 149, pp.1285-1288.

Rhodes GR, Dixon RH, & Silver D. (1973). Heparin induced thrombocytopenia with thrombotic and hemorrhagic manifestations. *Surg Gynecol Obstet*, 136, 3, (Mar 1973), pp.409-416.

Rice L, Attisha WK, Drexler A,& Francis JL. (2002). Delayed-onset heparin-induced thrombocytopenia. *Ann Intern Med*, 136, 3, (Feb 2002), pp.210-215.

Rota E, Bazzan M, & Fantino G. (2008). Fondaparinux-related thrombocytopenia in a previous low-molecular-weight heparin (LMWH)-induced heparin-induced thrombocytopenia (HIT). *Thromb Haemost*, 99.4, (Apr 2008), pp.779-781.

Salzman EW, Rosenberg RD, Smith MH, Lindon JN, & Favreau L. (1980). Effect of heparin and heparin fractions on platelet aggregation. *J Clin Invest*, 65, 1, (Jan 1980), pp.64-73.

Schmitt BP, & Adelman B. (1993). Heparin-associated thrombocytopenia: a critical review and pooled analysis. *Am J Med Sci*, 305, 4, (Apr 1993), pp.208-215.

Shantsila E, Lip GY, & Chong BH. (2009). Heparin-induced thrombocytopenia. A contemporary clinical approach to diagnosis and management. *Chest*, 135, 6, (June 2009), pp.1651-1664.

Sheridan D, Carter C, Kelton JG. (1986). A diagnostic test for heparin-induced thrombocytopenia. *Blood*, 67, 2, (Jan 1986), pp.27-30.

Strauss R, Wehler M, Mehler K, Kreutzer D, Koebnick C, et al. (2002). Thrombocytopenia in patients in the medical intensive care unit: bleeding prevalence, transfusion requirements, and outcome. *Crit Care Med*, 30, 2, (Aug 2002), pp.1765–1771.

Suh JS, Aster RH, & Visentin GP. (1998). Antibodies from patients with heparin-induced thrombocytopenia/thrombosis recognize different epitopes on heparin: platelet factor 4. *Blood*, 91, 1, (Feb 1998), pp.916-922.

Suh JS, Malik MI, Aster RH, & Visentin GP. (1997). Characterization of the humoral immune response in heparin- induced thrombocytopenia. *Am J Hematol*, 54, 3, (Mar 1997), pp.196-201.

Tardy B, Lecompte T, Boelhen F, Tardy-Poncet B, Elalamy I, et al. (2006). Predictive factors for thrombosis and major bleeding in an observational study in 181 patients with heparin-induced thrombocytopenia treated with lepirudin. *Blood*, 108, 5, (Sep 2006), pp.1492–1496.

Tardy-Poncet B, Tardy B, Reynaud J, Mahul P, Mismetti P, et al. (1999). Efficacy and safety of danaparoid sodium (ORG 10172) in critically ill patients with heparin-associated thrombocytopenia. *Chest*, 115, 6, (Jun 1999), pp.1616–1620.

Toyohira H, Nakamura K, Kariyazono H, Yamada K, Moriyama Y, et al. (1995). Significance of combined use of anticoagulants and antiplatelet agents in the early stage after prosthetic valve replacement. *Kyobu Geka*, 48, 9, (Aug 1995), pp.749-755.

Visentin GP, Ford SE, Scott JP, & Aster RHJ. (1994). Antibodies from patients with heparin-induced thrombocytopenia/thrombosis are specific for platelet factor 4 complexed with heparin or bound to endothelial cells. *Clin Invest*, 93, 1, (Jun 1994), pp.81-88.

Walenga JM, Jeske WP, & Messmore HL. (2000). Mechanisms of venous and arterial thrombosis in heparin-induced thrombocytopenia. *J Thromb Thrombolysis*, 10, (Suppl), pp.S13-S20.

Walenga JM, Jeske WP, Prechel MM, & Bakhos M. (2004). Newer insights on the mechanism of heparin-induced thrombocytopenia. *Semin Thromb Hemost*, 30, (Suppl1), (Feb 2004), pp.S57-S67.

Wallis DE, Workman DL, Lewis BE, Steen L, Pifarre R, et al. (1999). Failure of early heparin cessation as treatment for heparin-induced thrombocytopenia. *Am J Med*, 106, 6, (Jun 1999), pp.629-635.

Warkentin TE, & Bernstein RA. (2003). Delayed-onset heparin-induced thrombocytopenia and cerebral thrombosis after a single administration of unfractionated heparin [letter]. *N Engl J Med*, 348, 11, (Mar 2003), pp.1067-1069.

Warkentin TE, & Greinacher A. (2004). Heparin-induced thrombocytopenia: recognition, treatment, and prevention. *Chest*, 126, (suppl 3), (Sep 2004), pp.311S-337S.

Warkentin TE, & Heddle NM. (2003). Laboratory diagnosis of immune heparin-induced thrombocytopenia. *Curr Hematol Rep*, 2, 2, (Mar 2003), pp.148-157.

Warkentin TE, & Kelton JG. (1990). Heparin and platelets. *Hematol Oncol Clin North Am*, 4, 1, (Feb 1990), pp.243-264.

Warkentin TE, & Kelton JG. (1996). A 14-year study of heparin-induced thrombocytopenia. *Am J Med*, 101, pp.502-507.

Warkentin TE, & Kelton JG. (2001a). Temporal aspects of heparin-induced thrombocytopenia. *N Engl J Med*, 344, 17, (Apr 2001), pp.1286-1292.

Warkentin TE, & Kelton JG. (2001b). Delayed-onset heparin-induced thrombocytopenia and thrombosis. *Ann Intern Med*, 135, 7, (Oct 2001), pp.502-506.

Warkentin TE, Aird WC, & Rand JH. (2003b). Platelet-endothelial interactions: sepsis, HIT, and antiphospholipid syndrome. *Hematology (Am Soc Heamtol Educ Prog)*, pp.497-519.

Warkentin TE, Chong BH, & Greinacher A. (1998).Heparin-induced thrombocytopenia: towards consensus. *Thromb Haemost*, 79, 1, (Jun 1998), pp.1-7.

Warkentin TE, Cook RJ, Marder VJ, Sheppard JA, Moore JC, et al. (2005). Anti-platelet factor 4/heparin antibodies in orthopedic surgery patients receiving antithrombotic prophylaxis with fondaparinux or enoxaparin. *Blood*, 106, 12, (Dec 2005), pp.3791-3796.

Warkentin TE, Elavathil LJ, Hayward CP, Johnston MA, Russett JI, et al. (1997). The pathogenesis of venous limb gangrene associated with heparin-induced thrombocytopenia. *Ann Intern Med*, 127, 9, (Nov 1997), pp.804-812.

Warkentin TE, Greinacher A, Koster A, & Lincoff AM; American College of Chest Physicians. (2008a). Treatment and prevention of heparin-induced hrombocyotopenia. American College of Physicians evidence-based clinical practice guidelines (8th edition). *Chest*, 133, (suppl 6), (Jun 2008), pp.340S-380S.

Warkentin TE, Hayward CP, Smith CA, Kelly PM, Kelton JG. (1992). Determinants of donor platelet variability when testing for heparin-induced thrombocytopenia. *J Lab Clin Med*, 120, 3, (Sep 1992), pp.371-379.

Warkentin TE, Levine MN, Hirsh J, Horsewood P, Roberts RS, et al. (1995a). Heparin-induced thrombocytopenia in patients treated with low-molecular-weight heparin or unfractionated heparin. *N Engl J Med*, 332, 20, (May 1995), pp.1330-1335.

Warkentin TE, Roberts RS, Hirsh J, & Kelton JG. (2003a). An improved definition of immune heparin-induced thrombocytopenia in postoperative orthopedic patients. *Arch Intern Med*, 163, 20, (Nov 2003), pp.2518-2524.

Warkentin TE, Sheppard J, Moore J, Sigouin CS, & Kelton J. (2008b). Quantitative interpretation of optical density measurements using PF4-dependent enzyme-immunoassays. *J Thromb Haemost*, 6, 8, (Aug 2008). pp.1304-1312.

Warkentin TE, Sheppard JA, Horsewood P, Simpson PJ, Moore JC, et al. (2000). Impact of the patient population on the risk for heparin-induced thrombocytopenia. *Blood*, 96, 5, (Sep 2000), pp.1703-1708.

Warkentin TE. (1996a). Heparin-induced thrombocytopenia: IgG-mediated platelet activation, platelet microparticle generation, and altered procoagulant/ anticoagulant balance in the pathogenesis of thrombosis and venous limb gangrene complicating heparin-induced thrombocytopenia. *Transfus Med Rev*, 10, 4, (Oct 1996), pp.249-258.

Warkentin TE. (1996b). Heparin-induced skin lesions. *Br J Haematol*, 92, 2, (Feb 1996), pp.494-497.

Warkentin TE. (1999). Generation of platelet-derived microparticles and procoagulation activity by heparin-induced thrombocytopenia IgG/serum and other IgG platelet agonists: a comparison with standard platelet agonists. *Platelets*. 10, 5, (1999), pp.319-326.

Warkentin TE. (2000). Laboratory testing for heparin-induced thrombocytopenia. *J Thromb Thromblysi*, 10, (suppl 1), (Nov 2000), pp.S35-S45.

Warkentin TE. (2001). Laboratory testing for heparin-induced thrombocytopenia. In: Warkentin TE. Greinacher A. eds. Heparin-induced thrombocytopenia. 2nd ed. New York, NY: Marcel Dekker Inc; pp.231-269.

Warkentin TE. (2002). Platelet count monitoring and laboratory testing for heparin-induced thrombocytopenia. *Arch Pathol Lab Med*, 126, 11, (Nov 2002), pp.1415-1423.

Warkentin TE. (2003). Heparin-induced thrombocytopenia: pathogenesis and management. *Br J Haematol*, 121, 4, (May 2003), pp.535-555.

Warkentin TE. (2004a). Clinical picture of heparin-induced thrombocytopenia. In: Warkentin TE. Greinacher A. eds. Heparin-induced thrombocytopenia. 3rd ed. New York, NY: Marcel Dekker, pp.53-106.

Warkentin TE. (2004b) Laboratory testing for heparin-induced thrombocytopenia. In: Warkentin TE. Greinacher A. eds. Heparin-induced thrombocytopenia. 3rd ed. New York, NY: Marcel Dekker, pp.271-311.

Warkentin TE. (2007). Clinical picture of heparin-induced thrombocytopenia. In: Warkentin TE. Greinacher A. eds. Heparin-induced thrombocytopenia. 4rd ed. New York, NY: InformaHealthcare USA, pp.21-66.

Ziporen L, Li ZQ, Park KS, Sabnekar P, Liu WY, Arepally G, et al. (1998). Defining an antigenic epitope on platelet factor 4 associated with heparin-induced thrombocytopenia. *Blood*, 92, 9, (Nov 1998), pp.3250–3259.

Zwicker JI, Uhl L, Huang WY, Shaz BH, Bauer KA. (2004). Thrombosis and ELISA optical density values in hospitalized patients with heparin-induced thrombocytopenia. *J Thromb Haemost.* 12, 2, (Dec 2004), pp.2133-2137.

10

The Ubiquitin-Proteasomal System and Blood Cancer Therapy

Xinliang Mao and Biyin Cao
Cyrus Tang Hematology Center, Soochow University
P.R.China

1. Introduction

The ubiquitin-proteasomal system (UPS) is critical for the regulation of protein homeostasis and is composed of the protein ubiquitination system and proteasomal degradation system. Protein ubiquitination is referred to the process that the small protein ubiquitin is covalently tagged to a specific substrate protein. Once a protein is ubiquitinated, its structural conformation, cellular location, and biological function will change accordingly, or it will be delivered into the 26S proteasome complex for degradation by specific proteases. The UPS is extensively involved in nearly all the important cell biological activities, such as cell metabolism, cell proliferation, glycogen synthesis, immunological process, organogenesis, etc. (Ciechanover, 1998; Haglund and Dikic, 2005; Kirkin and Dikic, 2010).

The UPS system is also widely associated with various diseases, such as inflammation, arthritis, heart disease and cancers (Ciechanover et al., 2000). For example, the proteasome has emerged as a milestone target for cancer therapy, which was further demonstrated by the discovery of the proteasome inhibitor bortezomib for the therapy of multiple myeloma (Kisselev and Goldberg, 2001; Richardson et al., 2003). Recently, in addition to the proteasome, the protein ubiquitination pathway is also being developed as a novel target for anti-cancer drugs (Bedford et al., 2011 ; Colland, 2010). In this chapter, we will discuss the UPS system, its biological implications, and associated targeted drug discovery for hematological malignancies.

2. The ubiquitin-proteasomal system (UPS)

The UPS is composed by at least 6 components, including ubiquitin (Ub), ubiquitin-activating enzymes (UBA, E1), ubiquitin-conjugating enzymes (UBC, E2), ubiquitin ligases (E3), proteasomes, and deubiquitinases (Dub) (Figure 1). The substrate proteins are first tagged with a ubiquitin chain under the guidance of E1, E2 and E3, and the produced polyubiquitinated proteins are then transferred to 26S proteasomes where it is degraded by the 20S core particles.

2.1 Ubiquitination

Ubiquitin is a ubiquitinously expressed small protein composed of 76 amino acids and it plays a central role in the UPS system. It can be linked to a substrate protein with the

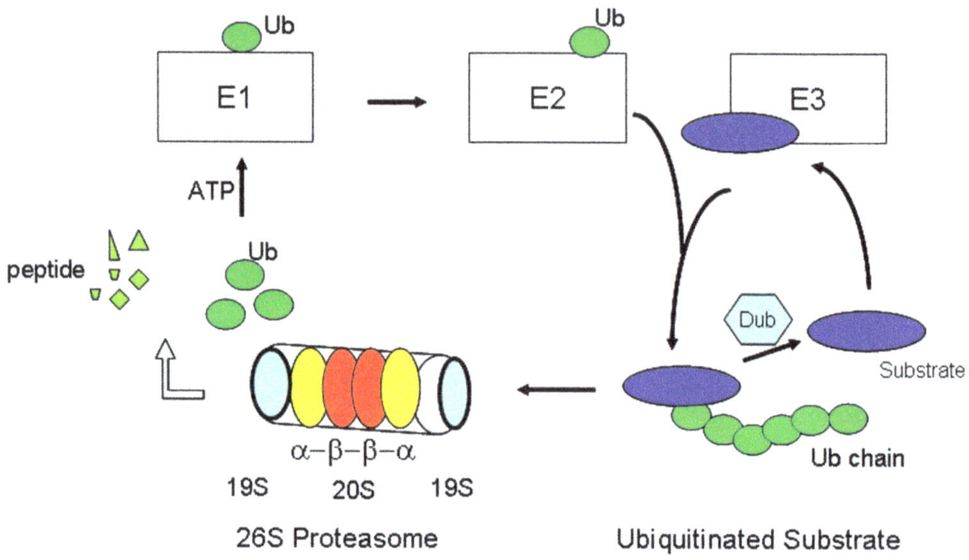

Fig. 1. The ubiquitination-proteasomal system (UPS). The UPS is composed of 6 components, including ubiquitin (Ub), ubiquitin-activating enzyme (E1), ubiquitin-conjugating enzyme (E2), ubiquitin ligase (E3), deubiquitinases (Dub) and proteasomes.

assistance of E1, E2, and E3, and can be removed from the target protein by Dubs. Ubiquitin is highly conserved and is expressed in most species but it is only found in eukaryotic organisms. This strong sequence conservation suggests that ubiquitin plays a very fundamental role in maintaining cell function and in species evolution. Actually, ubiquitin is involved in all aspects of cell biology and activities by regulating its extensive substrate proteins. Proteins will undergo turnover, translocation or conformational changes after they are covalently attached a ubiquitin, which is called ubiquitination, one of the most important post-translational modifications of proteins, where the carboxylic acid of the terminal glycine from the di-glycine motif in the activated ubiquitin forms an amide bond to the epsilon amine of the lysine in the substrate proteins (Ciechanover et al., 2000). In the 76 amino acids, there are 6 lysine residues (K) including K6, K11, K27, K29, K33, K48, and K63 as shown in Figure 2. These lysine residues are responsible for ubiquitin attachment to the target proteins. Theoretically, any lysine residues in a protein could be linked a ubiquitin, including ubiquitin itself, however, the biological function may differ and it depends on the ubiquitination status (Haglund and Dikic, 2005).

Ubiquitination can be categorized into three classes based on the tagged ubiquitin (Haglund and Dikic, 2005; Ye and Rape, 2009): i) monoubiquitination: proteins are bound to a single ubiquitin, ii) multiubiquitination or poly-monoubiquitination: proteins are tagged with several single ubiquitin molecules; iii) polyubiquitination: proteins are attached with poly-ubiquitin chains. These differences of ubiquitination on target proteins will regulate a variety of cellular processes, including protein degradation, signal transduction, membrane trafficking, DNA repair, chromatin remodelling, peroxisome biogenesis and viral budding (Ye and Rape, 2009). For example, polyubiquitin chain occurring at the 11th (K11) and 48th

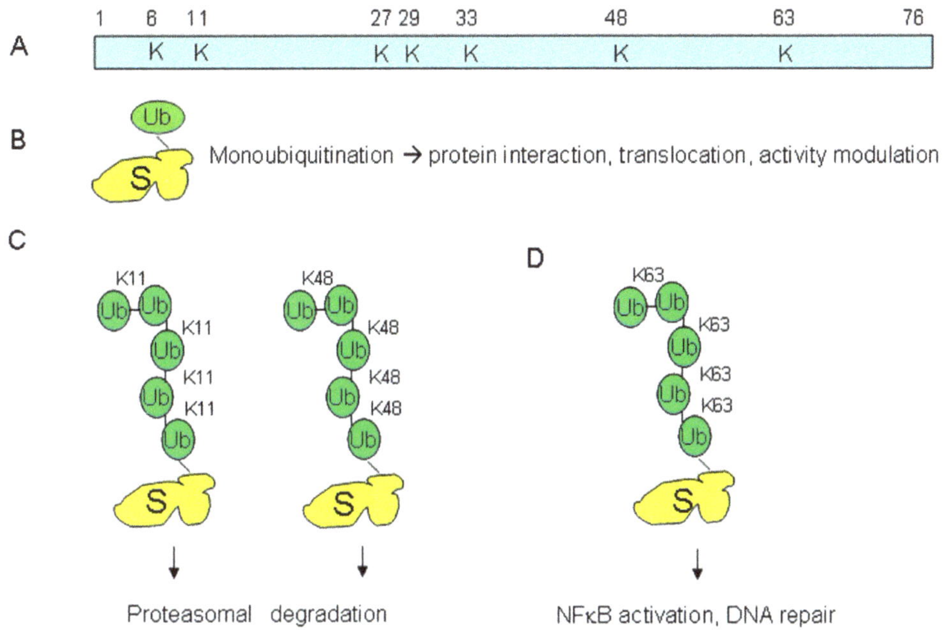

Fig. 2. Protein ubiquitination and functional modulation. There are 7 lysine (K) residues in 76 amino acids of ubiquitin and each could be further conjugated to a specific protein (A). Monoubiquitination (B) regulates protein conformation, cellular localization and protein interaction. Proteins tagged with polyubiquitin-chains occurring at K11 or K48 (C) are subject to degradation in the 26S proteasome. Polyubiquitination at K63 (D) activates NFκB function and is involved in DNA repair.

lysine (K48) of ubiquitin is mainly involved in protein degradation, but the K63 polyubiquitination is mainly responsible for modification of protein function and involved in signal transduction, including regulation of NFκB signal pathway, DNA repair and targeting to the lysosome (Ye and Rape, 2009). For other proteins polyubiquintinated at K6, 27, 29 or 33, whether they are involved in protein degradation or DNA repair is largely unknown (Ye and Rape, 2009)(Figure 2).

2.2 Ubiquitining enzymes

The ubiquitination process is an ATP-dependent enzymatic reaction and requires at least 3 types of enzymes, including E1, E2 and E3 as described earlier, thus the ubiquitination process is alternatively known as the E1-E2-E3 cascade. In the process of ubiquitination, ubiquitin is first activated by E1 using ATP as an energy source to form a ubiquitin-adenylate intermediate. Subsequently, the ubiquitin is transferred to the cysteine residue, the E1 active site, resulting in a thioester linkage between the C-terminal carboxyl group of ubiquitin and the E1 cysteine sulfhydryl group. Secondly, the activated ubiquitin is transferred from E1 to the cysteine of an E2 via a trans(thio)esterification reaction. Finally, the ubiquitination cascade creates an isopeptide bond between a lysine of the target protein and the C-terminal glycine of ubiquitin with the coordination of an E3 which identifies specific recognition modules in the target protein and is capable of interaction with both E2 and substrate (Ye and Rape, 2009).

In human genome, there are only two genes encoding E1, whilst E2 is encoded by 60-100 genes, and there are ~ 1000 different E3 genes (Deshaies and Joazeiro, 2009; Schulman and Harper, 2009). E1 activates ubiquitin at the top level, and transfers activated ubiquitin to different E2. E3s identify individual substrates and specifically ligate E2-Ub complex to a certain target protein. These enzymes form a hierarchical structure (Figure 3) and control the whole ubiquitination process. In this ubiquitination cascade, E1 binds to dozens of E2s, which bind to hundreds of E3s, and E3s specifically target thousands of substrate proteins.

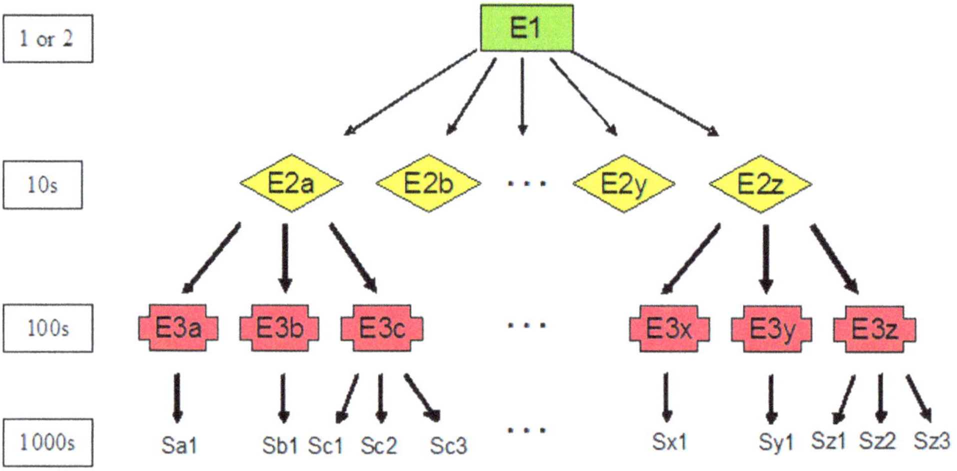

Fig. 3. E1, E2 and E3 form an enzymatic cascade for protein ubiquitination. One single E1 initiates the whole ubiquitination process, by activating Ub and transferring it to E2. There are around 100 E2s in human. Each E2 will deliver activated Ub to one or several E3s which are a large family of around 1000 members. E3s specifically identify target proteins (substrates) and attach Ub to individual proteins.

There are around 100 Dubs in human cells which cleave the ubiquitin-protein bonds thus regulating ubiquitin-dependent metabolic pathways (Colland, 2010). Polyubiquitinated proteins are deubiquitinated by Dubs immediately before degradation in the proteasome. In addition to ubiquitin recycling, Dubs are also involved in processing of ubiquitin precursors, in proofreading of protein ubiquitination and in disassembly of inhibitory ubiquitin chains.

2.3 The proteasome system

The 26S proteasome is a large protein complex with molecular weight more than 2000 kilodalton and it is composed of one 20S core particle and two 19S regulatory particles, where the core particle is made up of two α units (at the two ends) and two β units (in the middle). Each of these units is composed of 7 ring-like subunits thus the total 28 subunits stack up to form a hollow cylinder (Figure 1). The α subunits N-termini form a gate and serve as docking domains for the regulatory particles that block unregulated access of substrates to the interior cavity (Smith et al., 2007). Proteins are lysed in the core particle but proteases are only found in the interior surface of the β units, especially β1, β2 and β5. Although these proteases share a common mechanism, each subunit dominants its distinctive catalytic activity due to interatomic contacts with local residues near the active sites of each subunit. β1, β2, and β5 mainly present caspase-like, trypsin-like, and chymotrypsin-like activity, respectively. Each catalytic β subunit also possesses a conserved lysine residue required for proteolysis. The proteasomes catalyze thousands of polyubiquitinated proteins, therefore, they are critical in regulatory protein function and cell activity.

3. The UPS is extensively involved in hematological malignancies

3.1 Protein ubiquitination in blood cancers

Heavy ubiquitination levels of proteins, associated with overactivation of E1, have been observed both in leukemia cell lines and primary acute leukemia cells compared with the normal blood cells (Bedford et al., 2011; Xu et al., 2010). Additionally, blood cancer-specific proteins are also regulated by the UPS. For example, multiple myeloma (MM) tumor cells are recurrently associated with several chromosomal translocations that result in overexpression of transcription factors involved in the UPS pathway such as c-Maf, MafB, and fibroblast growth factor receptor 3 (FGFR3), which converge dysregulation of D-cyclins (Bergsagel and Kuehl, 2005). All these proteins could be poly-ubiquitinated and degraded in proteasomes. D-type cyclins are ubiquitinated under the coordination of SCF E3 ligase complex. The fibroblast growth factor receptor FGFR3 could also be ubiquitinated. In chronic leukemia, FGFR3 undergoes ubiquitination by c-Cbl, a RING finger domain-containing E3 ligase. In chronic leukemia cells, the specific BAR-ABL fusion protein is ubiquitinated by c-CBL. Targeting at c-CBL, arsenic induces degradation of BCR-ABL (Mao et al., 2010).

3.2 Ubiquitination enzymes and blood cancers

E1 is responsible for the first step of the ubiquitination process by activating ubiquitin and is overexpressed in all leukemia and MM cell lines and primary samples. When E1 is knocked down, these leukemia and MM cells will go to apoptosis (Xu et al., 2010). Several E2s have been reported to be involved in MM development. For example, CDC34, the cell cycle regulator, is highly expressed in MM patient cells and cell lines in contrast to normal cells (Block et al., 2001). CDC34 has been implicated in the ubiquitination of p27 (Kip1), IκBα, Wee1, and MyoD, thus facilitating the degradation of these proteins by 26S proteasomes and modulating cell cycle progression. Inhibition of CDC34 enzymatic activity abrogates interleukin-6-induced protection against dexamethasone-induced MM cell apoptosis.

Ubiquitin ligase E3s are the largest family in the UPS system. Various E3s are involved in leukemia, myeloma and lymphomas (Bernassola et al., 2008). For example, XIAP, the representative of the RING finger family of E3s, and Mdm2, the primary E3 ligase for p53 ubiquitination (Jones et al., 2008), are overexpressed in various leukemic and myeloma cells and contribute to cell proliferation and anti-apoptotic activity. XIAP is also the most important enzyme that inhibits caspase-3, -6, and -7 activities and confers to drug resistance. Skp2 is another important E3 ligase. In CML cells, BCR-ABL fusion oncogene frequently up-regulate Skp2 expression via transcriptional activation, while treatment of Bcr-Abl kinase inhibitor imatinib led to G1 growth arrest accompanied with reduced Skp2 expression (Chen et al., 2011). SKP2 contributes to increased p27(Kip1) turnover, cell proliferation, and a poor prognosis in many tumor types (Zhan et al., 2007).

3.3 Deubiquitinases and blood cancers

Attached ubiquitin can be removed by a ubiquitin protease from targeted protein. USP9X is one of the most studied deubiquitinases and is probably involved in deubiquitination from oncoprotein MCL-1. Increased USP9X expression correlates with increased MCL1 protein in human follicular lymphomas and diffuse large B-cell lymphomas (Schwickart et al., 2010). Moreover, patients with multiple myeloma overexpressing USP9X have a poor prognosis. Knockdown of USP9X increases MCL1 polyubiquitination, which enhances MCL1 turnover and cell killing by the BH3 mimetic ABT-737, an inhibitor of MCL1 (Schwickart et al., 2010). Thus, USP9X has been identified as an effective prognostic and therapeutic target. Another important Dub is CYLD, which is a negative regulator of NFκB. CYLD is located in the 16q12 and its lower expression in MM cells is highly associated with deletion of 16q. In T cell leukemia, the Notch/Hes1 pathway sustains NFκB activation through CYLD repression. In MM cells highly expressing NFκB, both the DNA copy number and protein expression of CYLD are markedly decreased. On the other hand, when treated with proteasome inhibitors such as MG132, CYLD will be accumulated in MM cells. CYLD presents as a tumor suppressor deubiquitinase and restoration of CYLD will sensitize cancer cell apoptosis (Jin et al., 2008).

3.4 Proteasomes and blood cancers

Several lines of evidence have shown that proteasome subunits in both leukemia and MM cells are abnormally higher than those normal or untransformed counterparts (Kumatori et al., 1990). Immunohistochemical staining shows considerably increased concentrations of proteasomes in leukemic cells from the bone marrow of patients with various types of leukemia and the predominant localization of these proteasomes in the nuclei. Moreover, enzyme immunoassay and Northern blot analysis indicate that the concentrations of proteasomes and their mRNA levels are consistently much higher in a variety of malignant human hematopoietic cell lines than in resting peripheral lymphocytes and monocytes from healthy adults. Proteasome expression is also increased in normal blood mononuclear cells during blastogenic transformation induced by phytohemagglutinin; their expression increased in parallel with induction of DNA synthesis and returned to the basal level with progress of the cell cycle. These findings strongly suggest that proteasomes are associated with cell cycle progression. Later studies demonstrated that proteasomes regulate a serial of cell cycle proteins, including p27, pRb, cyclin D, p53, p27, pro-apoptotic Bcl-2 family members, as well as the most important transcription factor in cell proliferation, NFκB (Kisselev and Goldberg, 2001). Importantly, leukemia and myeloma cells are more sensitive to proteasome inhibitors. An early study found that the IC_{50} to inhibit cell proliferation in lymphoma is 5 times lower than normal T cells when treating cells with lactacystin, a classic and typical inhibitor of proteasomes (Delic et al., 1998). Another study indicated that B-CLL cells are about 10 times more sensitive to lactacystin than normal peripheral B lymphocytes. These results strongly suggest that proteasomes could be used as a drug target for myeloma and lymphoma therapy.

4. Discovery of bortezomib and its application in MM therapy

4.1 Discovery of bortezomib as a treatment for myeloma

Proteasomes are critical for cancer cells, therefore they could be used as a drug target for cancer therapy. Efforts are first made to develop such kinds of inhibitors for MM therapy. The seminal contribution came from Myogenic which developed a series of proteasome inhibitors, including MG132, one of the most common proteasome inhibitors currently used in research, and MG-341, which was renamed PS-341 and was further developed as a promising drug candidate for cancer therapy. PS-341 alone achieved an overall remission rate of 35% in refractory and/or relapse myeloma patients, when it was used in combination with other drugs such as cyclophosphamide and dexamethasone, the ORR could reach around 90% or greater. Following several large and multi-center clinical trials, PS-341 was approved by Food and Drug Administration of USA for MM in 2003, and for mantle cell lymphoma in 2006. PS-341 is now known as its general name bortezomib based on its chemical structure and is marketed as Velcade®. Recent studies also demonstrated that bortezomib might be particularly active against the active B cell-like diffuse large B cell lymphoma (ABC-DLBCL). ABC-DLBCL has a worse survival after upfront chemotherapy and is characterized by constitutive activation of the NFκB pathway, which can inhibit chemotherapy. Although bortezomib alone has no activities on ABC-DLBCL, when administrated with chemotherapeutics, such as R-CHOP or DA-EPOCH-B, it achieved a superior overall response and survival according to a clinical study of 49 patients. Although ABC-DLBCL and GCB-DLBCL have similar poor outcome by regular chemotherapeutics, ABC-DLBCLs are more sensitive to bortezomib. Bortezomib presented a high responsive rate (83% *vs* 13%) and median overall survival (10.8 *vs* 3.4 months) in ABC compared with GCB-DLBCL, respectively (Dunleavy et al., 2009). It is predictable that bortezomib as an inhibitor of NFκB pathway will be developed for other cancer therapy.

4.2 Molecular mechanisms of bortezomib in the treatment of myeloma

Bortezomib is a dipeptide containing phenylalanine and leucine in which the carboxylic group is replaced by a boronic acid group (-RB(OH)2) (Figure 4).

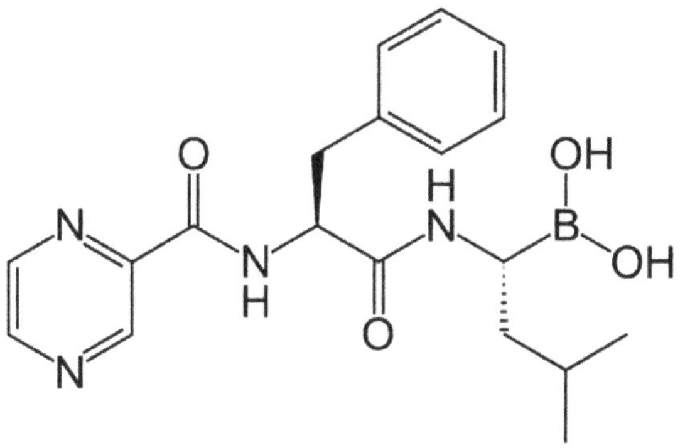

Fig. 4. The chemical structure of bortezomib. Bortezomib is a dipeptide made up of phenylalanine and leucine in which boronic acid group replaces the carboxyl group.

Bortezomib is a potent inhibitor of proteasomes. Mechanistically, its active boron acid group competitively and reversibly binds to the catalytic site of the 26S proteasome with high affinity and specificity. Specifically, the boric acid group of bortezomib binds to and blocks the catalytic threonine residue in the β subunits of the 20S core particle. Inhibition of proteasome results in accumulation of several important tumor suppressor proteins, including p21, p27, p53, PTEN, and IκBα. IκBα is an inhibitor of NFκB, the most important transcription factor in regulating cell proliferation. Normally, IκBα is bound to NFκB and inhibits its activity. The IκBα stability is regulated via the UPS pathway. Once IκBα is degraded, NFκB will be librated and translocated into the neucleus where it binds to the promoters of various genes and initiates their transcription and expression. IκBα/NFκB signaling plays a critical role in bortezomib-induced cell apoptosis. Bortezomib also interrupts the interaction of Mdm2 and its substrate p53, thus restoring p53 function and leading to cell apoptosis. Moreover, bortezomib directly acts on MM cells and alters cellular interactions and cytokine secretion in the bone marrow (BM) millieu to inhibit tumor cell growth, induce apoptosis, and overcome drug resistance. Specifically, bortezomib inhibits the paracrine growth of human MM cells by decreasing their adherence to bone marrow stromal cells (BMSCs) and related NFκB-dependent induction of interleukin-6 secretion in BMSCs, as well as inhibiting proliferation and growth signaling of residual adherent MM cells (Hideshima et al., 2001).

4.3 Pitfalls of bortezomib in MM treatment

Although bortezomib has made a great success in the treatment of MM and MCL, it is not a perfect drug, and some critical features prevent its application (Kumar and Rajkumar, 2008; Oerlemans et al., 2008). Firstly, it is unstable and it retains its activity for 4-8 hrs after reconstituted, thus having to be used within 8 hours. Secondly, the drug is administrated via *i.v.* injection which should be performed by a nurse at a clinic or in a hospital, which largely increases the cost of the health care system.

Thirdly, the therapeutic window of bortezomib is very narrow. The therapeutic dosage is 1.3 mg/m^2 body surface, it will produce dose-dependent toxicity when the dose reaches 1.5 mg/m^2. These adverse effects and toxicity include myelosuppression which leads to anemia, neutropenia and thrombocytopenia, and bortezomib-induced peripheral neuropathy, which occurs in more than 30% patients and this kind of neuropathy is sometimes even worse to affect patients' daily activity (Richardson et al., 2006). Although these kinds of adverse effects are recoverable when the drug is discontinued, some patients couldn't endure the severe effects. Recent studies suggest that some important genes (such as *RHOBTB2* and *SOX8*) involved in the development of the nervous system (especially the peripheral nervous system) are upregulated by bortezomib after one cycle therapy (Cavo et al., 2010).

Lastly, drug resistance is becoming an emerging issue. Although 35% of refractory and relapsed myeloma patients are generally responsive after bortezomib treatment, there are only 4% patients with a complete remission outcome and 65% had no response. There are several underlying issues for bortezomib resistance. Firstly, the resistance to bortezomib is associated with overexpression of β5 subunits of 20S core particles, which leads to impaired binding of bortezomib and decreased proteasome inhibition. For example, K562 cells with a high level of β5 are more resistant to bortezomib than other cell lines such as OCI-AML2 expressing low levels of β5 (Li et al., 2010). Secondly, bortezomib resistance is also associated with mutations in β5 gene. A DNA sequencing analysis in bortezomib-resistant cells revealed that the G322A mutation in PSMB5 gene leads to an Alanine→ Threonine change, which largely confers resistance because threonine is the target of bortezomib (Oerlemans et al., 2008). In a Jurkat cell model, mutations such as C323T and G326A are also reported (Lu et al., 2008). Thirdly, overexpression of other anti-apoptotic genes such as PSMD4 (Shaughnessy et al., 2010), a non-ATPase subunit of the proteosomal 19S regulator, and heat shock protein 27 (HSP27) (Chauhan et al., 2003), an important gene protecting cell against apoptosis, are also found to be associated with resistance to bortezomib. Recently, an siRNA screen identified several important molecular modulators that sensitize bortezomib-induced cell apoptosis, including proteasome subunits PSMA5, PSMB2, PSMB3, and PSMB7 (Zhu et a., 2011), this is quite reasonable because these genes directly modulate the proteasome function. To be noted, the Cyclin-dependent kinase 5 (CDK5) and other 11 genes were also identified from this screen, but their detailed roles in bortezomib-induced cell death are yet to be studied. A most recent study demonstrated that impaired bortezomib binding to mutant β5 subunit of the proteasome is the underlying basis for bortezomib resistance in leukemia cells, while proteasome subunit overexpression is an essential compensatory mechanism for the impaired catalytic activity of these mutant proteasomes (Franke et al., 2011).

5. Development of novel proteasomal inhibitors

Currently, several classes of novel proteasome inhibitors have been developed and some have been moved to advanced clinical trials for the treatment of various blood cancers, such as leukemia, lymphoma, and myeloma. Although they share some common features, these novel inhibitors of proteasomes could be classified as: highly selective and irreversible, orally active, non-competitive, and natural products. The details are shown in Table 1.

5.1 Highly selective and irreversible novel inhibitors of proteasomes

Several promising novel proteasomal inhibitors have been extensively investigated *in vivo*, *in vitro*, and in clinical settings. Compared with bortezomib, these agents are highly selective and irreversible, such as carfilzomib, NPI-0052, and PI-083.

5.1.1 Carfilzomib

Carflizomib, or PR-171, is a tetrapeptide epoxyketone and a selective and irreversible proteasome inhibitor that primarily targets the chymotrypsin-like (CT-L) subunits in both the constitutive proteasome (c20S, β5) and the immunoproteasome (i20S, LMP7) (Parlati et al., 2009). Inhibition of proteasome-mediated proteolysis results in an accumulation of polyubiquitinated proteins, which may lead to cell cycle arrest, induction of apoptosis, and inhibition of tumor growth. Compared with bortezomib, carfilzomib displays minimal cross reactivity on off-target enzymes, good tolerability and little side effects in multiple open-label clinical trials (O'Connor et al., 2009). In patients with relapsed or refractory multiple myeloma, twice-weekly consecutive-day single-agent carfilzomib 20 mg/m^2 , escalating to 27 mg/m^2 the second cycle was associated with a 54% overall response rate in bortezomib-naive patients and a 26% overall response rate in bortezomib and immunomodulatory drug refractory patients. The overall response rate is 20% higher than that with single bortezomib treatment. The U.S. Food and Drug Administration has granted fast track designation for carfilzomib to develop as a potential treatment of patients with relapsed and refractory multiple myeloma.

Drugs	Features	R&D Stage	Institutes
Highly selective and irreversible			
Carfilzomib (PR-171)	Epoxomicin analog Minimal activity against off-target enzymes Lymphoid neoplasms and multiple myeloma	Phase III for MM Phase I for solid tumors	Proteolix Onyx
Marizomib (NPI-0052 Salinospormide A)	Marine product, β-lactone-γ-lactam family More potent than Bortezomib MM, lymphomas, leukemias and solid tumors	Phase II for myeloma	Nereus Pharmaceuticals, Inc.
PI-083	From Streptomyces matensis Thr21,Gly47, Ala 49 of β5, Asp114 of β6 Cancer-selective proteasome inhibitor Myeloma, lung cancer, breast cancer	Preclinical	Moffitt Cancer Center
Orally active			
CEP-18770	Boronic-acid based More sustained Pharmacodynamics Competes with bortezomib Few side effects during treatment	Phase II for myeloma	Cephalon
PR-047	c20S, i20S >80% inhibition in most tissues High oral bioavailability		Proteolix
Non-comparative inhibitors on 20S proteasomes			
Clioquinol 5-Amino-8-hydroxyl-quine (5AHQ)	Binding to a subunits of 20S Non-competitive inhibition Overcome resistance to Bortezomib	Phase I	University Health Network
Natural Products			
Pristimerin	Isolated from Celastrus and Maytenus spp. Tripernoid family C6 of Pristimerin interacts with hydroxyl group of N-terminal Thr of c20S Inhibits IKK, suppresses NFκB, cyclin D	Preclicical	Mayo Clinic
EGCG (-)-epigallocatechin-3-gallate	From green tea Ester bond of EGCG attacked by N-terminal Thr of 20S Competitively inhibits Proteasome with Bortezomib	Preclinical	Not available

Table 1. Novel Proteasome inhibitors against blood cancers

5.1.2 Marizomib

Marizomib (NPI-0052 or salinosporamide A) is a structurally and pharmacologically unique β-lactone-γ-lactam proteasome inhibitor produced by a marine actinomycete *Salinispora tropica* (Macherla et al., 2005). Unlike bortezomib, marizomib irreversibly binds to proteasomes and inhibits all three protease activities, including chymotrypsin-like (CT-L, β5), trypsin-like (T-L, β2), and caspase-like (C-L,β1). This nature is responsible for its slower efflux, longer duration of action, and greater cytotoxicity (Obaidat et al.). Preclinical studies suggest that marizomib is a more potent inducer of apoptosis in myeloma cells than bortezomib, and demonstrates activity in bortezomib resistant cell lines as well. In addition to MM, marizomib has been evaluated in models for MCL, Waldenstrom's macroglobulinemia (WM), chronic and acute lymphocytic leukemia, glioma, colorectal and pancreatic cancers, and has exhibited synergistic activities in tumor models in combination with bortezomib, and various histone deacetylase inhibitors (B et al., 2011; Singh et al., 2010). Marizomib has been moved to Phase II clinical trials and achieved very good responses. In a Phase I study of 17 patients with relapsed and relapsed/refractory multiple myeloma, Drug- related adverse events have consisted principally of mild-to-moderate fatigue, nausea and diarrhea. More importantly, NPI-0052 does not appear to induce peripheral neuropathy or myelosuppression associated with bortezomib treatment (Hofmeister et al., 2009).

5.2 Orally active inhibitors of proteasomes: CEP-18770, PR-047 and ONX-0912

The *i.v.* administration of bortezomib largely increases the workload of the physicians and other medical staff and largely increases the healthcare budget. Therefore, orally active inhibitors of proteasomes are of great interest. Currently, several such orally active drugs have been developed, including CEP-18770, PR-047 and ONX-0912.

5.2.1 CEP-18770

CEP-18770 is a novel orally-active inhibitor of the chymotrypsin-like activity of the proteasome that down-modulates the NFκB activity (Piva et al., 2008). CEP-18770 induces apoptotic cell death in MM cell lines and in primary purified CD138-positive explant cultures from untreated and bortezomib-treated MM patients. Importantly, CEP-18770 exhibits a favorable cytotoxicity profile toward normal human epithelial cells, bone marrow progenitors, and bone marrow-derived stromal cells. Both intravenous and oral administration of CEP-18770 resulted in a sustained pharmacodynamic inhibition of proteasome activity in tumors relative to normal tissues, complete tumor regression of MM xenografts and improved overall median survival in a systemic model of human MM. In addition, CEP-18770 has a strong antiangiogenic activity *in vitro*, and potently represses RANKL-induced osteoclastogenesis. A recent study suggests that CEP-18770 enhances the anti-myeloma activity of bortezomib and melphalan which suggests a combinatorial regimen for MM therapy (Piva et al., 2008; Sanchez et al., 2010). This agent has moved to clinical trials for relapsed or refractory multiple myeloma (http://clinicaltrials.gov/ct2/show/NCT01348919) or for solid tumors and non-Hodgin's lymphomas (http://clinicaltrials.gov/ct2/show/NCT00572637).

5.2.2 PR-047

PR-047 is also an orally active inhibitor that selectively inhibits CT-L activity of both the constitutive proteasome (β5) and immunoproteasome (LMP7) and demonstrated an absolute bioavailability of up to 39% in rodents and dogs. It was well tolerated with repeated oral administration at doses resulting in >80% proteasome inhibition in most tissues and elicited an antitumor response equivalent to intravenously administered carfilzomib in multiple human tumor xenograft and mouse syngeneic models (Zhou et al., 2009). The favorable pharmacologic profile supports its further development for the treatment of malignant diseases.

5.2.3 ONX-0912

Like carfilzomib, ONX-0912 is also an epoxyketone compound with novel selective, irreversible inhibition activity to the immunopreteasome and constituent 20S particles. ONX-0912 displays great oral activity (Chauhan et al., 2010). Primary WM cells expressing higher level of 20S are more responsive to ONX-0912 (Roccaro et al., 2010). ONX-0912 induces WM cell apoptosis through c-JNK activation, NFκB inhibition, caspase cleavage, and initiation of the unfolded protein response. Moreover, ONX-0912 also reduce the secretion of BM-derived interleukin-6 (IL-6) and insulin-like growth factor 1 (IGF-1), thus inhibiting BM-induced Akt phosphorylation and phosphorylated extracellular signal-related kinase activation in WM cells. In addition to blood cancers, ONX-0912 also displays potent anticancer activity in solid tumors and a Phase I study of ONX 0912 administered orally in patients with advanced refractory or recurrent solid tumors is under evaluation (http://clinicaltrials.gov/ ct2/show/NCT01129349).

5.3 Non-classic inhibitors: Clioquinol and 5-amino-8-hydroxyl-quinoline

Most of the proteasomal inhibitors competitively bind to the β subunits of 20S proteasome, for example, MG-132, bortezomib, and carfilzomib. Recently, we found that a group of quinoline-based agents including clioquinol, chloroquine, 5-amino-8-hydroxyl quinoline (5AHQ), and metfloquinoline display potent inhibition on proteasomal catalytic activity by a non-competitive manner (Li et al., 2010; Mao et al., 2009). Further studies indicated that these agents bind to the α subunits other than β subunits of the 20S core particle as bortezomib or MG-132 does. In analysis of its binding to purified 20S archaeal proteasomes from *Thermoplasma acidophilium* by using nuclear magnetic resonance (NMR) technology, chloroquine binds to the α subunits with 260 Å distance from β active sites. Notably, chloroquine and MG132 can bind the proteasome simultaneously, further establishing that they exploit two completely separate binding pockets (Sprangers et al., 2008).

The interaction of 5AHQ with α_7– α_7 produced clear spectral changes localized to residues Ile159, Val113, Val87, Val82, Leu112, Val89, Val134, Val24 and Leu136, which are inside the antechamber. In contrast, MG132 which binds the proteolytic chamber produces shifts in the beta rings of the full proteasome. Binding to the α subunit, 5AHQ leads to a conformational change of the core particle and displays a non-competitive inhibition on proteasome. 5AHQ preferentially induced cell death in primary myeloma and leukemia cells compared with normal hematopoietic cells. More importantly, 5AHQ overcomes the resistance to bortezomib and is equally cytotoxic to human myelomonocytic leukemia THP1/BTZ500 cells which are 237-fold more resistant to bortezomib than wild-type THP1 cells because of the overexpression and mutation of the bortezomib-binding β5 subunits (Li et al., 2010). Therefore, a group of quinoline-based small molecules can inhibit proteasomal activity in a non-cannoical manner. Because of their low toxicity and novel inhibition mechanism, these compounds could be developed for MM and leukemia therapy. Currently, clioquinol has been moved to clinical trials for refractory acute myeloid leukemia.

5.4 Natural proteasomal inhibitors: Pristimerin and EGCG

Except for small chemical compounds or peptide reagents, several natural products have been identified and evaluated for MM treatment in both *in vivo* and *in vitro* assays. The most promising candidate could be NPI-0052 or marizomib isolated from a marine actinomycete *Salinispora tropica* as described above. Here we discuss two more agents in this category pristimerin and (-)-epigallocatechin-3-gallate (EGCG).

5.4.1 Prisitmerin

Pristimerin belongs to the tripernoid family and is isolated from a traditional Chinese medicine called *Celastrus* and *Maytenus spp*. Nucleophilic susceptibility and *in silico* docking studies show that C6 of pristimerin is highly susceptible towards a nucleophilic attack by the hydroxyl group of N-terminal threonine of the proteasomal chymotrypsin subunit. This interaction leads to an inhibition of the chymotrypsin-like activity of a purified rabbit 20S proteasome (Yang et al., 2008). Pristimerin displayed similar inhibition activity in purified rabbit 20S proteasomes and in human prostate cancer cell lysates (Tiedemann et al., 2009). The IC_{50}s are 2.2 and 3.0 μM *in vitro* and *in vivo*, respectively. The treatment of pristimerin in prostate cancer cells resulted in the accumulation of ubiquitinated proteins and three proteasome target proteins, Bax, p27 and IκBα. However, myeloma cells are more sensitive to pristimerin. Pristimerin potently inhibits both IKK and the proteasome in MM cells with an IC_{50} of 100 nM. Pristimerin causes overt suppression of constitutive NFκB activity in myeloma cells that may mediate its suppression of cyclin D, thus inducing myeloma cell apoptosis.

5.4.2 (-)-epigallocatechin-3-gallate (EGCG)

EGCG is one of the polyphenols found in green tea extract and inhibits proteasomal activity (Golden et al., 2009). The ester bond of EGCG is attacked by the N-terminal threonine residue of the proteasome, forming a covalent EGCG-proteasome complex which has been confirmed by high performance liquid chromatography (HPLC) analysis. Recent studies found that EGCG competitively inhibits proteasomal activity in a same manner as bortezomib does, thus neutralizing the inhibiting activity of bortezomib and other boronic acid-based proteasome inhibitors. Therefore, green tea polyphenols block the anticancer effects of bortezomib and green tea is not encouraged for myeloma patients who are using bortezomib (Golden et al., 2009). However, a recent study didn't find antagonism of bortezomib in preclinical *in vivo* experiments, where EGCG or ascorbic acid plasma concentrations are commensurate with dietary or supplemental intake and suggest that patients receiving bortezomib treatment do not need to avoid normal dietary consumption of green tea, vitamin C-containing foods, or EGCG or vitamin C dietary supplements (Bannerman et al., 2011).

6. Targeting at ubiquitination and deubiquitination systems for blood cancer treatment

Proteasomes are critical components of both cancer cells and normal tissues because they determine the fate of most of the proteins and therefore inhibition of proteasome will also lead to normal cell stress and apoptosis. Thus inhibition of proteasomes indiscriminately raises levels of hundreds of proteins regardless to their anticancer effect. Thus, proteasomal inhibitors are a double-edged sword because they kill cancer cells, simultaneously, kill normal cells. Because proteasome-coupled protein ubiquitination is more specific, inhibition of certain enzymes involved in protein ubiquitination will be a more pertinent target for cancer drug development. There are four kinds of enzymes, E1, E2, E3 and Dubs which contain thousands of members in total. Currently, with the exception of E2, inhibitors of these other enzymes have been identified and are being evaluated for the treatment of hematological malignancies.

6.1 Targeting at E1 for hematological malignancies

E1 or Ubiquitin-activating enzyme (UBA) controls the protein ubiquitination by activating ubiquitin using ATP as an energy supplier. Knockdown of E1 by small interfering RNA (siRNA) strategy decreases the abundance of ubiquitinated proteins in leukemia and myeloma cells and induced cell death (Xu et al., 2010). Blood cancer cells including leukemia and myeloma are more sensitive to E1 inhibitors. A small molecule PYZD-4409, an inhibitor of E1, can abolish protein ubiquitination, thus inducing endoplasmic reticulum (ER) stress, and leading to cancer cell apoptosis. PYZD-4409 also displayed ideal anti-leukemia activity *in vivo* without untoward toxicity by decreasing tumor volume and weight (Xu et al., 2010). However, the same concern may arise as that already seen in bortezomib because there is only a single E1 protein in humans.

6.2 Targeting at E3 for blood cancer therapies

The E3 ligases are the largest family in the UPS system. E3s are the primary determinant of substrate specificity and represent the largest and most diverse class of Ub/Ub-like regulatory enzymes. There are 600-1000 potential E3s responsible for E2 binding, substrate recognition, and regulatory functions. Targeting the ubiquitin ligases promises more specificity because most E3s tag only a few proteins for destruction. Such drugs can, in theory, block degradation of its specific substrate proteins. Currently, interfering with E3-substrate interaction is one of the leading strategies for anti-cancer drugs targeting at UPS.

One of the most promising E3s is Skp2, the F-box protein that controls degradation of p27, an important tumor suppressor gene (Zhan et al., 2007). Skp2 levels are abnormally high in leukemia and myeloma cells, therefore, blocking Skp2 activity might reasonably be expected to stop cancer cell proliferation. CpdA is such an inhibitor of Skp2 by preventing incorporation of Skp2 into the SCF Skp2 ligase, CpdA induces G1/S cell-cycle arrest as well as SCF Skp2- and p27-dependent cell killing (Chen et al., 2008). In models of MM, CpdA overcomes resistance to dexamethasone, doxorubicin, and melphalan, as well as to bortezomib, and also acted synergistically with this proteasome inhibitor. Importantly, CpdA is active against patient-derived plasma cells and both myeloid and lymphoblastoid leukemia blasts, and showed preferential activity against neoplastic cells while relatively sparing other marrow components (Chen et al., 2008).

Another interesting E3 is MdM2 which regulates p53 ubiquitination. Several inhibitors of MdM2 have been identified, such as Nutlins (Stuhmer et al., 2005) and MI-63 (Ding et al., 2006; Samudio et al., 2010). By disrupting the interaction of MdM2 and p53, both Nutlins and MI-63 can restore p53 which further tends to promote arrest of cell cycle and apoptosis. These drugs are effective in inducing apoptosis of MM cells which express wild-type p53, unfortunately, it won't work in cancer cells with mutated or deleted p53.

6.3 Targeting at deubiquitinases

Just like E3s, deubiquitinases play a tumor-suppressing or -promoting role dependent on its targeting protein. For example, USP9X is an oncoprotein enzyme that removes ubiquitin from the anti-apoptotic protein MCL-1 (Sun et al., 2011). MCL1 is overexpressed in most blood cancer cells, and is highly associated with cancer cell proliferation and protects cancer cells from apoptosis (Sun et al., 2011). MCL1 is degraded by proteasomes after poly-ubiquitination. High expression of USP9X is seen in leukemia and MM cells. A small molecule called WP1130 (Kapuria et al., 2010) has been identified as a partly selective Dub inhibitor by directly inhibiting activity of USP9x, USP5, USP14, and UCH37, which are known to regulate survival protein stability and 26S proteasome function. WP1130-mediated inhibition of tumor-activated Dubs results in downregulation of antiapoptotic and upregulation of proapoptotic proteins, such as Mcl-1 and p53, thus leading to cancer cell death (Kapuria et al., 2010).

Although large-scale inhibitors of ubiquitination enzymes are yet to fully develop, successful E3 and Dub inhibitors have established the proof-of-principle that inhibition of ubqitinating/deubiquitinating enzymes is novel and potentially powerful strategy to develop anti-blood cancer drugs and is surely an area that will expand greatly in the future.

7. Summary

The ubiquitin-proteasome system has been widely investigated in the association of hematological malignancies, it is extensively involved in the development and therapy of blood cancers, including leukemia, lymphoma and multiple myeloma. Targeting at the UPS specific genes/proteins, several novel drugs have been developed including the first-approved proteasome inhibitor-bortezomib in the treatment of myeloma and mantle cell lymphoma. The upcoming years will witness the introduction of more potent and more patient-friendly next generations of UPS inhibitors such as carfilozomib and inhibitors of ubiquitinating/deubiquitinating enzymes for the treatment of blood cancer patients.

8. Acknowledgment

This project was partly supported by the Priority Academic Program Development of Jiangsu Higher Education Institutions (PAPD).

9. References

B CP, M XA, K CA, Baritaki S, BerkFers C, Bonavida B, Chandra J, Chauhan D, C. Cusack J J, Fenical W, I MG, Groll M, P RJ, K SL, G KL, McBride W, D JM, C PM, S TCN, Oki Y, Ovaa H, Pajonk F, P GR, A MR, C MS, M AS, Valashi E, Younes A, & Palladino

MA (2011). Marizomib, a proteasome inhibitor for all seasons: preclinical profile and a framework for clinical trials. Current Cancer Drug Targets 11(3):254-284.

Bannerman B, Xu L, Jones M, Tsu C, Yu J, Hales P, Monbaliu J, Fleming P, Dick L, Manfredi M, Claiborne C, Bolen J, Kupperman E, & Berger A (2011) Preclinical evaluation of the antitumor activity of bortezomib in combination with vitamin C or with epigallocatechin gallate, a component of green tea. Cancer Chemotherapy and Pharmacology.

Bedford L, Lowe J, Dick LR, Mayer RJ, & Brownell JE (2011) Ubiquitin-like protein conjugation and the ubiquitin-proteasome system as drug targets. Nature reviews 10(1):29-46.

Bergsagel PL and Kuehl WM (2005) Molecular pathogenesis and a consequent classification of multiple myeloma. Journal of Clinical Oncology 23(26):6333-6338.

Bernassola F, Karin M, Ciechanover A, & Melino G (2008) The HECT family of E3 ubiquitin ligases: multiple players in cancer development. Cancer Cell 14(1):10-21.

Block K, Boyer TG, & Yew PR (2001) Phosphorylation of the human ubiquitin-conjugating enzyme, CDC34, by casein kinase 2. The Journal of Biological Chemistry 276(44):41049-41058.

Cavo M, Tacchetti P, Patriarca F, Petrucci MT, Pantani L, Galli M, Di Raimondo F, Crippa C, Zamagni E, Palumbo A, Offidani M, Corradini P, Narni F, Spadano A, Pescosta N, Deliliers GL, Ledda A, Cellini C, Caravita T, Tosi P , & Baccarani M (2010) Bortezomib with thalidomide plus dexamethasone compared with thalidomide plus dexamethasone as induction therapy before, and consolidation therapy after, double autologous stem-cell transplantation in newly diagnosed multiple myeloma: a randomised phase 3 study. Lancet 376(9758):2075-2085.

Chauhan D, Li G, Shringarpure R, Podar K, Ohtake Y, Hideshima T, & Anderson KC (2003) Blockade of Hsp27 overcomes Bortezomib/proteasome inhibitor PS-341 resistance in lymphoma cells. Cancer Research 63(19):6174-6177.

Chauhan D, Singh AV, Aujay M, Kirk CJ, Bandi M, Ciccarelli B, Raje N, Richardson P, & Anderson KC (2010) A novel orally active proteasome inhibitor ONX 0912 triggers in vitro and in vivo cytotoxicity in multiple myeloma. Blood 116(23):4906-4915.

Chen JY, Wang MC, & Hung WC (2011) Bcr-Abl-induced tyrosine phosphorylation of Emi1 to stabilize Skp2 protein via inhibition of ubiquitination in chronic myeloid leukemia cells. Journal of Cellular Physiology 226(2):407-413.

Chen Q, Xie W, Kuhn DJ, Voorhees PM, Lopez-Girona A, Mendy D, Corral LG, Krenitsky VP, Xu W, Moutouh-de Parseval L, Webb DR, Mercurio F, Nakayama KI, Nakayama K, & Orlowski RZ (2008) Targeting the p27 E3 ligase SCF(Skp2) results in p27- and Skp2-mediated cell-cycle arrest and activation of autophagy. Blood 111(9):4690-4699.

Ciechanover A (1998) The ubiquitin-proteasome pathway: on protein death and cell life. The EMBO Journal 17(24):7151-7160.

Ciechanover A, Orian A, & Schwartz AL (2000) The ubiquitin-mediated proteolytic pathway: mode of action and clinical implications. Journal of Cellular Biochemistry 34:40-51.

Colland F (2010) The therapeutic potential of deubiquitinating enzyme inhibitors. Biochemical Society Transactions 38(Pt 1):137-143.

Delic J, Masdehors P, Omura S, Cosset JM, Dumont J, Binet JL, & Magdelenat H (1998) The proteasome inhibitor lactacystin induces apoptosis and sensitizes chemo- and radioresistant human chronic lymphocytic leukaemia lymphocytes to TNF-alpha-initiated apoptosis. British Journal of Cancer 77(7):1103-1107.

Deshaies RJ and Joazeiro CA (2009) RING domain E3 ubiquitin ligases. Annual Review of Biochemistry 78:399-434. Ding K, Lu Y, Nikolovska-Coleska Z, Wang G, Qiu S, Shangary S, Gao W, Qin D, Stuckey J, Krajewski K, Roller PP, & Wang S (2006) Structure-based design of spiro-oxindoles as potent, specific small-molecule inhibitors of the 12MDM2-p53 interaction. Journal of Medicinal Chemistry 49(12):3432-3435.

Dunleavy K, Pittaluga S, Czuczman MS, Dave SS, Wright G, Grant N, Shovlin M, Jaffe ES, Janik JE, Staudt LM, & Wilson WH (2009) Differential efficacy of bortezomib plus chemotherapy within molecular subtypes of diffuse large B-cell lymphoma. Blood 113(24):6069-76.

Franke NE, Niewerth D, Assaraf YG, van Meerloo J, Vojtekova K, van Zantwijk CH, Zweegman S, Chan ET, Kirk CJ, Geerke DP, Schimmer AD, Kaspers GJ, Jansen G, & Cloos J (2011) Impaired bortezomib binding to mutant β5 subunit of the proteasome is the underlying basis for bortezomib resistance in leukemia cells. Leukemia Sept 23 [Epub ahead of print].

Impaired bortezomib binding to mutant β5 subunit of the proteasome is the underlying basis for bortezomib resistance in leukemia cells.

Golden EB, Lam PY, Kardosh A, Gaffney KJ, Cadenas E, Louie SG, Petasis NA, Chen TC, & Schonthal AH (2009) Green tea polyphenols block the anticancer effects of bortezomib and other boronic acid-based proteasome inhibitors. Blood 113(23):5927-5937.

Haglund K and Dikic I (2005) Ubiquitylation and cell signaling. The EMBO journal 24(19):3353-3359.

Hideshima T, Richardson P, Chauhan D, Palombella VJ, Elliott PJ, Adams J, & Anderson KC (2001) The proteasome inhibitor PS-341 inhibits growth, induces apoptosis, and overcomes drug resistance in human multiple myeloma cells. Cancer Research 61(7):3071-3076.

Jin W, Chang M, Paul EM, Babu G, Lee AJ, Reiley W, Wright A, Zhang M, You J, & Sun SC (2008) Deubiquitinating enzyme CYLD negatively regulates RANK signaling and osteoclastogenesis in mice. The Journal of Clinical Investigation 118(5):1858-1866.

Jones RJ, Chen Q, Voorhees PM, Young KH, Bruey-Sedano N, Yang D, & Orlowski RZ (2008) Inhibition of the p53 E3 ligase HDM-2 induces apoptosis and DNA damage--independent p53 phosphorylation in mantle cell lymphoma. Clinical Cancer Research 14(17):5416-5425.

Kapuria V, Peterson LF, Fang D, Bornmann WG, Talpaz M, & Donato NJ (2010) Deubiquitinase inhibition by small-molecule WP1130 triggers aggresome formation and tumor cell apoptosis. Cancer research 70(22):9265-9276.

Kirkin V and Dikic I (2010) Ubiquitin networks in cancer. Current Opinion in Genetics & Development 21(1):21-28.

Kisselev AF and Goldberg AL (2001) Proteasome inhibitors: from research tools to drug candidates. Chemistry & Biology 8(8):739-758.

Kumar S and Rajkumar SV (2008) Many facets of bortezomib resistance/susceptibility. Blood 112(6):2177-2178.

Kumatori A, Tanaka K, Inamura N, Sone S, Ogura T, Matsumoto T, Tachikawa T, Shin S, & Ichihara A (1990) Abnormally high expression of proteasomes in human leukemic cells. Proceedings of the National Academy of Sciences of the United States of America 87(18):7071-7075.

Li X, Wood TE, Sprangers R, Jansen G, Franke NE, Mao X, Wang X, Zhang Y, Verbrugge SE, Adomat H, Li ZH, Trudel S, Chen C, Religa TL, Jamal N, Messner H, Cloos J, Rose DR, Navon A, Guns E, Batey RA, Kay LE, & Schimmer AD (2010) Effect of noncompetitive proteasome inhibition on bortezomib resistance. Journal of the National Cancer Institute 102(14):1069-1082.

Lu S, Yang J, Song X, Gong S, Zhou H, Guo L, Song N, Bao X, Chen P, & Wang J (2008) Point mutation of the proteasome beta5 subunit gene is an important mechanism of bortezomib resistance in bortezomib-selected variants of Jurkat T cell lymphoblastic lymphoma/leukemia line. The Journal of Pharmacology and Experimental Therapeutics 326(2):423-431.

Macherla VR, Mitchell SS, Manam RR, Reed KA, Chao TH, Nicholson B, Deyanat-Yazdi G, Mai B, Jensen PR, Fenical WF, Neuteboom ST, Lam KS, Palladino MA, & Potts BC (2005) Structure-activity relationship studies of salinosporamide A (NPI-0052), a novel marine derived proteasome inhibitor. Journal of Medicinal Chemistry 48(11):3684-3687.

Mao JH, Sun XY, Liu JX, Zhang QY, Liu P, Huang QH, Li KK, Chen Q, Chen Z, & Chen SJ (2010) As4S4 targets RING-type E3 ligase c-CBL to induce degradation of BCR-ABL in chronic myelogenous leukemia. Proceedings of the National Academy of Sciences of the United States of America 107(50):21683-21688.

Mao X, Li X, Sprangers R, Wang X, Venugopal A, Wood T, Zhang Y, Kuntz DA, Coe E, Trudel S, Rose D, Batey RA, Kay LE, & Schimmer AD (2009) Clioquinol inhibits the proteasome and displays preclinical activity in leukemia and myeloma. Leukemia 23(3):585-590.

O'Connor OA, Stewart AK, Vallone M, Molineaux CJ, Kunkel LA, Gerecitano JF, & Orlowski RZ (2009) A phase 1 dose escalation study of the safety and pharmacokinetics of the novel proteasome inhibitor carfilzomib (PR-171) in patients with hematologic malignancies. Clinical Cancer Research 15(22):7085-7091.

Obaidat A, Weiss J, Wahlgren B, Manam RR, Macherla VR, McArthur K, Chao TH, Palladino MA, Lloyd GK, Potts BC, Enna SJ, Neuteboom ST, & Hagenbuch B (2011) Proteasome Regulator Marizomib (NPI-0052) Exhibits Prolonged Inhibition, Attenuated Efflux, and Greater Cytotoxicity than Its Reversible Analogs. The Journal of Pharmacology and Experimental Therapeutics 337(2):479-486.

Oerlemans R, Franke NE, Assaraf YG, Cloos J, van Zantwijk I, Berkers CR, Scheffer GL, Debipersad K, Vojtekova K, Lemos C, van der Heijden JW, Ylstra B, Peters GJ, Kaspers GL, Dijkmans BA, Scheper RJ, & Jansen G (2008) Molecular basis of bortezomib resistance: proteasome subunit beta5 (PSMB5) gene mutation and overexpression of PSMB5 protein. Blood 112(6):2489-2499.

Parlati F, Lee SJ, Aujay M, Suzuki E, Levitsky K, Lorens JB, Micklem DR, Ruurs P, Sylvain C, Lu Y, Shenk KD, & Bennett MK (2009) Carfilzomib can induce tumor cell death through selective inhibition of the chymotrypsin-like activity of the proteasome. Blood 114(16):3439-3447.

Piva R, Ruggeri B, Williams M, Costa G, Tamagno I, Ferrero D, Giai V, Coscia M, Peola S, Massaia M, Pezzoni G, Allievi C, Pescalli N, Cassin M, di Giovine S, Nicoli P, de Feudis P, Strepponi I, Roato I, Ferracini R, Bussolati B, Camussi G, Jones-Bolin S, Hunter K, Zhao H, Neri A, Palumbo A, Berkers C, Ovaa H, Bernareggi A, & Inghirami G (2008) CEP-18770: A novel, orally active proteasome inhibitor with a tumor-selective pharmacologic profile competitive with bortezomib. Blood 111(5):2765-2775.

Richardson PG, Barlogie B, Berenson J, Singhal S, Jagannath S, Irwin D, Rajkumar SV, Srkalovic G, Alsina M, Alexanian R, Siegel D, Orlowski RZ, Kuter D, Limentani SA, Lee S, Hideshima T, Esseltine DL, Kauffman M, Adams J, Schenkein DP, & Anderson KC (2003) A phase 2 study of bortezomib in relapsed, refractory myeloma. The New England Journal of Medicine 348(26):2609-2617.

Richardson PG, Briemberg H, Jagannath S, Wen PY, Barlogie B, Berenson J, Singhal S, Siegel DS, Irwin D, Schuster M, Srkalovic G, Alexanian R, Rajkumar SV, Limentani S, Alsina M, Orlowski RZ, Najarian K, Esseltine D, Anderson KC, & Amato AA (2006) Frequency, characteristics, and reversibility of peripheral neuropathy during treatment of advanced multiple myeloma with bortezomib. Journal of Clinical Oncology 24(19):3113-3120.

Roccaro AM, Sacco A, Aujay M, Ngo HT, Azab AK, Azab F, Quang P, Maiso P, Runnels J, Anderson KC, Demo S, & Ghobrial IM (2010) Selective inhibition of chymotrypsin-like activity of the immunoproteasome and constitutive proteasome in Waldenstrom macroglobulinemia. Blood 115(20):4051-4060.

Samudio IJ, Duvvuri S, Clise-Dwyer K, Watt JC, Mak D, Kantarjian H, Yang D, Ruvolo V, & Borthakur G (2010) Activation of p53 signaling by MI-63 induces apoptosis in acute myeloid leukemia cells. Leukemia & Lymphoma 51(5):911-919.

Sanchez E, Li M, Steinberg JA, Wang C, Shen J, Bonavida B, Li ZW, Chen H, & Berenson JR (2010) The proteasome inhibitor CEP-18770 enhances the anti-myeloma activity of bortezomib and melphalan. British Journal of Haematology 148(4):569-581.

Schulman BA, & Harper JW (2009) Ubiquitin-like protein activation by E1 enzymes: the apex for downstream signalling pathways. Nature Review Molecular Cell Biology 10(5):319-331.

Schwickart M, Huang X, Lill JR, Liu J, Ferrando R, French DM, Maecker H, O'Rourke K, Bazan F, Eastham-Anderson J, Yue P, Dornan D, Huang DC, & Dixit VM (2010) Deubiquitinase USP9X stabilizes MCL1 and promotes tumour cell survival. Nature 463(7277):103-107.

Shaughnessy JD, Jr., Qu P, Usmani S, Heuck CJ, Zhang Q, Zhou Y, Tian E, Hanamura I, van Rhee F, Anaissie E, Epstein J, Nair B, Stephens O, Williams R, Waheed S, Alsayed Y, Crowley J, & Barlogie B (2011) Pharmacogenomics of bortezomib test-dosing identifies hyperexpression of proteasome genes, especially PSMD4, as novel high-risk feature in myeloma treated with total therapy 3. Blood. May 31. [Epub ahead of print].

Singh AV, Palladino MA, Lloyd GK, Potts BC, Chauhan D, & Anderson KC (2010) Pharmacodynamic and efficacy studies of the novel proteasome inhibitor NPI-0052 (marizomib) in a human plasmacytoma xenograft murine model. British Journal of Haematology 149(4):550-559.

Smith DM, Chang SC, Park S, Finley D, Cheng Y, & Goldberg AL (2007) Docking of the proteasomal ATPases' carboxyl termini in the 20S proteasome's alpha ring opens the gate for substrate entry. Molecular cell 27(5):731-744.

Sprangers R, Li X, Mao X, Rubinstein JL, Schimmer AD, & Kay LE (2008) TROSY-based NMR evidence for a novel class of 20S proteasome inhibitors. Biochemistry 47(26):6727-6734.

Stuhmer T, Chatterjee M, Hildebrandt M, Herrmann P, Gollasch H, Gerecke C, Theurich S, Cigliano L, Manz RA, Daniel PT, Bommert K, Vassilev LT, & Bargou RC (2005) Nongenotoxic activation of the p53 pathway as a therapeutic strategy for multiple myeloma. Blood 106(10):3609-3617.

Sun H, Kapuria V, Peterson LF, Fang D, Bornmann WG, Bartholomeusz G, Talpaz M, & Donato NJ (2011) Bcr-Abl ubiquitination and Usp9x inhibition block kinase signaling and promote CML cell apoptosis. Blood 117(11):3151-3162.

Tiedemann RE, Schmidt J, Keats JJ, Shi CX, Zhu YX, Palmer SE, Mao X, Schimmer AD, & Stewart AK (2009) Identification of a potent natural triterpenoid inhibitor of proteosome chymotrypsin-like activity and NF-kappaB with antimyeloma activity in vitro and in vivo. Blood 113(17):4027-4037.

Xu GW, Ali M, Wood TE, Wong D, Maclean N, Wang X, Gronda M, Skrtic M, Li X, Hurren R, Mao X, Venkatesan M, Beheshti Zavareh R, Ketela T, Reed JC, Rose D, Moffat J, Batey RA, Dhe-Paganon S, & Schimmer AD (2010) The ubiquitin-activating enzyme E1 as a therapeutic target for the treatment of leukemia and multiple myeloma. Blood 115(11):2251-2259.

Yang H, Landis-Piwowar KR, Lu D, Yuan P, Li L, Reddy GP, Yuan X , & Dou QP (2008) Pristimerin induces apoptosis by targeting the proteasome in prostate cancer cells. Journal of Cell Biochemistry 103(1):234-244.

Ye Y and Rape M (2009) Building ubiquitin chains: E2 enzymes at work. Nature Review Molecular Cell Biology 10(11):755-764.

Zhan F, Colla S, Wu X, Chen B, Stewart JP, Kuehl WM, Barlogie B, & Shaughnessy JD, Jr. (2007) CKS1B, overexpressed in aggressive disease, regulates multiple myeloma growth and survival through SKP2- and p27Kip1-dependent and -independent mechanisms. Blood 109(11):4995-5001.

Zhou HJ, Aujay MA, Bennett MK, Dajee M, Demo SD, Fang Y, Ho MN, Jiang J, Kirk CJ, Laidig GJ, Lewis ER, Lu Y, Muchamuel T, Parlati F, Ring E, Shenk KD, Shields J, Shwonek PJ, Stanton T, Sun CM, Sylvain C, Woo TM, & Yang J (2009) Design and synthesis of an orally bioavailable and selective peptide epoxyketone proteasome inhibitor (PR-047). Journal of Medicinal Chemistry 52(9):3028-3038.

Zhu YX, Tiedemann R, Shi CX, Yin H, Schmidt JE, Bruins LA, Keats JJ, Braggio E, Sereduk C, Mousses S, & Stewart AK (2011) RNAi screen of the druggable genome identifies modulators of proteasome inhibitor sensitivity in myeloma including CDK5. Blood 117(14):3847-57.

11

Targeting the Minimal Residual Disease in Acute Myeloid Leukemia: The Role of Adoptive Immunotherapy with Natural Killer Cells and Antigen-Specific Vaccination

Sarah Parisi and Antonio Curti
Department of Hematology and Oncological Sciences "L. and A. Seràgnoli", University of Bologna, Bologna Italy

1. Introduction

Acute myeloid leukemia (AML) is a neoplastic disorder characterized by the clonal expansion of non-lymphoid hematopoietic progenitor cells with failure of normal hematopoiesis. Several biological and clinical parameters have been identified at diagnosis to classify different AML subtypes with different prognosis. In this view, genetic abnormalities confer the most important prognostic information. Therapeutic interventions based on conventional or high-dose chemotherapy have significantly improved the complete remission (CR) rates of acute leukemia. However, a significant portion of responding patients still harbors a minimal residual disease (MRD), which is often resistant to further pharmacological treatments and ultimately leads to disease relapse and progression. Although allogeneic stem cell transplantation may significantly improve the clinical results of AML patients who achieved complete remission, such approach has several and important limitations and is not applicable to all the patients. For these reasons, novel therapeutic approaches to improve the clinical outcome of AML patients are under investigation, and treatments with high compliance such as adoptive and active immunotherapy are desirable. Aim of the present work will be to focus the most relevant insights in the field. In particular, we will report about the use of natural killer (NK) cells as a means of adoptive immunotherapy against neoplastic cells, including AML. Moreover, we will discuss the role of vaccines against leukemia with particular emphasis on the immunogenicity of novel and promising leukemia-associated antigens.

2. Acute Myeloid Leukemia

Acute myeloid leukemia (AML) is a hematopoietic malignant disease rising from neoplastic transformation of myeloid stem cells. This causes the alteration of the normal cell differentiation and proliferation systems, resulting in the accumulation in bone marrow and peripheral blood of non-functional myeloid cells termed myeloblasts. AML may arise *de novo* or secondary to pre-existing myelodysplasia or previous chemotherapies.

Myeloblasts lack the normal proliferation systems and their over-proliferation and accumulation in bone marrow and peripheral blood cause lack of production of hematopoietic normal cells, this resulting in peripheral deficiency of platelets, neutrophils and hemoglobin.

Prognosis of AML depends on multiple factors: age at diagnosis (age>60 years is a poor prognostic factor), hyperleukocytosis, cytogenetic status and molecular specific characteristics are the most important ones.

AML can occur at every age, but its incidence increases with age (median age at presentation: 65 years). It has an annual incidence of 3.6 per 100,000. This incidence increases with age, rising to 16.3 per 100,000 per year in the over 65 age group. Older adults typically have a highly inferior prognosis and an increased risk of therapy-related toxicity and mortality.

Conventional treatment of AML is based on chemotherapy regimens and consists of several well-defined phases: the first one is the CR-induction cycle, based on the administration of 3 days-anthacycline associated with 7 days-cytarabine. Its aim is to 'empty' bone marrow and allow the normal hematopoietic cells repopulation.

Response rates with conventional chemotherapy range from 60% to 85% in young adults (age < 60 years), but more than 50% of these patients are going to relapse, with a five-year overall survival of 40%. Older patients with a diagnosis of AML have a poorer prognosis, with less than 10% of long survivers; this is due to biological unfavorable risk factors, such as unfavorable cytogenetics, which are more frequent in the elderly (Leith et al. 1997).

One of the main cause of relapse in patients who achieved complete remission after chemotherapy is the persistance of a small amount of leukemic cells termed MRD. Minimal residual disease detection became one of the main tasks for hematologists; immunophenotypical and molecular markers able to discriminate normal cells from blastic cells allow the detection of residual leukemic cells not detected by morphologic examinations.

After the induction therapy two or more consolidation cycles are needed in order to eradicate leukemic cells completely. Allogeneic stem cell transplantation is one of the most effective consolidation therapy, even if it is feasible only for fit patients and only if a suitable HLA-matched donor is available.

Moreover, allogeneic stem cell transplantation is highly effective if performed after obtaining first CR, while its efficacy is poor in case of relapsed/refractory patients.

Only young and fit patients can undergo stem cell transplantation because of its significantly high toxicity, mortality and morbidity rates.

Attempts to effectively prime and sustain anti-tumor immunity against leukemic cells have recently provided promising preclinical and clinical results. Results from allogeneic stem cell transplantation (SCT) represent the main evidence that leukemic cells are targets of the immune system. In fact, since the first clinical observation that allogeneic SCT offered a clinical advantage over autologous transplantation due to a graft-versus-leukemia (GVL) effect, much more attention has been given to the role of adoptive immunotherapy over conditioning regimen as a means to eradicate tumor cells. In particular, donor lymphocyte infusions (DLIs) are capable to restore a durable complete remission. Such results are the proof of principle of the crucial activity of anti-tumor immunity in controlling the growth of leukemic cells.

3. Adoptive immunotherapy with natural killer cells

Human NK cells are a subset of PB lymphocytes defined by the expression of CD56 or CD16 and the absence of the T-cell receptor (CD3) (Robertson et al, 1990). They recognize and kill transformed cell lines in an MHC-unrestricted fashion and play a critical role in the innate immune response. Several studies demonstrated that NK function, which is distinct from the MHC-restricted cytolytic activity of T cells, may be relevant for the immune control of tumor development and growth. Although NK cell killing is MHC-unrestricted, NK cells display a number of activating and inhibitory receptors that ligate MHC molecules to modulate the immune response (Lanier et al, 1998). NK cell receptors that recognize antigens at the HLA-A, -B, or -C loci are members of the immunoglobulin super family and are termed killer immunoglobulin receptors or KIRs (Farad et al, 2002). Engagement of these NK cell receptors results in stimulation or inhibition of NK cell effector function, which ultimately depends on the net effect of activating and inhibitory receptors (Figure 1).

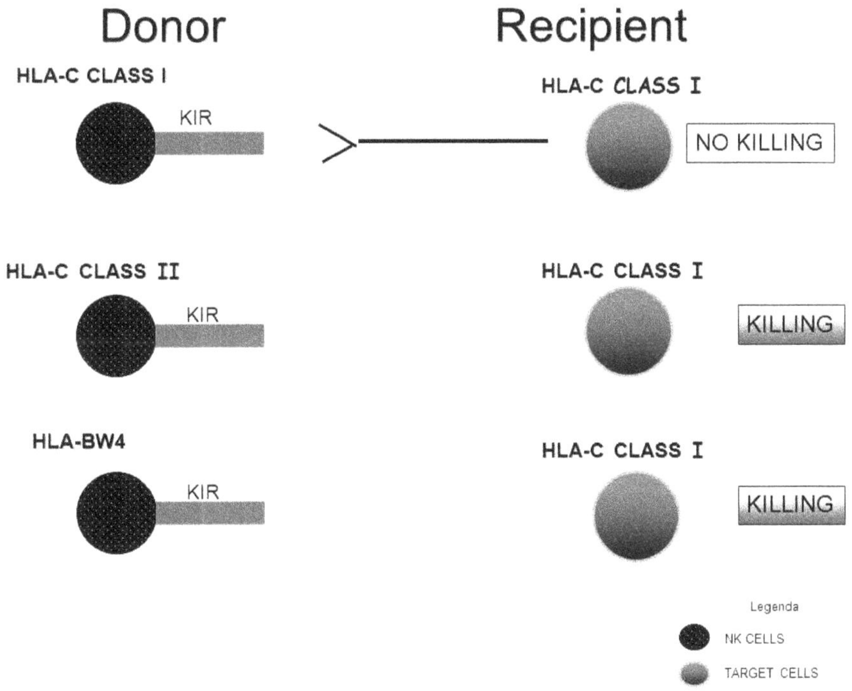

Clinical trials attempting to utilize the anti-tumor effect of NK cells have met only modest success due to the lack of understanding of receptors and ligands which determine whether NK cells will be activated or suppressed. On the contrary, data from haploidentical T-cell depleted transplantation suggest that KIR mismatch with tumor MHC may significantly impact on tumor cell killing, particularly in AML (Ruggeri et al, 2002). In fact, these studies show that AML patients with KIR ligand mismatch are significantly protected against leukemia relapse. In addition, preclinical and clinical investigations demonstrated that haploidentical KIR-mismatched NK cells play the main role as anti-leukemia effector cells and they exert their cytotoxic activity within 4-5 days (Ruggeri et al 2002, Ruggeri et al, 1999). In particular, high risk AML patients with a KIR-ligand mismatch in the graft-versus-host (GVDH) direction had a relapse rate of 0% compared to KIR-ligand matched patients who had a relapse rate of 75%. Given these results, haploidentical KIR-mismatch NK cells administered to AML patients as cell-based immunotherapy may induce NK cell-mediated killing of leukemia cells resulting in the elimination of residual disease in high risk AML patients. Furthermore, alloreactive mismatched NK cells facilitate hematopoietic engraftment after infusion of haploidentical stem cells, and inhibit the onset of GVHD by targeting host antigen-presenting cells (Ruggeri et al, 2002). Of note, the differential expression of activating ligands on hematopoietic and not hematopoietic tissues may provide an additional explanation for the observed GVL effect in the absence of GVHD.

Partially purified haploidentical NK cells have been already used clinically and labeled with ^{111}In to track, in vivo, their kinetics and organ distribution in patients with renal cancer (Brand et al, 2004). A seminal study demonstrated that up to 1.5 x 10^7/haploidentical NK cells/Kg can be safely infused in AML and cancer patients following Fludarabine/ Cyclophosphamide (Flu/Cy) immunosuppressive chemotherapy and, in some cases, clinical responses without GVHD had been observed (Miller et al, 2005). Interestingly, circulating haploidentical NK cells were found, in selected patients, up to 28 days after infusion especially when exogenous IL-2 was given for 9 doses. In vivo expansion of NK cells was correlated with a high IL-15 serum concentration. In particular, in this study, 19 poor risk AML patients were reported who had received a cell population containing a median of $8.5 \pm 0.5 \times 10^6$ and $1.75 \pm 0.3 \times 10^5$ NK and T cells, respectively. Five out of 19 patients achieved CR. NK cells adoptive immunotherapy was well tolerated and hematological and non hematological toxicity were mainly related to the immunosuppressive regimen and IL-2 administration. The maximum tolerated dose of NK cells was not achieved and GVHD was not observed despite the relatively high number of haploidentical T cells infused. However, it should be noted that NK cells were only partially purified after a single round of depletion of $CD3^+$ cells which resulted in less than 2 logs reduction of T cells.

More recently, a study of haploidentical KIR-HLA mismatched NK cell transplantation in childhood AML reported that NK cell therapy prolonged disease-free and overall survival (Rubnitz et al, 2010). In this pediatric cohort of AML patients, who underwent NK therapy after an immunosuppressive regimen, the 2-year event-free survival was 100%. Notably, all the children were considered at low-risk of relapse, with a significant fraction harboring good-prognosis cytogenetics. Furthermore, as children weigh less than adults, the median number of infused NK cells was significantly higher than in adult trial and the separation procedure consisted in highly purified NK cells. These differences may partially explain the discrepancy in clinical results and suggest that in adult patients the clinical effect of NK therapy may be implemented by increasing the number of infused NK cells.

We recently published the results of a clinical trial of adoptive immunotherapy with haploidentical KIR-mismatched NK cells in elderly patients with AML (Curti et al, 2011).

Thirteen AML patients, 5 with active disease, 2 in molecular relapse and 6 in morphological complete remission (CR);(median age 62 years, range 53-73) received highly purified $CD56^{+}CD3^{-}$ NK cells from haploidentical KIR-ligand mismatched donors after fludarabine/ cyclophosphamide immunosuppressive chemotherapy, followed by IL-2. The median number of infused NK cells was 2.74×10^{6}/Kg. T cells were under 10^{5}/Kg. No NK cell-related toxicity, including GVHD, was observed. One of the 5 patients with active disease achieved transient CR, whereas 4/5 patients had no clinical benefit. Both patients in molecular relapse achieved CR which lasted for 9 and 4 months, respectively. Three/6 patients in CR are disease-free after 34, 32 and 18 months. After infusion, donor NK cells were found in the peripheral blood of all evaluable patients (peak value on day 10). They were also detected in bone marrow in some cases. Donor-versus-recipient alloreactive NK cells were demonstrated *in vivo* by the detection of donor-derived NK clones that killed recipient's targets. Adoptively transferred NK cells were alloreactive against recipient's cells, including leukemia. Taken together, these data demonstrate that infusion of purified NK cells is feasible in elderly patients with high risk AML.

4. Vaccination against acute myeloid leukemia: WT1 as a novel promising antigen

During the last years a number of studies have demonstrated that tumor-associated antigens (TAA) may be recognized by the immune system leading to the activation of tumor-specific cytotoxic T lymphocytes (CTLs) with the potential to eradicate tumor cells. Moreover, during the last decade the role of dendritic cells (DCs) as natural adjuvants of immune response has been deeply elucidated. The identification of a wide number of TAA, together with new insights into the mechanisms underlying the activation of anti-tumor immune response, has led to the development of novel anti-tumor vaccination strategies which are currently under investigation in the clinical setting. In AML, some TAA, such as PRAME, Wilms' tumor gene (WT1), proteinase 3 have been recently identified. In particular, WT1, which is a zinc-finger transcription factor expressed during normal ontogenesis, is significantly over-expressed in acute and chronic myeloid leukemia and myelodysplastic syndromes and it appears as an attractive target for immunotherapy.

WT1-specific antibodies against the N-terminus portion of the WT1 protein have been found in the sera of AML patients, but not in healthy donors, suggesting that anti-WT1-specific immune response is present in these patients. Preclinical studies have clearly demonstrated that peptides from WT1 may be used to generate in vitro a WT1-specific cytotoxic response (Li et al, 2005; Pinilla-Ibarz et al, 2006; Oka et al, 2000). While a number of WT1-derived CD8 T-cell epitopes have been reported, two peptides, namely HLA-A0201-restricted peptide 126–134 and HLA-A24-restricted peptide 235–243, have been studied extensively. Since murine and human WT1 are similar, WT1 126 and WT1 235 have also been tested in animal models. B6 mice were injected with WT1 peptides and analyzed for the induction of a T-cell and B-cell mediated immune responses against WT1. This analysis revealed that WT1 vaccination induced WT1-specific immunity, which was also capable to delay in vivo the growth of tumor cell lines, naturally overexpressing WT1. Recently, a National Cancer Institute Pilot Project assigned to WT1 the position of best and most suitable target antigen for cancer immunotherapy, due to a number of characteristics, such as its therapeutic function, immunogenicity and expression level (Cheever et al, 2009)

These data have prompted several groups to investigate the role of WT1 as a tumor-antigen in the clinical setting of cancer immunotherapy. Particularly, Oka et al conducted phase I clinical trials using peptide WT1-235 (CMTWNQMNL) and its analogue (CYTWNQMNL) for patients with overt leukemia from MDS, MDS with myelofibrosis and AML (Oka et al, 2004). Vaccination was performed by injecting 0.3–3 mg of native or analogue peptide 235 emulsified with the adjuvant Montanide ISA51. The vaccination resulted in an increase in WT1-specific CTLs followed by a rapid reduction in leukemic blast cells. No serious toxicity was observed, but leukemic blasts relapsed after the vaccination was stopped. Recently, these investigators reported that biweekly injection of AML patients with either native or analogue peptide 235 along with Montanide and GM-CSF resulted in three patients remaining in CR for 4 years (Tsuboi et al, 2007). The WT1-235 peptide has also been shown to induce HLA-A0201-restricted CTL (Pinilla-Ibarz, 2006). Keilholz et al first reported that vaccination of a patient with recurrent AML, using HLA-A0201-restricted WT1 peptide 126 along with KLH as an adjuvant, induced CR (Mailander et al, 2004). No haematological or renal toxicities were observed. Rezvani et al reported a phase I clinical trial in patients with AML, CML and MDS, using combined HLA-A0201-binding peptide vaccines from PR1 169–177 and WT1 126–134. Their results show that the emergence of $PR1^+$ or $WT1^+CD8^+$ T cells in patients who received WT1 vaccine was associated with a decrease in WT1 mRNA expression, suggesting a vaccine-driven anti-leukemia effect (Rezvani et al, 2008). An analogue to WT1 peptide 126–134 was generated by substituting R for Y at the position 2 anchor motif (named WT1-A1) (Pinilla-Ibarz et al, 2006). This analogue peptide generated a more potent CD8 T-cell response which recognized and lysed $WT1^+$ leukemia cells in vitro. In addition to the HLA-A0201 and -A24 vaccines derived from WT1 protein, Asemissen et al identified a highly immunogenic HLA-A1-binding WT1 peptide (317–327) that is processed and able to induce a CD8 T-cell response in healthy donors and patients with haematological malignancies (Asemissen et al, 2006).

The German group reported about their phase 2 trial of WT1 peptide vaccination in patients with AML and MDS (Keilholz et al, 2009). Vaccination consisted of GM-CSF subcutaneously days 1 to 4, and WT1126-134 peptide and 1 mg keyhole limpet hemocyanin on day 3. Seventeen AML patients and 2 refractory anemia with excess blasts patients received a median of 11 vaccinations. Treatment was well tolerated. Objective responses in AML patients were 10 stable diseases (SDs) including 4 SDs with more than 50% blast reduction and 2 with hematologic improvement. An additional 4 patients had clinical benefit after initial progression, including 1 CR and 3 SDs. WT1 mRNA levels decreased at least 3-fold from baseline in 35% of patients. In 8 of 18 patients, WT1-tetramer$^+$ T cells increased in blood and in 8 over 17 patients in bone marrow, with a median frequency in bone marrow of 0.18% at baseline and 0.41% at week 18. This WT1 vaccination study provides immunologic, molecular, and preliminary evidence of potential clinical efficacy in AML patients, warranting further investigations.

Other approaches include the use of autologous DCs, generated from leukemia patients in CR and loaded with tumor antigens and/or the differentiation of leukaemia blasts into leukemic DCs. In particular, Van Tendeloo et al reported the results of a phase I/II clinical trial of WT1 vaccination based on antigen-loaded DCs with the induction of complete and molecular responses in some cases (Van Tendeloo et al, 2010). These results are promising. However, the clinical experience with DC-based vaccines targeting WT1 is far too limited and future studies are highly warranted to assess the role and the efficacy of these strategies of active immunotherapy in the clinical management of MRD in AML.

5. Conclusion

In conclusion, the clinical results of AML patients, especially if elderly, are particularly dismal, although the achievement of CR with MRD after combined chemotherapy appears as possible in the majority of patients. Unfortunately, the persistence of MRD leads to progression and patients ultimately die. For these reasons, alternative approaches for the prevention of relapse in CR patients are necessary and are currently under active investigation. In particular, the role of immunological therapies in the post-remission management of adult AML patients, such as NK therapy and active immunization against relevant tumor rejection antigens, including WT1, have been recently exploited with promising results in terms of immunological and clinical responses. Further studies (phase II-III) are highly warranted to really evaluate the role of such approaches and their impact on overall survival of AML patients.

6. References

[1] Asemissen A, U. Keilholz and S. Tenzer et al., Identification of a highly immunogenic HLA-A*01-binding T cell epitope of WT1, Clinical Cancer Research 12 (2006), pp. 7476–7482.

[2] Brand JM, Meller B, Von Hof K, et al. Kinetics and organ distribution of allogeneic natural killer lymphocytes transfused into patients suffering from renal cell carcinoma. Stem Cells and Development 2004; 13: 307-314.

[3] Cheever MA, Allison JP, Ferris AS, Finn OJ, Hastings BM, Hecht TT, Mellman I, Prindiville SA, Viner JL, Weiner LM, Matrisian LM.The prioritization of cancer antigens: a national cancer institute pilot project for the acceleration of translational research. Clin Cancer Res. 2009 Sep 1;15(17):5323-37.

[4] Curti A, Ruggeri L, D'Addio A, et al. Successful transfer of alloreactive haploidentical KIR ligand-mismatched natural killer cells after infusion in elderly high-risk acute myeloid leukemia patients. Blood. 2011 Jul 25. [Epub ahead of print]

[5] Farad SS, Fehniger T, Ruggeri L, et al. Natural killer cell receptors:new biology and insights into graft versus leukemia effect. Blood. 2002; 100: 1935-1947.

[6] Keilholz U, Letsch A, Busse A, Asemissen AM, Bauer S, Blau IW, Hofmann WK, Uharek L, Thiel E, Scheibenbogen C.A clinical and immunologic phase 2 trial of Wilms tumor gene product 1 (WT1) peptide vaccination in patients with AML and MDS. Blood. 2009 Jun 25;113(26):6541-8.

[7] Lanier LL. NK cell receptors. Annu Rev Immunol. 1998; 16: 359-393.

[8] Leith CP, Kopecky KJ, Godwin J, et al. Acute myeloid leukemia in the elderly: assessment of multidrug resistance (MDR1) and cytogenetics distinguishes biologic subgroups with remarkably distinct responses to standard chemotherapy. A Southwest Oncology Group study. Blood. 1997 May 1;89(9):3323-9.

[9] Li Z, Oka Y, Tsuboi A, Masuda T, Tatsumi N, Kawakami M, Fujioka T, Sakaguchi N, Nakajima H, Fujiki F, Udaka K, Oji Y, Kawase I, Sugiyama H. WT1(235), a ninemer peptide derived from Wilms' tumor gene product, is a candidate peptide for the vaccination of HLA-A*0201-positive patients with hematopoietic malignancies. Int J Hematol. 2005 Dec;82(5):458-459.

[10] Mailänder V, Scheibenbogen C, Thiel E, Letsch A, Blau IW, Keilholz U. Complete remission in a patient with recurrent acute myeloid leukemia induced by

vaccination with WT1 peptide in the absence of hematological or renal toxicity. Leukemia. 2004 Jan;18(1):165-166.
[11] Miller JS, Soignier Y, Panoskaltsis-Mortari A, et al. Successful adoptive transfer and in vivo expansion of human haploidentical NK cells in patients with cancer. Blood. 2005;105(8):3051-3057.
[12] Oka Y, Tsuboi A, Taguchi T, Osaki T, Kyo T, Nakajima H, Elisseeva OA, Oji Y, Kawakami M, Ikegame K, Hosen N, Yoshihara S, Wu F, Fujiki F, Murakami M, Masuda T, Nishida S, Shirakata T, Nakatsuka S, Sasaki A, Udaka K, Dohy H, Aozasa K, Noguchi S, Kawase I, Sugiyama H. Induction of WT1 (Wilms' tumor gene)-specific cytotoxic T lymphocytes by WT1 peptide vaccine and the resultant cancer regression. Proc Natl Acad Sci U S A. 2004 Sep 21;101(38):13885-13890.
[13] Oka Y, Udaka K, Tsuboi A, Elisseeva OA, Ogawa H, Aozasa K, Kishimoto T, Sugiyama H.Cancer immunotherapy targeting Wilms' tumor gene WT1 product. J Immunol. 2000 Feb 15;164(4):1873-1880.
[14] Pinilla-Ibarz J, May RJ, Korontsvit T, Gomez M, Kappel B, Zakhaleva V, Zhang RH, Scheinberg DA. Improved human T-cell responses against synthetic HLA-0201 analog peptides derived from the WT1 oncoprotein. Leukemia. 2006 Nov;20(11):2025-2033.
[15] Rezvani K, A.S.M. Young and S. Mielke et al., Leukemia-associated antigen specific T-cell responses following combined PR1 and WT1 peptide vaccination in patients with myeloid malignancies, Blood 111 (2008), pp. 236–242.
[16] Robertson MJ, Ritz J. Biology and clinical relevance of human natural killer cells. Blood. 1990; 76: 2421-2438.
[17] Rubnitz JE, Inaba H, Ribeiro RC, et al. NKAML: a pilot study to determine the safety and feasibility of haploidentical natural killer cell transplantation in childhood acute myeloid leukemia. J Clin Oncol. 2010;28(6):955-959.
[18] Ruggeri L, Capanni M, Casucci M, et al. Role of natural killer cell alloreactivity in HLA-mismatched hematopoietic stem cell transplantation. Blood. 1999; 94: 333-339.
[19] Ruggeri L, Capanni M, Urbani E, et al. Effectiveness of donor natural killer cell alloreactivity in mismatched hematopoietic transplants. Science. 2002; 295: 2097-2100.
[20] Tsuboi A, Oka Y, Nakajima H, et al. Long-term follow-up of three patients with acute myeloid leukemia with minimal residual disease who were treated with WT1 vaccination. In: Third international conference on WT1 in human malignancies, Berlin Sept 20-21, 2007.
[21] Van Tendeloo VF, Van de Velde A, Van Driessche A, et al. Induction of complete and molecular remissions in acute myeloid leukemia by Wilms' tumor 1 antigen-targeted dendritic cell vaccination Proc Natl Acad Sci U S A. 2010 Aug 3;107(31):13824-9.

12

Converting Hematology Based Data into an Inferential Interpretation

Larry H. Bernstein[1,*], Gil David[2], James Rucinski[3] and Ronald R. Coifman[2]
[1]*Triplex,*
[2]*Yale University Department of Mathematics,*
Program in Applied Mathematics, New Haven, CT,
[3]*New York Methodist Hospital-Weill-Cornell, Brooklyn, NY*
USA

1. Introduction

The most commonly ordered test used for managing patients worldwide is the hemogram, with or without the review of a peripheral smear. The measured features in a standard hemogram has undergone modification of the over the last 30 years with an expansion to the panel of tests. The initial hemogram was the hemoglobin, hematocrit, and total white cell count, to which platelet count, lymphocytes and neutrophils were added as the necessary vital dye stains and the resolution were substantially improved. The revolutionary Coulter principle used impedance of the cells passing through a narrow window. Newer instruments may used both impedance and/or flow cytometric principles. Yet the accurate identification of reticulocytes, measurement of cellular hemoglobin, measurement of immature granulocytes, lymphoid or myeloblasts, identification of clumped platelets interfering with identification of large platelets were all challenges to overcome. The hemogram provides a vital window to visualize the cellular changes associated with the production, release or suppression of the formed elements from the blood forming organ to the circulation. In this chapter, we shall not be concerned with the specific use of the hemogram in assessing disorders to the coagulation pathways or its use in detection of hematological and non-hematological tumors. Rather in the hemogram we can view data reflective of a broad spectrum medical conditions affecting most patients presenting to a physician who are then referred to a specialist for example in hematology-oncology or infectious diseases.

The theme of what we are about to present is that once we go beyond qualitative changes to the morphology of the cellular components of blood, we have also to consider their quantitative characteristics expressed as measurements of size, density, and concentration, which results in more than a dozen composite variables, including the mean corpuscular volume (MCV), mean corpuscular hemoglobin concentration (MCHC), mean corpuscular hemoglobin (MCH), total white cell count (WBC), total lymphocyte count, neutrophil count (mature granulocyte count and bands), monocytes, eosinophils, basophils, platelet count, and mean platelet volume (MPV), and flags to denote blasts, reticulocytes, platelet clumps, and so on. If you were to add the comprehensive metabolic panel, which includes monovalent and divalent cations and anions, total CO2, total protein and albumin, to name a few, there is a potential for information overload to the physician. These data in turn have to be comprehended in context with vital signs, key symptoms, and an accurate medical history. Consequently, the limits of memory and cognition are tested in medical practice on a daily basis. In this chapter we will discuss problems in the interpretation of data generated by automated laboratory diagnostic machinery, as experienced by the physician, and how through better design of the software (middleware) that presents this data the situation could be improved.

2. The current status of the physician-laboratory interface

The clinical laboratory has several divisions. Microbiology and anatomic pathology are the oldest, and they are the least automated, but they have rigorous definitions for their interpretation, as is true for immunohematology. Hematology and chemistry are the most automated, but their interpretations are more difficult than the other disciplines. To start with we will consider automated chemistry, hematology, and immunology with large high-throughput sample platforms. These analyzers have enhanced performance by interface with middleware, which have embedded rules to accept or reject a test result based on a result lying outside an assigned confidence limit, or based on a difference from a previous measurement within an assigned time interval in hours or days. A middleware is a minicomputer installed either between an instrument and a laboratory information system or between an instrument and a hospital information system. The middleware handles an enormous transaction rate of test workflow that would otherwise compete with physician interactions in trying to access the data output. The middleware also carries out on-line quality control checks, monitors the completion of panel accessions, and does "delta" checks for excessive differences between measurements taken in sequence. Further, depending on whether a test is measured from unclotted and unspun blood, or from plasma or serum fraction, hematology, chemistry and immunology testing are tested with different turnaround times (time from receipt to time to report). In all of these cases, tests from different core "instruments" or laboratory "facilities" of laboratory testing have to be interpreted without conflict in the production "silo" (the term refers to a separate mode of production that is separate from and not interoperable with other information sources).

3. Data overload and unstructured

The computer architecture that the physician uses to view the results is not open-architecture, and the middleware solutions used to overcome the problem are insufficient in that the data is not recombined from the rigid lists into a structured format that readily enables the physician to interpret the report. Consequently the results are more often than not presented as the designer would prefer, and not as the end-user would like. In order to optimize the interface for physician, the system would have a "front-to-back" design, with the call up for any patient ideally consisting of a dashboard design that presents the crucial information that the physician would likely act on in an easily accessible manner. The problem of the user having to adjust to what the system confronts them with is described by Didner (1) in an internal Bell Labs memo approved for external release. The key point being that each item used has to be closely related to a corresponding criterion needed for a decision. Currently, improved design is heading in that direction. In removing this limitation the output requirements have to be defined before the database is designed to produce the required output. The ability to see any other information, or to see a sequential visualization of the patient's course would be steps to home in on other views. In addition, the amount of relevant information, even when presented well, is a cognitive challenge unless it is presented in a disease- or organ-system structure. So the interaction between the user and the electronic medical record has a significant effect on practitioner time, ability to minimize errors of interpretation, facilitate treatment, and manage costs. This is a correction for a view from the mere transmission of a body of automated tests that are generated at sites not near to the patient, often with a high priority reporting required from the operating room, the emergency room, or the intensive care units in order to make triage decisions or to adjust fluids or make treatment decisions.

The reality is that clinicians are challenged by the need to view a large amount of data, with only a few resources available to know which of these values are relevant, or the need for action on a result, or its urgency. An approach (2,3), called the foresighted-practice guideline, aligned with concepts developed by Lawrence Weed (4). Weed emphasizes that the information infrastructure was lacking at the time of his writing (1997), and that tools are needed to extend the mind's capability to process large numbers of relevant variables. The challenge then becomes how fundamental measurement theory can lead to the creation at the point of care of more meaningful actionable presentations of results (5). WP Fisher (6) refers to the creation of a context in which computational resources for meeting the challenges will be incorporated into the electronic medical record. The one which he chooses is a probabilistic conjoint (Rasch) measurement model (7), which uses scale-free standard measures and meets data quality standards. He illustrates this by fitting a set of data provided by Bernstein (19)(27 items for the diagnosis of acute myocardial infarction (AMI) to a Rasch multiple rating scale model testing the hypothesis that items work together to delineate a unidimensional measurement continuum. The results indicated that highly improbable observations could be discarded, data volume could be reduced based on its internal consistency, and that consistency could be used to increase the ability of the care provider to interpret the data. The use of a computer-derived algorithm has been shown to aid the physician (8,9). A huge amount of progress has occurred regarding model construction and validation in the last 11 years. An ordinal regression (adjacent category logit model)(10) used on the AMI problem (11) is superceded by a Latent Class Model of Jay Magidson and Jeroen Vermunt (LatentGOLD, Statistical Innovations, Medford, MA)(12). The LatentGOLD has LC Cluster models, DFactor models, and LC Regression models and has the advantage of allowing performance of LC analyses on data containing more than just a few variables. It uses the fundamental methods of model fit (13,14) established as Alaike (AIC)(14,15,16) and Bayes (BIC)(14) information criteria. These have not been applied to classifying a large and complex medical data set.

4. Classified data a separate issue from automation

On the other hand, automation itself may not be as important as the critical value of the information provided. The disciplines required in blood banking and in microbiology have only been recently automated, but their importance is readily understood with the exception of an error in blood sample, or its contamination. To an extent, blood screening has become a large scale production to service the user population.

The classification of blood types emerged at the turn of the last century firstly as a result of the work of Paul Ehrlich (17) establishing a groundwork for immunology, and then later Karl Landsteiner's seminal work in laying the foundation for the blood groups (17). These works resulted in a well-defined classification of a set of identified blood group antigens and the absence of antibody in the individual's serum against the blood type, with the exception of auto-antibody reactions.

4.1 Microbiology classification

Microbiology classification has its origin in the taxonomic principles set down by Bergey's Manual of Determinative Bacteriology, which originated in 1857, and is maintained by Bergey's Trust. It is guided by observable features that are key for separating groups and subgroups. The kind of features that we readily identify are gram stain positivity, colonies on agar, cocciform or bacillary shape, outer capsule, motility, the clusters formed, the metabolic features in growth media, and even the expected antibiotic reactivity. Thus, we have an example: in Table 1.

GROUP 4
Description: Gram Negative, Aerobic/Microaerophilic rods and cocci
Key differences are: pigments/fluorescent, motility, growth requirements, denitrification,
morphology, and oxidase, read Genera descriptions
Examples: Acinetobacter, Pseudomonas, Beijerinckia
GROUP 5
Description: Facultatively Anaerobic Gram negative rods
Key differences are: growth factors, morph., gram rxn., oxidase rxn., read Genera descriptions
Examples: Family Enterobacteriaceae and Vibrionaceae
GROUP 17
Description: Gram-Positive Cocci
Key differences are: oxygen requirements, morph., growth requirements (45°C and supplements), read Genera descriptions
Examples: Micrococcus, Staphylococcus, Streptococcus, Enterococcus, Lactococcus

Table 1. Typical classes of bacteria

Table 1 does not further divide into subclasses, which requires metabolic differentiation in growth media.

4.2 Feature extraction

This further breakdown in the modern era is determined by genetically characteristic gene sequences that are transcribed into what we measure. Eugene Rypka contributed greatly to clarifying the extraction of features in a series of articles, which set the groundwork for the methods used today in clinical microbiology (18,19). The method he describes is termed S-clustering, and will have a significant bearing on how we can view hematology data. He describes S-clustering as extracting features from endogenous data that amplify or maximize structural information to create distinctive classes. The method classifies by taking the number of features with sufficient variety to map into a theoretic standard. The mapping is done by a truth table, and each variable is scaled to assign values for each: message choice. The number of messages and the number of choices forms an N-by N table. He points out that the message choice in an antibody titer would be converted from 0 + ++ +++ to 0 1 2 3. In looking at laboratory values the practitioner separates any test by low normal moderately-high high. Even though there may be a large number of measured values, the variety is reduced by this compression, even though there is risk of loss of information. Yet the real issue is how a combination of variables falls into a table with meaningful information. He describes how syndromic classification is uniquely valuable for clinical laboratory information by amplifying information in the course of making a pattern-identifiable syndromic classification. Rudolph, Bernstein and Babb (20) used it for the diagnosis of acute myocardial infarction.

5. Optimal weighting and value assigned to predictor variables

We are interested in classifying data as essential for determining optimal decision limits for tests, and for analyzing variable combinations that are essential and optimal for separating the groups that are separated with fewest errors. This is only possible by reducing data uncertainty. We are concerned with accurate assignment into uniquely variable groups by information in test relationships. One determines the effectiveness of each variable by its contribution to information gain in the system. The reference or null set is the class having no information. Uncertainty in assigning to a classification is only relieved by providing sufficient information. One determines the effectiveness of each variable by its contribution to information gain in the system. The possibility for realizing a good model for approximating the effects of factors supported by data used for inference owes much to the discovery of Kullback-Liebler distance or "information" (21), and Akaike (22) found a simple relationship between K-L information and Fisher's maximized log-likelihood function (23).

5.1 Advances in applied mathematics

Perhaps the current exponential growth of knowledge since the mapping of the human genome a decade ago has been enabled by parallel advances in applied mathematics, which has not been a part of the entrance competencies for premedical education, and is now taught to some extent in medical and postmedical education for a better understanding of modern clinical trials. The knowledge and use of the science of complexity in much of what we encounter is brought to account by Ray Kurzweill (24). In a univariate universe, we have significant control in visualizing data because we can be confident in separating unlike data by methods that rely on distributional assumptions, although errors in assignment can be substantial. The median (by rank order assignment is the best method of assignment under the circumstances). In reality, there is likely to be a different assignment of predictor values given an association with a different disease entity. In order to better define the target output another variable is necessary. As we attend to more associated outputs, the number of predictors is expanded. Now we begin to have multiple classes delineated by the confidence limits of the conjoint predictors. As the number of separate categories increases, the size of the database has to increase to limit the error in the so called model representation.

5.2 Complexity

As the complexity of models have increased to using several predictors for at least two outputs, and the dependencies are not clear, the models used for analysis of the data are derived by tables and use of the goodness of fit. The development of the Akaike Information Criterion (15,16,21,22,23) brought together two major disciplines that had separate developments, information theory and statistics. The powerful tools now available are not dependent on distributional assumptions, and allow classification and prediction. In fact modeling today has a primary goal of finding an underlying structure in studied data sets. A sequence of exploratory programs have been developed by Statistical Innovations, a Boston based company founded by Jay Magidson focused on classification problems with complex data sets, encompassing a mixture of nominal and continuous predictors, and where there is a high complexity with the data sample size may approach the number of predictors (COREXpress® , Latent GOLD® 4.5, LG-Syntax Module, Latent GOLD® Choice , SI-CHAID® , GOLDMineR). Many articles can be cited concerning these advances (25-32). Further, IBM has introduced a software program for Predictive Analytics available in 2011.

6. Prior experience in similarly developed taxonomies can be applied to hematology

We consider a novel approach to medical inference to have considerable parallel with work in bacterial taxonomy, or the rapidly growing work in genomics, proteomics, and translational medicine. In the diagnosis of anemia, we divide these into microcytic, normocytic and macrocytic. We also consider whether there is proliferation of marrow precursors, whether there is domination of a cell line, and whether there is a suppression of hematopoiesis. This gives us a two dimensional model. Then we consider another, the release into the blood of immature cells, for intermediate to the blast stage. Keep in mind that the thalassemias (and hemoglobin H disease) are characterized by moderate to severe microcytosis, and there is no anisocytosis (variation in size), and being a genetic disorder in production of globin chains, there is a high RBC count, whereas, iron deficiency anemia (IDA) differs by lack of iron incorporation into hemoglobin so that there is a low MCV, anisocytosis, and a low RBC count so that the ratio (Mentzer's index) of the MCV/RBC is very low with thalassemia, but not in IDA. We shall elaborate more on the creation of an evidence-based inference-engine that can substantially interpret the data at hand and convert it in real time to a "knowledge-based opinion", which is improvable from what exists today by incorporating clinical features and duration of onset into the model.

The evaluation of platelet abnormalities is somewhat more limited, but addresses the disorders of platelet numbers and of platelet size, and clumping. This does not discern abnormalities of platelet function (like von Willebrands, or drug induced). When platelets decrease abruptly with disseminated intravascular coagulation (DIC), as in sepsis or with massive trauma, the evidence is pretty good.

6.1 Hematopoiesis

Figure 1 is a pictorial diagram of hematopoietic cell lineages that are readily found in texts and cells are delineated further by identification of cell differentiation (CD) antigens. This lineage is expressly important for both the innate response and the humoral response to injury. Our knowledge of the innate response has become more and more intimately associated with long term metabolic effects, constitution, and chronic inflammation.

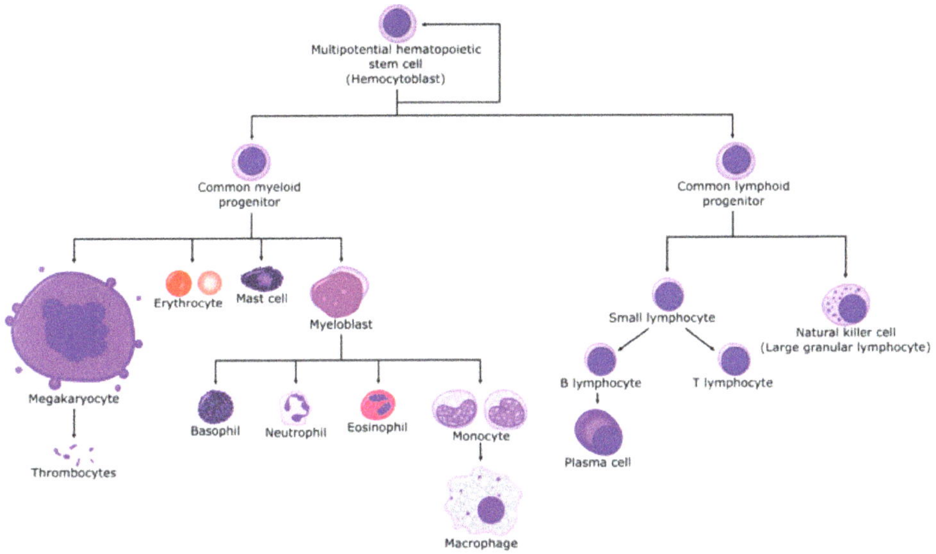

Fig. 1. A common depiction of the evolution of the myeloid and lymphoid cell lines from a multipotential hematopoietic stem cell. The platelets, red blood cells, mast cells and myeloid series are depicted as derived from a common myeloid progenitor cell. A branching from the myeloblast gives the granulocytic cells and the monocyte. Promyelocyte, metamyelocyte and myelocyte are intermediates not shown (band neutrophil is viewed as a neutrophil). The lymphocyte series is being more defined (as the myelocytic) that the naïve depiction by cell differentiation (CD) markers, and interactions are being investigated by cytokine, chemokine and cell signaling pathways.

Figure 1 shows a primary separation into a lymphocytic and a myeloid series. Note that the erythrocyte series and platelets are shown to be in lineage from a myeloid progenitor cell. It is conceivable that this picture is an oversimplification, but in clinical application, it is readily understood. This makes sense with respect to the uncommon evolution of myeloid metaplasia into erythroleukemia, but the diagram doesn't have an obvious connection for myelofibrosis, except for in the monocyte-macrophage linkage.

6.2 Peripheral smear

The peripheral smear is only viewed on the basis of flagged features seen on the hemogram. Blasts, indicative of release of very immature lymphocytes or myeloblasts are flagged and have to be reviewed by a pathologist before release, or done by the hematology supervisor and retained for pathologist review. In the case of children, there are numerous lymphocytes, and there may also be normoblasts and reticulocytes released from an active marrow. The presence of small mononuclear cells can be correctly identified by an experienced morphologist, but not necessarily by an automated cell counter. Consequently, proportionately more peripheral smears are evaluated for children than for adults. The greatest problem in the childhood age group is infection or sepsis. The lymphocyte and reticulocyte counts are very high in the infant, and the peak age for acute lymphocytic leukemia is at two years old. This makes it far more difficult to identify myelocytes and metamyelocytes (not shown in Figure 1), indicators of myeloid proliferation, in children than adults (33). The band neutrophil has been used to signify a left shift in myelopoiesis associated with sepsis, but it is quite variable and has been largely disregarded. This has accounted for the use of an automated cell counter that is also a flow cytometer for improved recognition of immature neutrophils below the band count. In the case of the red cell series (not shown) we classify first based on the RBC count, and then on the cell size. By these measures we have a decrease in mature red cell count based on WHO standards, adjusting for menstruation and pregnancy in women. We at the same time consider whether the RBC is normocytic, microcytic, or macrocytic and/or megaloblastic. What about increased or decreased production? Thalassemia is characterized by small cells that are neither hypochromic, or decreased in the peripheral circulation. Platelets may be large, they may be excessive in number, or they may be significantly decreased.

7. Extension of conditions and presentation to the electronic medical record (EMR)

We have published on the application of an automated inference engine (34) to the Systemic Inflammatory Response (SIRS), a serious infection, or emerging sepsis. We can report on this without going over previous ground. Of considerable interest is the morbidity and mortality of sepsis, and the hospital costs from a late diagnosis. If missed early, it could be problematic, and it could be seen as a hospital complication when it is not. Improving on previous work, we have the opportunity to look at the contribution of a fluorescence labeled flow cytometric measurement of the immature granulocytes (IG)(35), which is now widely used, but has not been adequatedly evaluated from the perspective of diagnostic usage. We have done considerable work on protein-energy malnutrition (PEM)(36-38), to which the automated interpretation is currently in review (39). Of course, the cholesterol, lymphocyte count, serum albumin provide the weight of evidence with the primary diagnosis (emphysema, chronic renal disease, eating disorder), and transthyretin would be low and remain low for a week in critical care. This could be a modifier with age in providing discriminating power.

7.1 Design of EMR

The current design of the Electronic Medical Record (EMR) is a linear presentation of portions of the record by services, by diagnostic method, and by date, to cite examples. This allows perusal through a graphical user interface (GUI) that partitions the information or necessary reports in a workstation entered by keying to icons. This requires that the medical practitioner finds the history, medications, laboratory reports, cardiac imaging and EKGs, and radiology in different workspaces. The introduction of a DASHBOARD, a visual panel of essential information on the computer screen that is widely used in business organizations, has allowed a presentation of drug reactions, allergies, primary and secondary diagnoses, and critical information about any patient the care giver needing access to the record. The advantage of this innovation is obvious. The startup problem is what information is presented and how it is displayed, which is a source of variability and a key to its success.

7.2 Dashboard

We are proposing an innovation that supercedes the main design elements of a DASHBOARD and utilizes the conjoined syndromic features of the disparate data elements. So the important determinant of the success of this endeavor is that it facilitates both the workflow and the decision-making process with a reduction of medical error. This has become extremely important and urgent in the 10 years since the publication "To Err is Human" (40), and the newly published finding that reduction of error is as elusive as reduction in cost. Whether they are counterproductive when approached in the wrong way may be subject to debate.

7.3 Syndromic classification

In order to clarify the concept of syndromic classification we make a distinction between lists of diseases that are assigned to abnormal test results and can be appended to test results. The oldest application has been in the identification of bacteria after culture isolation using growth in defined media that identify genetically determined metabolic pathways characteristic for each organism. A solid foundation in this work was elaborated by Rypka (18, 19). This was made less complicated by the genetic complement that defines its function. We introduce an AUTOMATED inference engine processing the data and making an interpretation available to the ordering physician and can anticipate an enormous impact on diagnosis and treatment. It addresses the complexity of inputs and enables rather than disables the practitioner. The method identifies outliers and combines data according to commonality of features. In some cases there may be conditions that are aggregated by similarity and dissimilarity into variants of the same condition with different treatment responses. How can we have confidence that we can successfully approach this problem in a new way? In the first place we are able to construct an interpretation of the composite data that is consistent with how a practitioner views multisystem pathophysiology in service of clinical decision-making.

8. A new inference methodology identifies and classifies anomalies

The main mathematical breakthroughs are provided by accurate patient profiling and inference methodologies in which anomalous subprofiles are extracted and compared to potentially relevant cases. Our methodologies organize numerical medical data profiles into demographics and characteristics relevant for inference and case tracking. As the model grows and its knowledge database is extended, the diagnostic and the prognostic become more accurate and precise.

As an example, inputs from test data such as hematology results are processed for anomaly characterization and compared with similar anomalies in a data base of 30,000 patients, provide diagnostic statistics, warning flags, and risk assessment. These are based on past prior experience, including: diagnostics and treatment outcomes (collective experience). The system was trained on this database of patients, built the learning knowledge base and used to analysis and diagnosis 5,000 new patients. Our system identified successfully the main risks with very high accuracy (more than 96%) and very low false rate (less than 0.5%)(34).

9. Representation and conclusion

The main benefit is a real time assessment as well as diagnostic options based on comparable cases, flags for risk and potential problems as illustrated in Figure 2. Figure 2 depicts the following case acquired on 04/21/10. The patient was diagnosed by our system with severe SIRS.

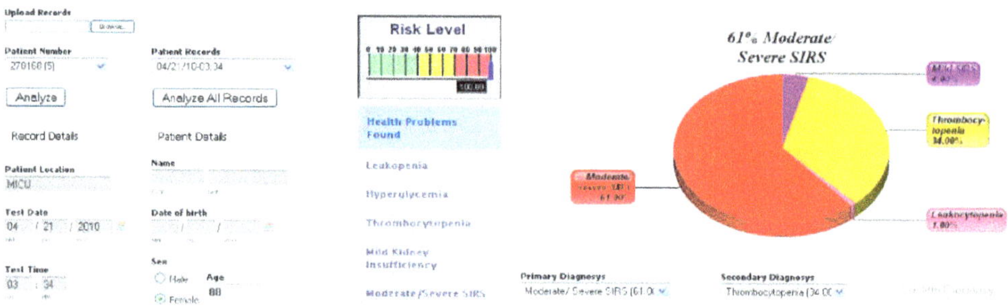

Fig. 2. The depiction of a patient diagnosed with severe systemic inflammatory response syndrome (SIRS), which may evolve into multiple organ failure (MODS), and death by circulatory collapse (systemic shock) if not arrested, depending on systemic functional reserve and successive stress. The far right is a pie chart of measured effects, and primary and secondary diagnoses. The middle lists the diagnoses found above which there is a scale with the risk. The left is patient demographics.

We anticipate that the effect of implementing this diagnostic amplifier would result in higher physician productivity at a time of great human resource limitations, safer prescribing practices, rapid identification of unusual patients, better assignment of patients to observation, inpatient beds, intensive care, or referral to clinic, shortened length of patients ICU and bed days.

10. References

[1] Didner RS. Back-to-Front systems design: A guns and butter approach. Unpublished research, 1979. Bell Laboratories, Piscataway, NJ 08854.

[2] Naegele TA, Wetzler HP. The foresighted practice guideline model: A win-win solution. http://www.swcp.com

[3] Naegele TA. Practice guidelines and clinical decision making. J Osteopath Med. March 1993:53-8.

[4] Weed L. New Connections between medical knowledge and patient care. Brit Med J 1997; 315:231-5.

[5] Haux R. Health information systems - past, present, future. Int J Med Inform. 2006; 75(3-4):268-81. Epub 2005 Sep 19.

[6] Fisher, W. P., Jr., Bernstein, L. H., Qamar, A., Babb, J., Rypka, E. W., & Yasick, D. (2002, February). At the bedside: Measuring patient outcomes. Advance for Administrators of the Laboratory, 11(2), 8, 10 [http://laboratory-manager.advanceweb.com/Article/At-the-Bedside-7.aspx].

[7] Fisher, W. P., Jr., & Burton, E. (2010). Embedding measurement within existing computerized data systems: Scaling clinical laboratory and medical records heart failure data to predict ICU admission. Journal of Applied Measurement, 11(2), 271-287.
[8] Linacre JM. Many-Facet Rasch Measurement. 1994. Mesa Press. Chicago,IL.
[9] Qamar A, McPherson C, Babb J, Bernstein LH, et al. The Goldman algorithm revisited: prospective evaluation of a computer-derived algorithm versus unaided physician judgement in suspected acute myocardial infarction. Amer Heart J 1999; 138:705-9.
[10] Goldman L, Weinberg M, Weisberg M, Olshen R, Cook EF, Sargent RK, Lamas GA, Dennis C, Wilson C, Deckelbaum L, Fineberg H, Stiratelli R. A computer-derived protocol to aid in the diagnosis of emergency room patients with acute chest pain. N Engl J Med 1982;307:588-596.
[11] Bernstein LH, Qamar A, McPherson R, Zarich S. Evaluation of a new graphical ordinal regression model (GOLDminer) in the diagnosis of myocardial infarction utilizing clinical features and laboratory data. http://www.statisticalinnovations.com/products/goldminer_tutorial2.html
[12] Magidson, J. and Vermunt, J.K. Latent class models for clustering: A comparison with K-means. Canadian Journal of Marketing Research, 2002; 20, 36-43.
[13] Browne MW, Cudeck R. Alternative ways of assessing model fit. In Testing Structural Equation Models (Bollen KA, Long JS, eds). 1993. Chapter 6. pages 1-34. SAGE Publishers, Inc. Newbury Park, CA. ISBN 0-8039-9507-8 (pbk).
[14] Raftery AE. Baysian model selection in structural equation models. In Testing Structural Equation Models (Bollen KA, Long JS, eds). 1993. Chapter 7. pages 163-179. SAGE Publishers, Inc. Newbury Park, CA. ISBN 0-8039-9507-8 (pbk).
[15] Akaike H. Factor analysis and AIC. Psychometrika 1987; 52:317-332.
[16] Bozdogen H. Model selection and Akaike's information criteria (AIC): the general theory and irs analytical extensions. Psychometrika 1987; 52:345-370.
[17] JW Goding. Emergence of the concept of complementarity and binding between antigen and antibodies: Contributions of Ehrlich and Landsteiner. In (JW Goding) Monoclonal Antibodies. Principles and Practice. Antibody Response. Elsevier Ltd 1996. Chapter 2. pages 7-25. (ISBN 978- 0 -12-287023-1).
[18] Rypka EW. Methods to evaluate and develop the decision process in the selection of tests. In Nakamura R. ed. Clinics in Laboratory Medicine.Phila.: WB Saunders Co.1992; 12(2):351-86.
[19] Rypka EW, Madar DA. A system for detecting emerging events: the systems-cybernetics approach. Presentation: Research Association of Medical and Biological Organizations (RAMBO). Biology department, University of New Mexico, Albuquerque, NM. July 17, 1996.
[20] Rudolph RA, Bernstein LH, Babb J. Information induction for predicting acute myocardial infarction. Clin Chem 1988; 34:2031-8.
[21] Kullback S, Liebler RA. On information and sufficiency. Annals of Math Statistics 1951; 22:79-86.
[22] Akaike H. Information theory as an extension of the maximum likelihood principle. In BN Petrov and F Csaki, Eds. Second International Symposium on Information Theory. Akdemiai Kiado, Budapest. 1973; 267-281.

[23] Fisher RA. On the Mathematical Foundations of Theoretical Statistics. Philosophical Transactions of the Royal Society of London. A. 1922; 222:309-368.
[24] Kurzweill R. The Singularity is Near: When Humans Transcend Biology. 2005. Viking Press. ISBN 0670033847.
[25] Jaynes ET. Bayesian Methods: General Background, ' In Maximum Entropy and Bayesian Methods in Applied Statistics.(Justice JH, ed). 1986, pp 1-26. Cambridge University Press.
[26] Skilling J. Classic maximum entropy. In Maximum Entropy and Bayesian Methods in Applied Statistics.Skilling J, ed. 1989. Pp 45-52. Kluwer Publishers, Norwell, MA.
[27] Burnham, K. P., and D. R. Anderson. 1998. Model selection and inference: a practical information-theoretic approach. Springer-Verlag, New York, New York, USA. 353 pp.
[28] Malakoff D. Bayes offers a 'new' way to make sense of numbers. Science 1999; 286:1460–64.
[29] Magidson J, Vermunt JK. Comparing Latent Class Factor Analysis with the traditional approach in Data Mining. In Bozdogan, ed. Statistical Datamining and Knowledge Discovery. 2004. Chapter 22, pg 373. CRC Press.
[30] Vermunt JK, Magidson. In Latent Class Models for Classification. Computational Statistics and Data Analysis. 2003:531-533.
[31] Magidson J. Latent Class (Finite Mixture) Segments. How to find themand what to do with them. Sensometrics, Rotterdam. 2010. Presentation.
[32] http://statisticalinnovations.com/products/latentgold_v4.html.
[33] Roehrl MH, Lantz D, Sylvester C, Wang JY. Age-dependent reference ranges for automated assessment of immature granulocytes and clinical significance in an outpatient setting. Arch Pathol Lab Med 2011; 135(4):471-77.
[34] David G, Bernstein L, Coifman RR. Generating evidence based interpretation of hematology screens via anomaly characterization. The Open Clinical Chemistry Journal 2011; 4:101-6.
[35] Bernstein LH, Rucinski J.Measurement of Granulocyte Maturation May Improve the Early Diagnosis of the Septic State. Clin Chem Lab Med 2011; 49 (in press) Doi 10.1515/CCLM.2011688
[36] Brugler L, DiPrinzio MJ, Bernstein L. The five year evolution of a malnutrition treatment program in a community hospital. J Comm J Qual Improv 1999; 25(4):191-206.
[37] Brugler L, Stankovic A, Bernstein L, Scott F, OSullivan-Maillet J. The role of visceral protein markers in protein calorie malnutrition. Clinical Chemistry and Laboratory Medicine 2002; 12:1360–1369.
[38] Brugler L, Stankovic AK, Schlefer M, Bernstein L. A simplified nutrition screen for hospitalized patients using readily available laboratory and patient information. Nutrition 2005; 21:650–658.
[39] David G, Bernstein L, Coifman RR. The Automated Malnutrition Assessment. Nutrition Nut-11-00351 (Elsevier) in review
[40] Executive Summary. To Err Is Human. (Kohn LT, Corrigna JM, Donaldson MS, eds.) Committee on Quality of Healthcare in America. IOM. National Academy Press 2000. Washington, DC. http// www.nap.edu/books/0309068371/html. ISBN 978-0-309-06837-6.

13

Physiological Factors in the Interpretation of Equine Hematological Profile

K. Satué[1], A. Hernández[1] and A. Muñoz[2]
[1]*Department of Animal Medicine and Surgery, School of Veterinary Medicine, Cardenal Herrera-CEU University, Valencia*
[2]*Department of Animal Medicine and Surgery, Equine Sport Medicine Centre, School of Veterinary Medicine, University of Córdoba*
Spain

1. Introduction

Cellular components of the blood reflect specific changes in an organ or body system or more often, a general response of the individual to some physiological or pathological conditions. In this chapter, we will review the main physiological factors that should be considered when interpreting equine hematological profiles. The interpretation of the hematological profile in conjunction with history and physical findings directs the clinician in the selection of other diagnostic, imaging and sampling techniques. Additionally, a hematological profile provides invaluable information concerning the severity of the disease and the response to a treatment, and it helps in establishing a prognosis. Further, horses can have different hematological disorders, making hematology important in equine medicine. A special consideration should be made for equine athletes, since the assessment of a hematological profile is pivotal in the diagnosis of a reduced performance.

2. Erythron

2.1 Introduction and specific characteristics of the equine erythrocytes

The term erythron refers to red cell precursors, the tissues in which production takes place and mature erythrocytes themselves and its functional unit, the red blood cell (RBC). The erythron is assessed from peripheral blood samples, by calculating the number of circulating RBC, hemoglobin concentration (HB), packed cell volume (PCV), volumetric indices, such as mean corpuscular volume (MCV), mean corpuscular hemoglobin (MCH) and mean corpuscular hemoglobin concentration (MCHC), a morphological examination at microscopic level (Messer, 1995; Kramer, 2000) and sometimes, examination of the bone marrow (Lording, 2008). When interpreting an equine hematological profile, some specific characteristics of this species should be kept in mind.

PCV unstable. The horse is somewhat unique compared to most other mammalians in that the spleen is a very capacious organ, storing between 6 and 12 L of red-cell-rich blood at rest (Persson, 1967; McKeever et al., 1993). Large numbers of RBCs temporally sequestered in the spleen can be rapidly transferred into the circulation in response to excitement (handling, venipuncture, loss blood, twitching, and pain) and intense exercise (Persson, 1967; 1983). This response is induced by the release of catecholamines and therefore, the resting PCV in horses should be carefully assessed under different excitation levels (Persson, 1967; Schalm and Carlson, 1982). By contrast, tranquilizers and anesthetics decreased circulating RBCs, because of splenic sequestration (Jain, 1986). Comparable changes are not found in splenectomized horses following excitement and strenuous exercise or tranquilization (Kunugiyama et al., 1997).

The intensity of changes in circulating RBC in relation to spleen activity depends on individual variations, age, breed and fitness level and in the case of exercise, duration and intensity. The time required for RBCs to return to resting values is dependent on the degree of the excitement, and it can vary from 40 to 60 minutes to up to several hours (Jain, 1986).

Rouleaux formation and erythrocyte sedimentation rate. Rouleaux formation is the result of the aggregation of RBCs in linear stacks and depends on the number of RBCs and their tendency to aggregate. Rouleaux formation is a characteristic finding in healthy horses, as a result of weak surface changes on RBC membranes (Brockus et al., 2003). There is a positive correlation between the rate of rouleaux formation and the rate of setting of RBCs in anticoagulated blood (erythrocyte sedimentation rate). Rouleaux formation is accentuated in some diseases associated with hyperproteinemia, because high concentrations of plasma proteins, particularly fibrinogen and immunoglobulins, have an insulating effect that reduces the RBC surface membrane charge, promoting RBC aggregation (Schalm and Carlson, 1982; Brockus et al., 2003).

Autoagglutination can be seen in some horses without hemolysis as a result of cold antibodies, with a maximal activity at 4-20°C or as a result of unfractioned heparin treatment (Monreal et al., 1995). Macroscopically, agglutination has a granular appearance and microscopically, appears as grape-like clusters of RBCs. It should be differentiate from rouleaux by using the saline dilution test. Typically a 1:2 dilution will disperse rouleaux but not the autoagluttinated RBCs. Infrequently, a higher dilution (up to 1:10) may be needed to disperse rouleaux. Agglutination causes erroneous MCV values and RBC numbers determined by impedance, because the aggregates may interfere with the electronic or optical evaluation of the erythrocytes. Pre-treating cell suspensions from agglutinated heparin-treated horses with trypsin might reverse the agglutination, improving the accuracy of cell counts (Grondin and Dewitt, 2010).

Absence of peripheral signs of regeneration. Life span of equine RBC in the circulation is approximately 140 to 150 days (Schalm and Carlson, 1982). RBCs are released from bone marrow as mature cells and the horse is unique in failing to release reticulocytes into peripheral blood when there is a regenerative response to hemorrhage or hemolysis. Therefore, morphological features indicative of regeneration, such as reticulocytes and polychromasia are rare in equine blood films. Reticulocyte counts may be performed on marrow aspirates in anemic horses. Values greater than 5% are consistent with accelerated erythropoiesis. Further, in those cases where anemia derives from decreased erythropoiesis, bone marrow examination may identify the cause and enable to carry out a definitive diagnosis (Schalm and Carlson, 1982).

The only indication of maximally stimulated erythropoiesis in routine hematology data is anisocytosis and increased MCV (by up to 10 to 15 fl above baseline levels for an individual horse) (Jain, 1986). Other way to evaluate regeneration is to interpret RBC distribution width or RDW. It is a coefficient of the degree of anisocytosis of circulating RBCs. This parameter will be increased in anemias with significant macrocytosis and/or microcytosis. The RDW is wider in healthy horses than in other species, and normal values range between 14 and 25% (Kramer, 2000). Similarly, assays of RBC creatine concentrations enable a more accurate evaluation of the erythropoietic response in horses. Mean RBC creatine concentration is significantly higher in young RBC populations (Wu et al., 1983), it shows a positive correlation with the reticulocyte count in bone marrow aspirates and a negative correlation with myeloid-erythroid ratio (Lording, 2008). However, it is not a common clinical procedure.

The response to hemolysis is greater than following hemorrhage, although the regenerative capability of horses is relatively poor compared with other species (Brockus et al. 2003). Complete recovery from very severe hemolytic or hemorrhagic anemia may take approximately 1 to 2 months and 2 to 3 months respectively (Lumsden et al., 1975a,b).

Howell-Jolly bodies. They are nuclear remnants of DNA that occasionally are seen in healthy equine peripheral blood films. They are small, round, purple inclusions. Increased number can be seen with enhanced erythropoiesis and with decreased or compromised splenic function (Schalm and Carlson, 1982; Kramer, 2000; Grondin and Dewitt, 2010).

RBC morphology. Equine RBC is relatively small compared to other animal species, with a mean diameter of 5-6 µm and a MCV of approximately 40 to 52 fl (Lassen and Swardson, 1995; Kramer, 2000; Grondin and Dewitt, 2010). They exhibit a mild degree of anisocytosis and RBC size may differ between horse breeds. Breeds dedicated to sport, such as Thoroughbred racehorses or Standardbred horses have an MCV lower than other breeds. Because HB is spread over a larger number of cells, the total surface of the red cell mass is increased. This adaptation of sport equine breeds appears to be a mean to achieve an easier gas exchange during exercise (Allen and Powell, 1983; Kramer, 2000).

2.2 Physiological factors influencing erythron in horses

2.2.1 Sampling handling

In relation to the anticoagulant used, blood parameters in horses are not altered after anticoagulation in heparin-lithium or EDTA. On the contrary, when using sodium citrate, most hematological parameters significantly decrease, compared with the other anticoagulants (Sharif et al., 2010).

Once the blood sample has been taken, another parameter to consider is the time to conduct the blood test. This should be done as soon as possible, preferably within the first 6 hours after collection, in order to avoid the damage caused by storage. The most common change associated with storage is an increase in the RBC size, a fact that artefactually leads to increased MCV and PCV (Allen et al., 1988). However, within limitations in some hematological parameters, equine blood samples stored in EDTA at 4°C for a maximum of 72 hrs may be adequate for blood tests (Sharif et al., 2010).

Exposure of the sample to high temperatures or direct sunlight can cause hemolysis, resulting in altered RBC values (Rose and Hodgson, 1994).

2.2.2 Accuracy of measurements

The accuracy of the determinations results from the characteristics of the equipment of analysis. Therefore, it is very important to know the sources of errors according to the type of equipment. It has been recommended to conduct repeated measurements, allowing a more reliable interpretation of the results (Persson, 1975; Jain, 1993; Rose and Hodgson, 1994). In fact, Persson (1975) described a variation of up to 30% in baseline HB in three Standardbred horses in which blood samples were obtained in 7 consecutive days.

2.2.3 Attitude and degree of excitement of the horse

Another aspect that might influence the interpretation of RBC parameters is the attitude and the degree of excitement the horse has before and during blood withdrawal (Rose and Hodgson, 1994). Excitement leads to a rise in circulating RBC, HB and PCV. This is the result of the splenic contraction produced by the release of adrenaline and noradrenaline (Kurosawa et al., 1998). The main limiting factor is the time to collect the blood sample. Venipuncture for longer than 30 sec significantly alters the hemograma, as it involves splenic mobilization, resulting from the actions of the sympathetic-adrenal and hypothalamic-pituitary axis (Persson, 1967; Kurosawa et al., 1998).

There are many physiological factors that cause stress in the horse, such as exercise (whether in training or competition), adverse environmental conditions, particularly high heat and humidity, but also dust and very cold or windy weather, long-distance transport, insufficient rest between athletic events, lack of sleep at shows (e.g. late night events or activity in the boarding barn, stall too small for the horse to lie down and rest comfortably), new experiences during training or competition, confinement, removal from familiar environment and social group, changes in daily routine when traveling and at shows, strange environments (e.g. boarding at shows), presence and activity of strange horses and people at shows and increased stress levels in the handlers and rider and weaning, among others (Friend, 2001).

2.2.4 Method of venipuncture

An early study showed that the use of vacuum tubes for blood collection can cause cell damage (Archer, 1977). The use of higher gauge needles leads to satisfactory results according to most of the authors (Jeffcott, 1977; Messer, 1995). In our experience, additional care should be having in blood samples taken in maximally exercised horses in order to avoid hemolysis. Recently, it has been demonstrated that there are not significant differences when comparing hematological parameters obtained using two different methods: venipuncture and intravenous catheter (May et al., 2010).

2.2.5 Feeding

Another factor to take into account when interpreting equine erythrogram is the food and the time of blood sampling in relation to time of feeding. Significant increases in PCV and total plasma proteins (TPP) are found in animals after be fed. This fact has been associated with loss of fluids through the saliva and other gastrointestinal fluids, as well as fluid shifts from the circulation to the gastrointestinal system (Kerr and Snow, 1982). Similarly, there are variations in RBC parameters in horses subjected to different nutritional regimes (Greppi et al., 1996), as well as in animals which common salt is added to the food, supplied 8 hrs before blood collection. In main lines, it is recommended to avoid collecting blood samples within 3 hrs of feeding a large concentrate meal or hay ration or at least ensure that samples are collected at the same time each day.

2.2.6 Circadian biological rhythms

RBC parameters exhibit diurnal infradian, circadian and ultradian rhythms, both in athletic and sedentary horses (Gill and Rastawicka, 1986). Gill and Rastawicka (1986) described elevations in PCV and HB overnight in comparison to light time. Hauss (1994) relates this variation to the influence exerted by alternation between periods of light and darkness on erythropoiesis. After that, Greppi et al. (1996) corroborated these results, and they also found a significant effect of biological rhythms in TPP.

2.2.7 Gender

Hematological differences linked to gender seem to have limited importance in horses. Indeed, minor differences between adult females and males have been reported. However, the results of research in this field are subjected to controversy. Males have slightly higher RBC, HB and PCV, while females have higher MCH and MCHC (Jain, 1986; Hernández et al., 2008; Satué et al., 2009). By contrast, Gill and Rastawicka (1986) observed in Thoroughbred racehorses and Quarter Horses that RBC, PCV and HB were higher in mares than in males. Persson and Ullberg (1974) had reported that baseline hematologic values were higher in stallions than in mares and geldings, probably because of the effect of androgens on erythropoiesis. However, this feature was not seen during exercise in this paper. The authors explained these results indicating that mares and geldings established a hypokinetic circulation with increased oxygen uptake by active muscle during exercise (Persson and Ullberg, 1974).

2.2.8 Season

Season is an exogenous factor that modulates the dynamic of blood components in horses, both in cycling and pregnant mares (Gill and Wanska, 1978; Gill and Kownacka, 1979; Satué, 2004; Satué et al., 2011). Indeed, the patterns of seasonal changes on RBC, HB and PCV in Thoroughbreds and Arabian horses have showed decreased values in winter (Gill and Wanska, 1978; Gill et al., 1979). In Carthusian mares, Satué et al. (2011) confirmed these results. RBC, PCV and MCV in summer were significantly higher than in spring, autumn and winter. However, HB in spring was significantly higher and MCV and MCH in spring and summer were significantly lower than in other seasons, without modifications in MCHC (Satué et al., 2011). These variations could be related to the effect of some factors, such as the breeding season (Satué et al., 2011). Furthermore, these patterns could be subjected to a different degree of tolerance to the cold, and dissimilar changes in ambient temperatures in different locations (Ruiz et al., 2004). It has been suggested that intense cold decreases RBC due to the reduction in the half-life (Ruiz et al., 2004).

2.2.9 Altitude

Horses subjected to high altitude have significantly higher RBC, HB and PCV values, compared to animals that live at less altitude. It is considered a compensatory mechanism for the lower content of oxygen in the atmospheric air, which is proportionally reduced to the altitude (Wickler and Anderson, 2000).

2.2.10 Age

The influence of age on hematological parameters have been evaluated in different horse breeds (Ralston et al., 1988; McFarlane et al., 1998; Cebulj-Kadunc et al., 2002; 2003; Satué, 2004; Hernández et al., 2008; Satué et al., 2009). Most of the studies on age with hematology have focused on foals from birth to 4 years of age (Harvey et al., 1984; Jain, 1993), even though geriatric horses have received much attention recently, probably because of the increase of the age population (McFarlane et al., 1998).

Newborn foals have RBCs of fetal origin, large size and high RBC, HB and PCV. These parameters are reduced sharply within 12-24 hrs of life, then decline more gradually over the subsequent 2 weeks, and after that, they remain in the lower limit of the adult reference internal during the first year of life (Jain, 1986; Harvey, 1990; Grondin and Dewitt, 2010). The initial hematological changes in foals at birth are thought to be due to the increase in fetal RBC destruction, inadequate iron supplementation, needed for HB synthesis, catecholamine release and expansion of plasma volume as adjustments of fluid balance as a result of the osmotic effect of colostral immunoglobulins. Declines in these values are attributed to decreased RBC survival time, decreased iron delivery to the bone marrow, decreased stimulus for erythropoietin production as a result of higher HB saturation, increased blood oxygen content, and enhanced delivery of oxygen to the tissues due to lower 2,-3 diphosphoglycerate concentrations (Harvey, 1990). Normal adult hematological values are attained at 1-2 years of age. MCV are high at birth and then decrease, reaching its lowest values at 3-5 months of age (Jain, 1986; Harvey, 1990). They do not increase to adult values until approximately 1 year of age (Harvey, 1990). Microcytosis in foals has been attributed to a decrease in serum iron as a result of increased demand for growth. These RBCs may be too small to be recognized as erythrocytes by some impedance counts, hence generating erroneous MCV, RBC and PCV values. Mild anisocytosis is also a typical finding in young foals (Harvey, 1990). MCHC remains constant after birth and is similar to adult values (Harvey, 1990).

Stewart et al. (1970) found that PCV and HB were lower in foals younger than 2 years. Between 3 and 4 years of age, there was a gradual increase in MCV and MCH and since HB and PCV remained unchanged during this period, the increase in MCV was accompanied by a slight reduction in RBC. In Carthusian pregnant mares and in Spanish Purebred horses, Hernández et al. (2008) and Satué et al. (2009) found a reduction of RBC with a compensatory increase in MCV and MCH associated with aging. These results agree with those presented for other equine breeds, such as Standardbreds (Jain, 1986; Ralston et al., 1988), Lipizziano (Cebulj-Kadunc et al., 2002) and wild horses (Plotka et al., 1988). However, McFarlane et al. (1998) found a decreasing trend in geriatric horses, without achieving statistical significance. This fact was linked to a reduced regenerative capacity of the bone marrow (McFarlane et al., 1998).

As indicated before, increased MCV appears to be a common finding associated with aging in the horse (Ralston et al., 1988; McFarlane et al., 1998; Satué, 2004) and it has been explained as the result of changes in the dynamics of maturation of the RBCs (McFarlane et al., 1998).

2.2.11 Breed

Breed in horses exerts a significant effect on the erythron. Light horse breeds or 'hot-blooded breeds' have higher RBC, HB and PCV and blood volume compared to draft horses or 'cold-blooded breeds' (Jain, 1993; Kramer, 2000; Grondin and Dewitt, 2010). Thus, PCV as low as 24% can be found in healthy draft horses and pony breeds. Further, Thoroughbreds have smaller MCV than draft horses. Breeds ancestrally closer have minor differences in HB, MCH and MCHC (Jain, 1986). American miniature horses have lower RBC, HB and PCV but higher MCV, MCH and MCHC than other breeds (Harvey et al., 1984). Donkeys have similar RBC, HB and PCV than ponies, but much higher MCV (Jeffcott, 1977).

2.2.12 Exercise

Exercise has variable effects on the erythrogram, depending on exercise duration and intensity (short-term high intensity or maximal exercise and long-term low intensity or submaximal prolonged exercise), fitness and training levels and environmental conditions. In main lines, exercise results in increased RBC, HB and PCV. At the onset of the exercise, this rise derives from the mobilization of splenic RBC under the influence of the catecholamines. The direct effect of this increased RBC is a greater oxygen transport capacity and therefore, aerobic performance. Both the intensity and the duration of the exercise determine the magnitude of the catecholamine response (Kurosawa et al., 1998). The extent of the increase in PCV is a function of the exercise intensity in maximal exercises and in increasing-intensity exercises and a linear relationship between PCV and speed has been described (Persson, 1983; Muñoz et al., 1998; 1999). This relationship is maintained until the maximum PCV is achieved (60-65%) (Persson, 1983).

Even though the majority of the increase in PCV in high-intensity exercises is due to the splenic contraction, exercise-induced fluid shifts also have a role. A decrease of 5-10% in plasma volume is expected in short-term and in incremental-intensity exercises (McKeever et al., 1993; Muñoz et al., 1998). This reduction is attributed to the loss of sweat in order to dissipate heat produced by muscle contraction and to the exchange of fluids between the different body compartments, because of changes in blood pressure (McKeever et al., 1993; Muñoz et al., 1998; 1999).

The rise in PCV during exercise is linked to higher HB and RBC. If we consider the importance of increased HB in the oxygen transport capacity, it is plausible to think that increased PCV, HB and RBC leads to higher aerobic capacity and therefore, exercise performance (Muñoz et al., 1997). Indeed, several studies carried out in splenectomized horses have demonstrated a marked reduction in exercise performance (McKeever et al., 1993; Kunugiyama et al., 1997). On the other hand, there is a close relationship between increased PCV and blood viscosity. As a consequence, there should be a limit in the elevation of PCV that offsets improved oxygen-carrying capacity (Muñoz et al., 1997). This fact has been implied in the loss of performance of horses with red cell hypervolemia (Funkquist et al., 2000).

Other changes associated with brief maximal exercises are small increases in MCV and decreases in MCH and MCHC. Additionally, RBC in blood samples obtained after this type of exercise seems to be more resistant to osmotic stress (Smith et al., 1989), although a later study found a reduced RBC deformability (Geor et al., 1992).

On the other hand, prolonged submaximal exercise or endurance exercise leads to moderate increase in PCV, associated with loss of fluids because of the quantitative importance of sweating. In this case, the increased PCV, HB and RBC are good indices of dehydration. We have found that endurance horses with PCV higher than 50% are disqualified from competition and some of them require intensive intravenous fluid therapy (Muñoz et al., 2010; Trigo et al., 2010). The increase in PCV should be equal to the increase in TPP. In these cases where PCV increases and TPP remains unchanged, other reasons different from dehydration should be considered in order to explain these results. In fact, we found that the most rapid endurance horses in competitions can have higher PCV than the slower horses. Other reason that can lead to increased PCV in endurance horses is pain. We studied 13 endurance horses that had increased PCV (PCV> 52%) with non-increased TPP (TPP<7.2 g/dl) during a competition. One of them had laminitis, 2 had heart arrhythmias, 2 had colic, 3 were retired from competition by the owners and the remaining 5 were able to finish the competition (Trigo et al., 2010).

2.2.13 Training

Although training has limited effects on RBC parameters at rest, some differences are found between horses undergoing high-intensity and endurance training. Speed-trained horses have higher RBC, HB and PCV, which is considered an adaptation for a greater demand for oxygen uptake, stimulating RBC production. However, it is very difficult to obtain a 'true' basal blood sample in these horses, because of their demeanor and nervous temperament. The increased excitability of a horse as it gets fitter could result in elevations of RBC, HB and PCV values (McKeever et al., 1993). On the other hand, regular monitoring of the hemogram during training has little value for assessing the fitness of the horse, but it is very helpful in order to detect subclinical problems that can significantly reduce exercise performance. Decreases in PCV have been reported as a consistent finding in horses with viral respiratory tract disease and in gastric ulcers (McGowan, 2008; Nieto et al., 2009).

In Standardbred trotters, prolonged and/or intensive training can result in an excessive increase in red cell mass, phenomenon known as red cell hypervolemia, which results in a significant reduction of racing performance. Some authors have related the hypervolemia with overtraining (Golland et al., 2003). It has been hypothesized that increased blood viscosity leads to reduced capillary perfusion and inadequate utilization of oxygen by contracting muscles.

By contrast, endurance-trained horses have lower resting RBC, PCV and HB than sprint-trained horses (Muñoz et al., 2010; Robert et al., 2010; Trigo et al., 2010). In fact, in our experience, is very common to find PCV as low as 30-32% in endurance healthy horses with good performance (Muñoz et al., 2010). There are two main reasons to explain these results. Firstly, it has been indicated that feeding fibrous diets might increase water consumption and then plasma volume (Robert et al., 2010). The second reason is the effect of a greater release of aldosterone, which promotes water and electrolyte-conserving mechanisms in the kidneys and gastrointestinal tract (McKeever et al., 2002). These changes appear at the beginning of the training program, with retention of water and electrolytes after only 3 days of endurance training (McKeever et al., 2002). The advantage of plasma expansion in endurance horses is to provide extra total body water for the maintenance of cardiovascular and thermoregulatory stability during prolonged exercise in order to compensate the significant losses associated with sweating (McKeever et al., 2002; Robert et al., 2010). Despite these results, it is clear that hematological measurements are of little value in assessing the fitness or progress of endurance horses in training.

2.2.14 Reproductive status

The researchers that have evaluated the hematological changes resulting from pregnancy in the mare have provided controversial results. Studies in Thoroughbred, Arabian, Carthusian, Brazilian and Breton pregnant mares have described a significant increase in RBC parameters during pregnancy (Berlink et al., 2000; Satué, 2004; Satué et al., 2008). There is not a reasonable explanation to justify these results, although it has been hypothesized that the increased fetal metabolic requirements might condition this response (Satué, 2004). In an early study, a mild anemia appeared at the end of pregnancy (Trum, 1952). This result agrees with studies carried out in pregnant women (Bailit et al., 2007) and other animal species (Steinhardt et al., 1994; Zvorc et al., 2006). The decrease of RBC parameters in pregnancy has been associated with an absolute gain of plasma, RBC and HB. As the increase in RBC and HB is slower than the rise in plasma, a relative oligocythemia is found, despite the increased erythropoietin concentration probably derived from placental prolactin. The hypervolemia of pregnancy has been associated with water and sodium retention after an activation of the renin-angiotensin-aldosterone axis, stimulated by estrogens (Satué and Domingo, 2008). The hypervolemia of pregnancy is necessary in order to meet the demands of the gravid uterus, to protect the mother and the fetus from the harmful effects of decreased venous return and to prevent the mother from suffering the adverse effects of blood loss during delivery (McMullin et al., 2003).

It has been suggested that iron deficiency anemia is common in the pregnant mare. Detlef (1985) studied the effect of iron supplementation in pregnant mares compared with untreated control mares. In the treated mares, RBC and HB were not changed during pregnancy, whereas a decline in RBC parameters was found in the control group. Additionally, the foals born from supplemented mothers had higher HB and RBC than the foals born from the untreated mares (Detlef, 1985).

Near the parturition, RBC parameters do not change (Taylor-Macallister et al., 1997). After delivery, RBC parameters increase slightly, until the total blood volume is restored by releasing the attachments and fetal fluids. On the other hand, lactation induces a reduction in RBC, HB and PCV (Harvey et al., 1994; 2005).

2.2.15 Administration of sedatives-tranquilizers

The administration of tranquilizing compounds, such as phenothiazine derivatives (acepromazina, chlorpromazine…) and adrenergic α-2 agonists (xylazine, romifidine, detomidine…) significantly affect the RBC parameters. These drugs lead to a relaxation of the smooth muscle in the splenic capsule, promoting the storage of RBC (Jeffcott, 1977). Further, these drugs, after an initial short phase of hypertension, have a prolonged hypotensive effect. Hypotension leads to increased plasma volume, with the subsequent hemodilution and reduced RBC parameters at rest (Jain, 1986).

3. Leukon

The term leukon refers to the set of data derived from total and differential count of white blood cells (WBC) and the analysis of WBC morphology (Grondin and Dewitt, 2010). Circulating WBC represents the outcome of the dynamic production of the bone marrow, the release of the cells to the peripheral blood and, the storage in different organs or pools.

Cells can coexist in different stages of maturation, being fully mature cells (neutrophils, NEU, eosinophils, EOS, monocytes, MON, lymphocytes, LYM and basophils, BAS) and immature (band neutrophils, metamyelocytes, myelocytes and progranulocytes) (Messer, 1995; Welles, 2000; Grondin and Dewitt, 2010).

3.1 Neutrophils

The release of NEU from the bone marrow into the circulated depends on the tissue demands and the production of different humoral substances. After passing into the blood, NEU can be in the circulating pool or stored in the marginal pool (in the endothelium of several organs, such as lungs or intestine). Three main locations of the NEU can be described: 1) Bone marrow. There is a proliferating population of NEU, including promyelocytes, myelocytes, metamyelocytes, and mature ENU, prepared for release into peripheral blood; 2) Blood. In the blood compartment, mature NEU appear as round cells, 10-15 µm of diameter, with clear cytoplasm, neutral or granules stain pink and with the nucleus polymorphic and segmented and the chromatin arranged in the form of knots; 3) Tissues. In inflammatory processes, there is a release of chemotactic substances that promotes NEU migration from the vascular bed into the tissues. Marginal pool of NEU adheres to the vascular endothelium, mainly in the small vessels. This fact facilitates the migration to the tissues, while serving as a reserve, so there is a continuous exchange between circulating and marginal pools (Lassen and Swardson, 1995; Grondin and Dewitt, 2010; Smith, 2000; Welles, 2000).

Barr bodies (sex chromatin lobe/ drumstick) can be recognized in females and resemble a small purple body attached to the nucleus by a thin chromatin strand. Further, in peripheral blood, both mature and immature or band NEU can be found. Equine band NEUs are less frequently seen because horses do not exhibit marked left shifts during inflammatory insults compared to dogs and cats. In cases of bacterial infection, the band NEUs might represent between 1 and 10% of the total WBC differential count (Welles, 2000). Band NEUs have a polymorphic nucleus, without constrains, with a less condensed chromatic pattern than the segmented NEUs. The cytoplasm is similar to this of the mature NEU (Jain, 1993; Welles, 2000). Hypersegmented NEUs are rarely seen in healthy and they have five or more lobes separated by filaments. Prolonged storage of blood may lead to the artefactual development of hypersegmented NEUs. Idiopathic hypersegmentation of NEUs have been described in Quarter Horses that lacked evidences of clinical disease. Hyposegmented NEUs have also been reported in apparently healthy Arabian horses, which were diagnosed as Pelger-Huët anomaly (Grondin et al., 2007).

Circulating NEUs have a half-life of 10.5 hours, renewing approximately 1.5 times per day (Lassen and Swardson, 1995; Welles, 2000). Then, they leave the bloodstream and migrate into the tissues. It is a unidirectional movement, because they do not return to the peripheral circulation. In the tissues, NEUs are functional for 1 to 2 days, and then, they are fagocyted by the monocyte-macrophage system or by the mucosal surfaces (Welles, 2000).

3.2 Lymphocytes

LYM are the second largest population of circulating WBCs, after NEUs and the main components of the immune system. They are smaller than NEUs and the other granulocytes, with a dark-staining nuclei, coarse chromatin pattern and scant amount of blue cytoplasm. The mature cell has a diameter of 7-12 µm, an eccentric, round nucleus with a notch on some occasions (Latimer and Rackich, 1992). LYMs are made up to 38-66% T cells, 17-38% B cells with the remaining being null cells (Tizard, 2009). Occasionally, larger LYMs are present, and they have smooth chromatin patterns and large amounts of pale blue cytoplasm (Jain, 1986). Reactive LYMs or immunocytes are rarely seen in health. They are slightly larger than small LYMs, with scalloped nuclear margins, moderately aggregated chromatin, scant to moderate amounts of intensely basophilic cytoplasm and sometimes, they have a pale-staining Golgi zone (Latimer, 1999; Grondin and Dewitt, 2010).

The half-life of LYMs varies between 20 and 200 days (Schalm and Carlson, 1982), with a mean duration of transit through the blood of 30 hrs. Blood LYMs have the ability to recirculate in the blood, lymphatic channels, lymphoid and peripheral tissues and they are able to have mitosis, allowing amplification of the immune response (Jain, 1986; Latimer, 1999; Welles, 2000). Most of the LYMs are originated in the peripheral lymphoid tissues, and only a small percentage comes from central lymphoid tissues, i.e. bone marrow and thymus. The circulation time depends on the LYM subtype and the tissue of origin. T cells circulate more rapidly than B cells and migration through the splenic parenchyma is faster than through the lymph nodes (Hopkins and McConnell, 1984).

3.3 Eosinophils

EOS are cells slightly larger than neutrophils that contain large, reddish-orange granules in the cytoplasm, often obscuring the nuclei and giving a raspberry-like appearance, with a pale blue cytoplasm (Kramer, 2000; Smith, 2000). The lobulated nucleus seldom shows fine filamentation. Degranulated EOSs are vacuolated and are rarely seen in health (Latimer, 1999; Grondin and Dewitt, 2010). The amount of EOS in peripheral blood is low, because most of these cells migrate into tissues, such as the bronchial mucosa, gastrointestinal tract…The half-life of circulating EOS is about 2 to 12 hrs (Latimer, 1999; Young, 2000).

3.4 Monocytes

MON are the largest WBC in circulation, with a large, broad, variable in shape nuclei (oval, bilobed, horseshoe) with lacy chromatin and gray-blue cytoplasm with small azurophilic granules. The cytoplasm can also have a few clear vacuoles of variable size, located in the cell periphery and with a foamy appearance (Jain, 1993; Bienzle, 2000). After their production in the bone marrow, MON are released into the bloodstream. In circulation, they distributed between the circulating and marginal pools, with a ratio of 1/3.5 between them. This ratio remains constant in different physiological states and in response to disease. The mean circulating MON life is about 8.4 hrs, and there is not exchange at the tissue level and blood. In the tissues, the MONs mature into macrophages, a transformation that is accompanied by changes in ultrastructure, in the appearance of cellular receptors or by metabolic changes. The half-life of macrophages ranges from several days to months (Bienzle, 2000; Welles, 2000).

3.5 Basophils

BAS are cells slightly larger than the NEUs, with a lobulated nucleus, although to a lesser extent than NEUs, a cytoplasm from blue to gray, with large amounts of granules distributed irregularly, and with an intense purple stain that vary in size and shape and can mask the nucleus (Jain, 1993; Kramer, 2000).

3.6 Physiological factors influencing leukogram in horses

There are two main WBC responses, physiological leukocytosis and stress leukocytosis. Physiological leukocytosis refers to changes in circulating WBC associated with the intervention of the sympathetic-adrenal axis resulting from splenic contraction in cases of fear, excitement, or high intensity exercise. There is a mobilization of the marginal pool of NEUs and/or LYM, because of a reduction in NEU adherence capacity, increased blood flow through the microvasculature and splenic contraction (Latimer, 1999). These events result in leukocytosis with mature neutrophilia and/or lymphocytosis. In some cases, eosinophilia and monocytosis are also found (Snow et al., 1983; Welles, 2000). These changes are transient and the marginal pool of NEUs is restored again in 20-30 min after the onset of the response and the LYM counts returned to baseline after 1 hr (Rossdale et al., 1982).

Stress leukocytosis is associated with cortisol release under certain stressful situations. This hormone induces neutrophilia without left shift, lymphopenia and eosinopenia. Neutrophilia derives from the mobilization from the marginal pool, the reduced ability to migrate from the blood to the peripheral tissues and the increased mobilization of the population of bone marrow reserve. Lymphopenia is the result of LYM sequestration from lymphoid tissues and the eosinophenia derives from the marginalization of EOS in the blood vessels and the decreased release from the bone marrow (Caracostas et al., 1981; Welles, 2000). This response appears between 2 and 4 hours after the elevation of the endogenous cortisol concentrations or after exogenous administration of corticoids (Rossdale et al., 1982; Burguez et al., 1983). Normal values are recovered in 24 hrs. This response has been also found after an endurance exercise and in response to a great variety of pathological processes (Welles, 2000).

3.6.1 Breed

Minor differences have been found among equine breeds in relation to WBC, with the hot-blooded horses having higher WBC compared to cold-blooded horses (Jain, 1986; Harvey et al., 1984). Thoroughbreds and Arabian have a mean NEU/LYM ratio of 1.0, whereas cold-blooded horses and miniature horses have ratios of 1.7 and 0.67, respectively (Jain, 1986).

3.6.2 Time of the day

In Thoroughbred racing horses, Allen and Powell (1983) described that LYM count has higher in the evenings and lower in the mornings. These findings have been attributed to the circadian variations in the release of endogenous corticoids. It is well known that maximum cortisol concentrations appear in the morning (McKeever, 2011).

3.6.3 Gender

WBC and granulocytes are higher in females than in stallions, as recently found in Spanish Purebred horses (Hernández et al., 2008; Satué et al., 2009). On the contrary, previous researchers performed in warm-blooded horse breeds reported higher values in males and in females (Lassen and Swardson, 1995; Cebulj-Kadunc et al., 2002). Other study failed to find significant differences between sexes (Lacerda et al., 2006).

3.6.4 Age

NEU number is low in the fetus (<1,500/µl, before 300 days of gestation), increases after birth in response to cortisol (8,000/µl) and then decrease to mean adult values (4000/µl) at about 4-6 months of age. Band NEU do not exceed 150/µl in healthy foals (Harvey, 1990; Allen et al., 1998). Foals born at term have higher NEU count than foals born prematurely. LYM numbers in foals are low at birth (average 1,400/µl), increase to 5,000/µl at 3 months of age, and reach adult values at 1 year of age (Jain, 1986; Harvey, 1990). LYMs further decline during adulthood while NEU count remains the same, resulting in a higher NEU/LYM ratio in aged horses compared to foals (Jain, 1986). The ratio NEU/LYM reaches values of 2/1 in geriatric horses (Jain, 1993; Lassen and Swardson, 1995; Hernández et al., 2008). The progressive trend towards lymphopenia in geriatric horses is characterized by a reducing in B cells CD4+ and CD8+, in relation to immune senescence (Smith et al., 2002; Hernández et al., 2008; Satué et al., 2010).

EOSs are not routinely detected in the fetus and in foals at birth, achieving a mean of 400/µl by 4 months of age (Harvey, 1990). EOSs count increases with aging due to prolonged exposure to allergens through life (Jain, 1993; Satué et al., 2009). However, McFarlane et al. (1998), Cebulj-Kadunc et al. (2003) and Hernández et al. (2008) did not found differences in EOS count between young and adult horses. Band NEU, MON and BAS do not seem to change with aging in horses (Harvey, 1990; Jain, 1993; Lassen and Swardson, 1995; Cebulj-Kadunc et al., 2003; Satué, 2004; Hernández et al., 2008).

3.6.5 Exercise

WBC show different responses according to the type of exercise. Sprint exercise is associated with leukocytosis because of neutrophilia but mainly because of lymphocytosis, with a decrease in NEU/LYM ratio. These changes are likely secondary to catecholamine release and splenic contraction. At 3 hr after exercise, there is an increase in NEU/LYM ration, because the increase of NEU and decrease in LYM associated with cortisol concentrations. The NEU/LYM ratio returns to baseline values by 6 hrs after exercise (Snow et al., 1983).

Endurance exercise is associated with leukocytosis, resulting from a neutrophilia and lymphopenia (Snow et al., 1982). Probably this is combined effect of increased circulating corticosteroids and splenic contraction. Horses that completed an endurance event at a faster speed have higher NEU/LYM ration than slower horses (Trigo et al., 2010). Additionally, it has been demonstrated that exhausted endurance horses had left shift in the NEUs and significantly lymphopenia (Trigo et al., 2010).

3.6.6 Training

Total WBC is unchanged during training for racing and for endurance events. In addition, there are no alterations in the proportions of the different WBC populations. Some overtrained horses develop eosinophenia together with clinical signs of disease, and this result has led to the hypothesis that EOSs may be a more sensitive indicator of training stress than other types of WBCs (Tyler-McGowan et al., 1999). It is important to take into account that decreased NEU count and later, increased LYM count is consistent with systemic or respiratory disease, that are common causes of loss of performance in trained horses (McGowan, 2008).

3.6.7 Reproductive status

Although in main lines, estrous cycle and pregnancy do not change substantially the leukogram (Berlink et al., 2000; Da Costa et al., 2003), some studies have found a reduction in WBC, NEU and EOS counts during pregnancy (Satué, 2004; Satué et al., 2010). The reduction in WBC in Thoroughbred mares appears during the first 4 months of pregnancy, with a trend toward increase from half of pregnancy and it is maintained until the time of delivery (Gill et al., 1994). During delivery, leukocytosis with neutrophilia, lymphopenia and eosinopenia appear, in association with the hypothalamic-pituitary-adrenal stimulation and glucocorticoid release (Silver et al., 1984; Harvey et al., 1994). However, this idea has not been confirmed by all the authors (Taylor-Macallister et l., 1997). Finally, lactation induces leucopenia with an intensity proportional to the degree of stress during the period of maximum milk production (Harvey et al., 1994).

4. Platelets

Platelets or thrombocytes are cytoplasmic fragments of megakariocytes. Equine platelets stain very lightly with Wright-Giemsa stain and sometimes can be difficult to discern on blood films. They are round, oval or elongate, measuring 2.5-3.5 µm in diameter, with light blue cytoplasm with fine azurophilic granules (Kramer, 2000). The survival time of equine platelets in circulating blood is 4-7 days (Jain, 1993). Equine platelet concentrations are some of the lowest reported for mammals. Finding 6-10 platelets/field of high resolution in a peripheral blood film indicates an adequate platelet concentration. Mean platelet volume (MCV) and mean platelet mass have been reported in horses: 4.3-5.6 fl and 0.47-0.96 10^6/fl respectively (Boudreaux and Ebbe, 1998).

Morphologically, giant platelets, greater than the diameter of a RBC, are associated with accelerated thrombocytopoiesis. Platelet clumping indicates platelet activation and aggregation during blood collection, and might lead to erroneously low platelet concentrations. EDTA-dependent pseudo thrombocytopenia has been reported in a Thoroughbred gelding (Hinchcliff et al., 1993).

4.1 Physiological factors influencing platelets in horses

4.1.1 Anticoagulant

The use of EDTA as anticoagulant, although it can produce aggregation in normal situations, it is more common in patients with severe gastrointestinal disease due to platelet activation by circulating endotoxins and formation of aggregates of platelets and leukocytes (Hinchliff et al., 1993; Saigo et al., 2005).

4.1.2 Blood sample collection and analytical time

Repeated venipuncture, alterations in blood flow or delay in carrying out the analysis alter platelet count. It is advisable to perform the analysis within the first 2 hrs after collection, as MPV can be altered if the EDTA-sample is kept refrigerated. On the other hand, it is interesting to use sodium citrate as an anticoagulant in order to measure platelet size (Sellon, 1998; Seghatchian, 2006).

4.1.3 Breed

In Quarter Horses, Jeffcott (1977) found that the number of platelets in this breed was higher than in other equine breeds. A clear explanation for this result is lacking, although factors others than the breed should be taken into consideration.

4.1.4 Age

Platelet numbers in foals do not change during the first year of life. In adult horses, age determines a progressive decrease in platelet count (Ralston et al., 1988; Jain, 1993; Satué, 2004; Satué et al., 2009), as well as in other species (Zinkl et al., 1990). By contrast, other studies in horses did not agree with these results (McFarlane et al., 1998).

4.1.5 Exercise and training

The effect of exercise on platelet parameters seems to be intensity dependent. Short brief or maximal exercise results in significant increases in platelet numbers, whereas moderate exercise does not appear to alter platelet numbers (Bayly et al., 1983). Further, some studies reported reduced platelet aggregability in response to high-intensity exercise (Bayly et al., 1983), but other authors described increased aggregability and activation of platelets (Kingston et al., 2002). One possible explanation for the diverse results is the modifications in blood pH and hemoconcentration, with changes in ionized calcium concentrations and platelet activity. In addition, and given many of the methodological and technical problems when working with equine platelets, it is unknown if training alters platelet function.

4.1.6 Reproductive status

In human beings, laboratory animals and female elephants, a marked activation of the megakaryopoiesis has been found at the end of pregnancy. This fact continues during the initial weeks after delivery, possibly in association with high concentrations of estrogen, progesterone and other steroid hormones (Jackson et al., 1992). In the mare, most of the studies concluded that pregnancy does not exert significant effects on circulating platelets (Harvey et al., 1994; Berlink et al., 2000). However, Satué (2004) and Satué et al. (2010) described a progressive decline in platelet numbers during pregnancy in Carthusian broodmares. Hormonal dynamic during pregnancy, coupled with increased levels of thromboxane B2 produced by the placenta, chorion and amnion.

While in other species delivery leads to thrombocytosis (Suárez et al., 1988; Jackson et al., 1992), mares during delivery do not develop significant changes in platelet numbers (Harvey et al., 1994). This response is attributed to the combined effect of stress and increased release of estrogen, progesterone and other steroid hormones. Finally, lactation does not exert evident influence of circulation platelet numbers in mares (Harvey et al., 1994; Satué, 2004).

5. Conclusion

Hematological profile is frequently used in horses as an aid for the diagnosis and/or consequences of systemic, infectious and some parasitic diseases. It can also provide significant information about the response to treatment, the severity of the process and the metabolic state of an animal. Despite the wide use of hematology, interpretation is challenging because many exogenous and endogenous factors significantly modify blood parameters. The present chapter reviews the current knowledge of the influence of physiological factors on erythrocytes, leukocytes and platelets in horses.

6. References

Allen, A.L., Myers, S.L., Searcy, G.P. & Fretz, P.B. (1998). Hematology of equine fetuses with comparison to their dams. *Veterinary Clinical Pathology.,* Vol. 27, (September 1998), pp. 93-100, ISSN: 0275-6382.

Allen, B.V. & Powell, D.G. (1983). Effects of training and time of day of blood sampling on the variation of some common haematological parameters in the normal throroughbred racehorses. In: *Equine Exercise Physiology.* Snow, D.H., Persson, S.G.B. & Rose, R.J. (eds.), pp. 328-335, Granta Editions, ISBN: 0-7020-2857-6, Cambridge, England.

Allen, B.V. (1988). Relationships between the erythrocyte sedimentation rate, plasma proteins and viscosity, and leucocyte counts in thoroughbred racehorses. *Veterinary Record.,* Vol. 1, N° 22, (April 1988), pp. 329-332, ISSN: 2042-7670.

Archer, R.K. (1977). Technical methods. In: *Comparative Clinical Haematology.* Archer, R.K. & Jeffcott, L.B. (eds.), pp. 537-586, Blackwell Scientific Publications, ISBN: 1078-8956, Oxford.

Bailit, J.L., Doty, E. & Todia, W. (2007). Repeated hematocrit measurements in low risk pregnant women. *Journal of Reproduction Medicine,* Vol. 52, N° 7, (July 2007), pp. 619-622, ISSN: 0024-7758.

Bayly, W.M., Meyers, K.M., Keck, M.T., Huston, L.J. & Grant, B.D. (1983). Exercise-induced alterations in haemostasis in thoroughbreds horses. In: *Equine Exercise Physiology.* Snow, D.H., Persson, S.G.B., Rose, R.J. (eds.), pp. 336-343, Granta Editions, ISBN: 0-7020-2857-6, Cambridge, England.

Berlink, B., Correa, J., Evangelista, A., Peixoto, R. & Penteado, C. (2000). Constituintes hematimétricos do sangue de éguas gestantes de raça árabe. *Veterinaria Noticias,* Vol. 6, N° 1, (Marzo 2000), pp. 51-55, ISSN: 0104-3463.

Bienzle, D. (2000). Monocytes and macrophages. In: *Schalm´s Veterinary Hematology.* Feldman, B.F., Zinkl, J.G., Jain, N.C. (eds.), pp. 318-320, Lippincott Williams & Wilkins, ISBN: 978-0-8138-1798-9, Iowa, U.K.

Boudreaux, M.K. & Ebbe, S. (1998). Comparison of platelet number, mean platelet volume and platelet mass in five mammalian species. *Comparative Haematolology International,* Vol. 8, n° 1, (March 1998), pp. 16-20, ISSN: 0938-7714.

Brockus, C.W. & Anderasen, C.B. Erythrocytes. In: *Duncan and Prasse´s Veterinary Laboratory Medicine: Clinical Pathology.* Latimer, K.S., Mahaffey, E.A. & Prasse, K.W. (eds.), pp. 3-45, Iowa State Press, ISBN 0813820146, Iowa, U.K.

Burguez, P.N., Ousey, J., Cash, R.S. & Rossdale, P.D. (1983). Changes in blood neutrophil and lymphocyte counts following administration of cortisol to horses and foals. *Equine Veterinary Journal,* Vol. 15, N° 1, (January 1983), pp. 58-60, ISSN: 2042-3306.

Caracostas, M.C., Moore, W.E. & Smith, J.E. (1981). Intravascular neutrophilic granulocyte kinetics in horses. *American Journal of Veterinary Research,* Vol. 42, N° 4, (April 1981), pp. 623-625, ISSN: 0002-9645.

Cebulj-Kadunc, N., Bozic, M., Kosec, M. & Cestnik, V. (2002). The influence of age and gender on haematological parameters in Lipizzan horses. *Journal of Veterinary Medicine Serie A, Physiology, Pathology and Clinic Medicine,* Vol. 49, N° 4, (May 2002), pp. 217-221, ISSN: 0931-184X.

Cebulj-Kadunc, N., Kosec, M. & Cestnik, V. (2003). The variations of white blood cell count in Lipizzan horses. *Journal of Veterinary Medicine Serie A, Physiology, Pathology and Clinic Medicine,*Vol. 50, N° 5, (June 2003), pp. 251-253, ISSN: 0931-184X.

Da Costa, R.P., Carvalho, H., Agrícola, R., Alpoim-Moreira, J., Martins, C. & Ferreira-Dias, G. (2003). Peripheral blood neutrophil function and lymphocyte subpopulations in cycling mares. *Reproduction in Domestic Animals,* Vol. 38, N° 6, (December 2003), pp. 464-469, ISSN: 1439-0531.

Detlef, C. (1985). Untersuchungen uber das rote blutbild und der eisenversorgunganzei genden parameter bei stuten und deren fohlen im peripartalen abschnitt unter besonderer berucksichtigung einer eisensubstitution. *Inaugural Dissertation zur Erlangung des Doktorgrades bei dem Fachbereich* Veterinarmedizin und Tierzucht der Justus-Liebig-Universitat zu Gieben.

Friend, T.H. (2001). Dehydration, stress and water consumption of horses during long-distance commercial transport. *Journal of Animal Science,* Vol. 78, N° 10, (October 2000), pp. 2568-2580, ISSN 0021-8812.

Funkquist, P., Nyman, G. & Persson, S.G. (2000). Haemodynamic response to exercise in Standardbred trotters with red cell hypervolaemia. *Equine Veterinary Journal,* Vol.32, No.5 (September 2000), pp. 426-431, ISSN 2042-3306.

Geor, R.J., Weiss, D.J., Burris, S.M. & Smith, C.M. (1992). Effects of furosemide and pentoxifylline on blood flow properties in horses. *American Journal of Veterinary Research,* Vol.53, No.11 (November 1992), pp. 2043-2049, ISSN 0002-9645.

Gill, J. & Kownacka, M. (1979). Seasonal changes in erythrocyte, hemoglobin and leukocyte indexes in pregnant mares of thoroughbred horses. *Bulletin of the Academy Polish Science and Biology,* Vol. 27, N° 2, (June 1979), pp. 143-148, ISSN 0001-4141.

Gill, J. & Rastawicka, M. (1986). Diurnal changes in the hematological indices in the blood of racing Arabian horses. *Polskie Archiwum Weterynaryjne.,* Vol. 26, N° 1 (November 1986), pp. 169-179, ISSN 0079-3647.

Gill, J. & Wanska, E. (1978). Seasonal changes in erythrocyte, hemoglobin and leukocyte indexes in barren mares of thoroughbred horses. *Bulletin of the Academy Polish Science and Biology,* Vol. 26, N° 5, pp. 347-53, ISSN 0001-4141.

Gill, J., Flisinska-Bojanowska, A. & Grzelkowska, K. (1994). Diurnal and seasonal changes in the WBC number, neutrophil percentage and lysozyme activity in the blood of barren, pregnant and lactating mares. *Advances in Agricultural Sciences.,* Vol. 3, N° 1, pp. 15-23, ISSN 0021-8596.

Gill, J., Szwarocka-Priebe, T., Krupska, U. & Peplowska, Z. (1979). Seasonal changes in haematological indices, protein and glycoprotein levels and in activity of some enzymes in Arabian horses. *Bulletin of the Academy Polish Science and Biology,* Vol. 26, N° 10, (Feb 1979), pp. 719-723, ISSN 0001-4141.

Golland, L.C., Evans, D.L., McGowan, C.M., Hodgson, D.R. & Rose, R.J. (2003). The effects of overtraining on blood volumes in Standardbred racehorse. *Equine Vet. J.,* Vol. 165, N° 3, (May 2003), pp. 228-232, ISSN 2042-3306.

Greppi, G.F., Casini, L., Gatta, D., Orlandi, M. & Pasquini, M. (1996). Daily fluctuations of haematology and blood biochemistry in horses fed varying levels of protein. *Equine Veterinary Journal,* Vol. 28, N° 5, (September 1996), pp. 350-353, ISSN 2042-3306.

Grondin, T.M. & Dewitt, S.F. (2010). Normal hematology of the horse and donkey. In: *Schalm´s Veterinary Hematology.* Weiss, D.J. & Wardrop, K.J. (eds.), pp. 821-828, Wiley Blackwell Inc., ISBN 978-0-8138-1798-9, Ames, I.A.

Grondin, T.M., Dewitt, S.E. & Keeton, K.S. (2007). Pelger-Hüet anomaly in an Arabian horse. *Veterinary Clinical Pathology.,* Vol. 36, N° 3, (September 2007), pp. 306-310, ISSN 0275-6382.

Harvey, J.W. (1990). Normal hematologic values. In: *Equine Clinical Neonatology.* Koterba, A.M., Drummond, W.H. & Kosch, P.C. (eds.), pp. 561-570, Lea & Febiger, ISBN 0812111842, Philadelphia.

Harvey, J.W., Asquith, R.L., Pate, M.G., Kipivelto, J., Chen, C.L. & Ott, E.A. (1994). Haematological findings in pregnant, postparturient and nursing mares. *Comparative Hematology International,* Vol. 4, N° 1, (April, 1994), pp. 25-29, ISSN 0938-7714.

Harvey, J.W., Pate, M., Kivipelto, J. & Asquith, R. (2005). Clinical biochemistry of pregnant and nursing mares. *Veterinary Clinical Pathology,* Vol. 34, N° 3, (September 2005), pp. 248-254, ISSN 0275-6382.

Harvey, R.B., Hambright, M.B. & Rowe, L.D. (1984). Clinical biochemical and hematologic values of the American Miniature Horse: reference values. *American Journal of Veterinary Research,,* Vol. 45, N° 5, (May 1984), pp. 987-990, ISSN 0002-9645.

Hauss, E. (1994). Chronobiology of circulating blood cells and platelets. In: *Biological Rhythms in Clinical and Laboratory Medicine.* Touitou, Y. & Hauss, E. (eds.), pp. 504-526, Springer-Verlag, ISBN 9783540544616, N.Y.

Hernández, A.M., Satué K.; Lorente, C.; Garcés, C. & O`connor J.E. (2008). The influence of age and gender on haematological parameters in Spanish Horses. *Proceeding of Veterinary European Equine Meeting - XIV SIVE Congress,* Venice (Italy).

Hinchcliff, K.W., Kociba, G.J. & Mitten, L.A. (1993). Diagnosis of EDTA-dependent pseudothrombocytopenia in a horse. *Journal of American Veterinary Medical Association,* Vol. 203, N° 12, (December 1993), pp. 1715-1716, ISSN 0003-1488.ç

Hopkins, J. & McConnell, I. (1984). Immunological aspects of lymphocyte recirculation. *Veterinary Immunology and Immunopathology,* Vol. 6, N° 1, (May 1984), pp. 3-33, ISSN 0165-2427.

Jackson, C.W., Steward, S.A., Ashmun, R.A. & McDonald, T.P. (1992). Megakaryocytopoiesis and platelet production are stimulated during late pregnancy and early postpartum in the rat. *Blood,* Vol. 79, N° 7, (April 1992), pp. 1672-1678, ISSN 0006-4971.

Jain, N.C. (1986). The horse. Normal haematologic with comments on response to disease. In: *Schalm's Veterinary Hematology.* Jain N.C. (ed.), pp. 140-177, Lea & Febiger, ISBN 0812109422 9780812109429, Philadelaphia, USA.

Jain, N.C. (1993). Comparative hematology of common domestic animals. In: *Essentials of Veterinary Hematology,* Jain N.C. (ed.), pp. 19-53, Lea & Febiger, ISBN 0-6121-1437-X, Philadelphia.

Jeffcott, L.B. (1977). Clinical haematology of the horse. In: *Comparative Clinical Haematology.* Archer, R.K. & Jeffcott, L.B. (eds.), pp. 161-213, Blackwell Scientific Publications, ISBN 1618-5641, Oxford, U.K.

Kerr, M.G. & Snow, D.H. (1982). Alterations in haematocrit, plasma proteins and electrolytes in horses following the feeding of hay. *Veterinary Record*, Vol. 110, pp. 538-540, ISSN 0042-4900.

Kingston, J.K., Bayly, W.M., Sellon, D.C., Meyers, K.M. & Wardrop, K.J. (2002). Effects of formaldehyde fixation on equine platelets using flow cytometric methods to evaluate markers of platelet activation. *American Journal of Veterinary Research*, Vol. 63, N° 6, (June 2002), pp. 840-844, ISSN 0002-9645.

Kramer, J.W. (2000). Normal hematology of the horse. In: *Shalm's Veterinary Hematology*. Feldman, B.F., Zinkl, J.G. & Jain, N.C. (eds.), pp. 1069-1074, Williams & Wilkins, ISBN: 978-0-8138-1798-9, Philadelphia, UK.

Kunugiyama, I., Ito, N., Narizuka, M., Kataoka, S., Furukawa, Y., Hiraga, A., Kai, M. & Kubo, K. (1997). Measurement of erythrocyte volumes in splenectomized horses and sham-operated horses at rest and during maximal exercise. *Journal of Veterinary Medical Science*, Vol. 59, N° 9, (September 1997), pp. 733-737, ISSN 0916-7250.

Kurosawa, M., Nagata, S., Takeda, F., Mima, K., Hiraga, A., Kai, M. & Taya, K. (1998). Plasma catecholamine, adrenocorticotropin and cortisol responses to exhaustive incremental treadmill exercise of the thoroughbred horse. *Journal of Veterinary Medical Science*, Vol. 9, N° 1, (December 1998), pp. 9-18, ISSN 0737-0806.

Lacerda, L., Campos, R., Sperb, M., Soares, E.; Barbosa, E., Rerreira, R., Santos, V. & González, F.H. (2006). Hematological and biochemical parameters in three high performance horse breeds from southern Brazil. *Archives of Veterinary Science.*, Vol. 11, N° 2, (October 2006), pp. 40-44, ISSN 1517-784X.

Lassen, E.D. & Swardson, C.J. (1995). Hematology and hemostasis in the horse: normal functions and common abnormalities. *Veterinary Clinics of North America: Equine Practice*, Vol. 11, N° 3, (Dec 1995), pp. 351-389, ISSN 0749-0739.

Latimer, K.S. & Rakich, P.M. (1992). Peripheral blood smears. In: *Cytology and Hematology of the Horse*. Cowell, R.L. & Tyler, R.D. (eds.), pp. 191-235, American Veterinary Publications, ISBN 0-323-01317-1, California, USA.

Latimer, K.S. (1999). Leukocytic hematopoiesis. In: *Equine Medicine and Surgery*. King, C. (ed.), pp. 1992-2001, Mosby, ISSN 9780815117438, St. Louis, USA.

Lording, P.T. (2008). Erythrocytes. *Veterinary Clinics of North America: Equine Practice*, Vol. 24, N° 2, (August 2008), pp. 225-237, ISSN 0749-0739.

Lumsden, H.J., Valli, V.E., McSherry, B.J., Robinson, G.A. & Claxton, M.J. (1975, a). The kinetics of hematopoiesis in the light horse III. The hematological response to hemolytic anemia. *Canadian Journal of Comparative Medicine*, Vol. 39, N° 3, (July 1975), pp. 332-339, ISSN 0008-4050.

Lumsden, H.J., Valli, V.E., McSherry, B.J., Robinson, G.A. & Claxton, M.J. (1975, b). The kinetics of hematopoiesis in the light horse II. The hematological response to hemorrhagic anemia. *Canadian Journal of Comparative Medicine,*, Vol. 39, N° 3, (July 1975), pp. 324-331, ISSN 0008-4050

May, M.L., Nolen-Walston, R.D., Utter, M.E. & Boston, R.C. (2010). Comparison of hematologic and biochemical results on blood obtained by jugular venipuncture as compared with intravenous catheter in adult horses. *Journal of Veterinary Internal Medicine*, Vol.24, No.6, (November-December 2010), pp. 1462-1466, ISSN 1939-1676.

McFarlane, D., Sellon, D.C. & Gaffney, D. (1998). Hematologic and serum biochemical variables and plasma corticotropin concentration in healthy aged horses. *American*

Journal of Veterinary Research, Vol. 59, N° 9, (October 1988), pp. 1247-1251, ISSN 0002-9645.

McGowan, C. (2008). Clinical pathology in the racing horse: the role of clinical pathology in assessing fitness and performance in the racehorse. *Veterinary Clinics of North America: Equine Practice*, Vol.24, No.2, (August, 2008), pp. 405-421, ISSN 0749-0739.

Mckeever, K.H. (2011). Endocrine alterations in the equine athlete: an update. *Veterinary Clinics of North America: Equine Practice*, Vol. 27, N° 1, (April 2011), pp. 197-218, ISSN 0749-0739.

McKeever, K.H., Hinchcliff, K.W., Reed, S.M. & Robertin, J.T. (1993). Role of decreased plasma volume in haematocrit alterations during incremental treadmill exercise in horses. *American Journal of Physiology* Vol. 265, N° 2, (August 1993), pp. 404-408, ISSN 0363-6135.

McKeever, K.H., Scali, R., Geiser, S. & Kearns, C.F. (2002). Plasma aldosterone concentration and renal sodium excretion are altered during the first days of training. *Equine Veterinary Journal*, Vol.32, N°34, (September 2002), pp. 524-532, ISSN 2042-9645

McMullin, M.F., White, R., Lappin, T., Reeves, J. & Mackenzie, G. (2003). Haemoglobin during pregnancy: relationship to erythropoietin and haematinic stats. *European Journal of Haematology*, Vol. 71, N° 1, (July 2003), pp. 44-50, ISSN 1600-0609.

Messer, NT. (1995). The use of laboratory tests in equine practice. *Veterinary Clinics of North America: Equine Practice*, Vol. 11, N° 3, (December 1995), pp. 345-350, ISSN 0749-0739.

Monreal, L., Villatoro, A.J., Monreal, M., Espada, Y., Anglés, A.M. & Ruiz-Gopegui, R. (1995). Comparison of the effects of low - molecular - weight and unfractioned heparin in horses. *American Journal of Veterinary Research.*, Vol. 56, N° 10, (October 1995), pp. 1281-1285, ISBN 0002-9645.

Muñoz, A., Riber, C., Trigo, P., Castejón-Riber, C., Castejón, F.M. (2010). Dehydration, electrolyte imbalances and renin-angiotensin-aldosterone-vasopressin axis in successful and unsuccessful endurance horses. *Equine Veterinary Journal*, Vol.42, No.38, (November 2010), pp, 83-90, ISSN 2042-3306.

Muñoz, A., Santisteban, R., Rubio, M.D., Agüera, E.I., Escribano, B.M. & Castejón, F.M. (1998). Locomotor, cardiocirculatory and metabolic adaptations to training in Andalusian and Anglo-Arabian horses. *Research in Veterinary Science*, Vol.66, No.1, (February 1998), pp. 25-31, ISSN 0034-5288.

Muñoz, A., Santisteban, R., Rubio, M.D., Riber, C., Agüera, E.I. & Castejón, F.M. (1999). Locomotor response to exercise in relation to plasma lactate accumulation and heart rate in Andalusian and Anglo-Arabian horses. *Veterinary Research Communications*, Vol.23, No6, (October, 1999), pp. 369-384, ISSN 0165-7380.

Muñoz, A., Santisteban, R., Rubio, M.D., Vivo, R., Agüera, E.I., Escribano, B.M. &, Castejón, F.M. (1997). The use of functional indexes to evaluate fitness in Andalusian horses. *Journal of Veterinary Medical Science*, Vol.59, No.9, (September 1997), pp. 747-752, ISSN 0916-7250.

Nieto, J.E., Snyder, J.R., Vatistas, N.J. & Jones, J.H. (2009). Effect of gastric ulceration on physiologic responses to exercise in horses. American *Journal of Veterinary Research*, Vol.70, No.6, (June 2009), pp. 787-795, ISSN 0002-9645.

Persson, S.G.B. & Ullberg, L. (1974). Blood volume in relation to exercise tolerance in trotters. *Journal of South African Veterinary Association*, Vol. 45, N° 4, pp. 293-299, ISSN 0038-2809.

Persson, S.G.B. (1967). On blood volume and working capacity in horses. *Acta Physiologica Scandinava, Suppl.*, Vol. 19, pp. 1-189, ISSN 0302-2994.

Persson, S.G.B. (1975). The circulatory significance of the splenic red cell pool. *Proceeding of the 1st International Symposium on Equine Hematology*, Michigan State University, East Lansing.

Persson, S.G.B. (1983). Evaluation of exercise tolerance and fitness in the performance horse. In: *Equine Exercise Physiology*. Snow, D.H., Persson, S.G.B. & Rose, R.J. (eds.), pp. 441-447, ISBN 1478-0615, Granta Editions, Cambridge, U.K.

Plotka, E.D., Eagle, T.C., Gaulke, S.J., Tester, J.R. & Siniff, D.B. (1988). Hematologic and blood chemical characteristics of feral horses from three management areas. *Journal of Wild Diseases*, Vol. 24, N° 2, (April 1988), pp. 231-239, ISSN 0090-3558.

Ralston, S.L., Nockels, C.F. & Squires, E.L. (1988). Differences in diagnostic test results and haematologic data between aged and young horses. *American Journal of Veterinary Research*, Vol. 49, N° 8, (August 1988), pp. 1387-1392, ISSN 0002-9645.

Robert, C., Goachet, A.G., Fraipont, A., Votion, D.M., Van Erck, E. & Leclerc, J.C. (2010). Hydration and electrolyte balance in horses during an endurance season. *Equine Veterinary Journal*, Vol.42, No.38, (November 2010), pp, 98-104, ISSN 2042-3306.

Rose, R.J. & Hodgson, D.R. (1994). Hematology and biochemistry. In: *The Athletic Horse: Principles and Practice of Equine Sports Medicine*. Hodgson, D.R. & Rose, R.J. (eds.), pp. 63-76, ISBN 0721637590, W.B. Saunders Company, Philadelphia.

Rossdale, P.D., Burguez, P.N. & Cash, R.S. (1982). Changes in blood neutrophil-lymphocyte ratio related to adrenocortical function in the horse. *Equine Veterinary Journal*, Vol. 14, N° 4, (October 1982), pp. 293-298, ISSN 2042-3306.

Ruiz, G., Rosenmann, M. & Cortes, A. (2004). Thermal acclimation and seasonal variations of erythrocyte size in the Andean mouse Phyllotis xanthopygus rupestres. *Comparative Biochemistry and Physiology A*, Vol. 139, N° 4, (December 2004), pp. 405- 409, ISSN 1095-6433.

Saigo, K., Sakota, Y. & Masuda, Y. (2005). EDTA-dependent pseudothrombocytopenia: clinical aspects and laboratory tests. *Rinsho Byor.*, Vol. 53, N° 7, (July 2005), pp. 646-653, ISSN 0047-1860.

Satué, K. & Domingo, R. (2008). Microhematocrit values, total proteins and electrolytes concentrations in Spanish Purebred mares during pregnancy. *Proceedings of 10th Annual Congress of the European Society of Veterinary Clinical Pathology (ESVCP) and the 8th Biennial Congress of the International Society for Animal Clinical Pathology (ISACP), European Society of Veterinary Clinical Pathology*, 30 september-3 october, CAB Abstracts, Barcelona (Spain).

Satué, K. & Domingo, R. (2011). Longitudinal study of the renin-angiotensin-aldosterone system in purebred Spanish broodmares during pregnancy. *Theriogenology*, Vol.75, No.7, (April 2011), pp. 1185-1194, ISSN 0093-691X.

Satué, K. (2004). Hematología en la yegua Pura Raza Española de Estirpe Cartujana. *Doctoral Thesis.* Departament of Animal Medicine and Surgery. CEU-Cardenal Herrera University.

Satué, K., Blanco, O. & Muñoz, A. (2009). *Age-related differences in the hematological profile of Andalusian broodmares of Carthusian strain.* Veterinarny Medicine, *Vol. 54, N° 4, (April 2009), pp. 175–182, 2009, ISSN 8750-7943.*

Satué, K., Hernández A. & Lorente, C. (2008). Erythrocyte parameters in Spanish horse: influence of age and gender. *Proceedings of 10th Annual Congress of the European Society of Veterinary Clinical Pathology (ESVCP) and the 8th Biennial Congress of the International Society for Animal Clinical Pathology (ISACP), European Society of Veterinary Clinical Pathology,* 30 september-3 october, CAB Abstracts, Barcelona (Spain).

Satué, K., Hernández, A., Lorente, C. & O´Coonor, J.E. (2010). *Immunophenotypical characterization in Andalusian horse: variations with age and gender.* Veterinary Immunology and Immunopathology, *Vol. 133, N° 2, (February 2010), pp. 219-227, ISSN 0165-2427.*

Satué, K., Muñoz, A. & Montesinos, P. (2011). Seasonal variations in the erythrogram in pregnant Carthusian mares. *Proceeding of 13th conference of the ESVCP/ECVCP, 9TH conference of AECCP, 12TH ACCP and ASVCP,* 31 Aug-3 Sept, Dublin (Ireland).

Schalm, O.W. & Carlson, G.P. (1982). The blood and the blood forming organs. In: *Equine Medicine and Surgery.* pp. 377-414, American Veterinary Publications.

Seghatchian, J. (2006). A new platelet storage lesion index based on paired samples, without and with EDTA and cell counting: comparison of three types of leukoreduced preparations. *Transfusion Apher. Science,* Vol. 35, N° 3, (December 2006), pp. 283-292, ISSN 1473-0502.

Sellon, D.C. (1998). Thrombocytopenia in horses. *Equine Veterinary Education,* Vol. 10, N° 3, (June 1998), pp. 133-139, ISSN 0957-7734.

Sharif, M., Ameri, M., Moshfeghi, S., Sharifi, H., Mohammad, S. & Mohsen, S. (2010). Artifactual changes in haematological variables in equine blood samples stored at different temperatures and various anticoagulants. *Comparative Clinical Pathology,* pp. 1-4, (October 2010), ISSN 1618-565X.

Silver, M., Ousey, J.C. & Dudan, F.E. (1984). Studies on equine prematurity 2: post natal adrenocortical activity in relation to plasma adrenocorticotrophic hormone and catecholamine levels in terms and premature foals. *Equine Veterinary Journal,* Vol. 16, N° 4, (July 1984), pp. 278-286, ISSN 2042-3306.

Smith, G.S. (2000). Neutrophils. In: *Schalm´s Veterinary Hematology. Feldman,* B., Zinkl, J. & Jain, N. (eds.), pp. 281-298, Williams & Wilkins, ISBN: 978-0-8138-1798-9, Philadelphia, UK.

Smith, J., Erickson, H. & Debowes, R. (1989). Changes in circulating equine erythrocytes induced by brief, high speed exercise. *Equine Veterinary Journal,* Vol. 21, N° 6, (November 1989), pp. 444-446, ISSN 2042-3306.

Smith, J.E., Erickson, H.H., Debowes, R.M. & Clark, M. (1989). Changes in circulating equine erythrocytes induced by brief, high-speed exercise. *Equine Veterinary Journal,* Vol.21, No6, (November 1989), pp. 444-446, ISSN 2042-3306.

Smith, R. III, Chaffin, K., Cohen, N. & Martens, R.J. (2002). Age-related changes in lymphocyte subset in Quarter Horse foals. *American Journal of Veterinary Research,* Vol. 63, N° 4, (April 2002), pp. 531-536, ISSN 0002-9645.

Snow, D.H., Kerr, M.G., Nimmo, M.A. & Abbott, E.M. (1982). Alterations in blood, sweat, urine and muscle composition during prolonged exercise in the horse. *Veterinary Record*, Vol. 110, N° 16, (April 1982), pp. 377-384, ISSN 0042-4900.

Snow, D.H., Ricketts, S.W. & Douglas, T.A. (1983). Post-race biochemistry in thoroughbreds. In: *Equine Exercise Physiology*. Snow, D.H., Persson, S.G.B., Rose, R.J. (eds.), pp. 389-399, Granta Editions, ISBN: 0-7020-2857-6, Cambridge, England.

Steinhardt, M., Thielscher, H.H. von Horn, T., von Horn, R., Ermgassen, K., Ladewig, J. & Smidt, D. (1994). The hemoglobin concentration in the blood of dairy cattle of different breeds and their offspring during the peripartum period. *Tierärztliche Practice*, Vol. 22, N° 2, (April 1994), pp. 129-135, 1994, ISSN 0303-6286.

Stewart, G.A., Clarkson, G.T. & Steel, J.D. (1970). Hematology of the race horse and factors affecting interpretation of the blood count. *Proceeding of the Annual Convention of the American Association of Equine Practitioners,* pp 70, . pp: 17. COMPLETAR ANA ¡¡¡¡.

Suárez, C.R., Gonzalez, J., Menéndez, C., Fareed, J., Fresco, R. & Walenga, J. (1988). Neonatal and maternal platelets: activation at time of birth. *American Journal of Hematology,* Vol. 29, N° 1, (September 1988): 18-21, ISSN 0361-8609.

Taylor-Macallister, C., Macallister, C.G., Walker, D. & Aalseth, D. (1997). Haematology and serum biochemistry evaluation in normal postpartum mares. *Equine Veterinary Journal,* Vol. 29, N° 3, (May 1997), pp. 234-235, ISSN 2042-3306.

Tizard, J.R. (2009). *Veterinary Immunology: an introduction* (8th ed.), Saunders Elsevier, ISBN 0721601367, St. Louis, Missouri.

Trigo, P., Castejón, F.M., Riber, C. & Muñoz, A. (2010). Use of biochemical parameters to predict metabolic elimination in endurance rides. *Equine Veterinary Journal,* Vol.42, No.38, (November 2010), pp, 142-146, ISSN 2042-3306.

Trum, B.F. (1952). Normal variances in horse blood due to breed, age, lactation, pregnancy and altitude. *American Journal of Veterinary Research,* Vol. 13, N° 49, (October 1952), pp. 514-519, ISSN 0002-9645.

Tyler-McGowan, C.M., Golland, L.C., Evans, D.L., Hodgson, D.R. & Rose, R.J. (1999). Haematological and biochemical responses to training and overtraining. *Equine Veterinary Journal. Suppl.*, Vol. 30, N°, (October 1999), pp. 621-625, ISSN 2042-3306.

Welles, E. (2000). Clinical interpretation of equine leucograms. In: *Schalm´s Veterinary Hematology*. Feldman, D.F., Zinkl, J.G., Jain, N.C. (eds.), pp. 405-410, Williams & Wilkins, ISBN: 978-0-8138-1798-9, Philadelphia, UK.

Wickler, S.J. & Anderson, T.P. (2000). Hematological changes and athletic performance in horses in response to high altitude (3.000 m). *American Journal of Physiology Regulatory Integrative Comparative Physiology,* Vol. 279, N° 4, (November 2000), pp. 1176-1181, ISSN 1522-1490.

Wu, M.J., Feldman, B.F. & Zinkl, J.G. (1983). Using red blood cell creatinine concentration to evaluate the equine erythropoietic response. *American Journal of Veterinary Research,* Vol. 44, N° 8, (August 1983), pp. 1427-1432, ISSN 0002-9645.

Young, K.M. (2000). Eosinophils. In: *Schalm´s Veterinary Hematology*. Feldman, D.F., Zinkl, J.G., Jain, N.C. (eds.), pp. 297-307, Williams & Wilkins, ISBN: 978-0-8138-1798-9, Philadelphia, UK.

Zinkl, J., Mae, D., Guzmán, P., Farver, T. & Humble, J. (1990). Reference ranges and the influence of age and sex on hematological and serum biochemical values in donkeys (*Equus asinus*). *American Journal of Veterinary Research,* Vol. 51, N° 3, (March 1990), pp. 408-413, ISSN 0002-9645.

Zvorc, Z., Mrljak, V., Susic, V. & Gotal, J.P. (2006). Haematological and biochemical parameters during pregnancy and lactation in sows. *Veterinarski Arhives,* Vol. 76, N° 3, (June 2006), pp. 245-253, ISSN 0372-5480.

14

The Effects of Splenectomy and Autologous Spleen Transplantation on Complete Blood Count and Cell Morphology in a Porcine Model

Nina Poljičak-Milas[1], Anja Vujnović[2], Josipa Migić[3], Dražen Vnuk[4] and Matko Kardum[1]

[1]*Faculty of Veterinary Medicine, Department of Pathophysiology, University of Zagreb*

[2]*Croatian Veterinary Institute*

[3]*Pliva d.o.o.*

[4]*Faculty of Veterinary Medicine, Surgery, Orthopedics and Ophthalmology Clinic, University of Zagreb*

Croatia

1. Introduction

Spleen, as a part of hematopoietic and immune system, plays an important role in the life cycle of blood cells. There are three major functions of the spleen and these are handled by three different tissues within the spleen. Reticuloendothelial tissue is responsible for removing old or damaged erythrocytes and cell debris from the blood stream. This same tissue may participate in hematopoiesis when there is an increased need for red blood cells and is a place where young erythrocytes produced in bone marrow undergo the process of maturation before releasing into the blood stream. Venous sinusoids along with the ability of the spleen to contract, provides a means for expelling the contained blood to meet increased circulatory demands in certain animals. White pulp provides lymphocytes and a source of plasma cells and hence antibodies for the cellular and humoral specific immune defenses (Dyce et al., 2002; Teske, 2000).

Splenectomy is a surgical removal of the spleen that may be carried out in patients whose spleen has been ruptured by trauma or damaged by other pathological processes such as cancer, infections or some autoimmune diseases (Tillson, 2003). However, total removal of the spleen may lead to side effects such as postsplenectomy infections and sepsis, due to the decreased production of antibodies and phagocytes or thrombosis, due to elevated platelet count in blood (Bessler et al., 2004; Khan et al., 2009; Miko et al., 2003; Timens & Leemans, 1992). Also, many studies report increased count of morphologically abnormal erythrocytes, immature red blood cells and pathologic erythrocyte inclusions in the peripheral blood of various species following splenectomy as a result of the loss of splenic filtrating function (Haklar et al., 1997; Resende et al., 2002; Traub et al., 1987). In addition, it has been reported that removal of the spleen causes significantly higher increase of reticulocyte count than other surgeries. This suggests that spleen may somehow hormonally regulate the release of red blood cells into circulation, thus after removal of spleen bone marrow releases more red blood cells as well as more immature erythrocytes into the blood stream (Knežević et al., 2002; Lorber, 1958). Splenectomy also causes changes in number of white blood cells with subsequent leukocytosis (Bessler et al., 2004; Karagülle et al., 2007). Initial transient neutrophilia is followed by the persistent lymphocytosis and monocytosis. Increased leukocytosis accompanied by the significant left shift is found in patients, and often there are myelocytes or other precursor in the granulocytic series in their peripheral blood (Labar & Hauptmann, 1998; Tang et al., 2003; Zhang et al., 2002).

Severe postoperative infections after removal of the spleen prompted a development of alternative methods to conserve functions of the spleen. Autologous spleen transplantation is a method of choice after total splenectomy in order to preserve splenic immune and hematopoietic functions (Marques et al., 2003; Patel et al., 1981). The effectiveness of splenic autotransplant depends on many factors and is still controversial (Theodorou et al., 2007). Studies done on rats, mice, rabbits and men report that autotransplantat's capability of recovering its primary function highly depends on the volume of transplanted spleen tissue (Karagülle et al., 2007; Miko et al., 2003; Resende & Petroianu, 2003; Tang et al., 2003).

In the recent years there is a close cooperation between Faculty of Veterinary Medicine and Medical faculty in University of Zagreb. Because of close interests that both faculties have, combined projects and seminars have been established. One of the best examples was education of Medical faculty surgeons for laparoscopic cholecystectomy, liver lobectomy, laminectomy, and for experimental wounds surgery on our faculty, in the Clinic for Surgery, Orthopedics and Ophthalmology. These operative procedures were carried out on pigs because of its similarity in organs size. In recent years, a xenotransplantation of pig organs to nonhuman primates is being investigated. In order to prolong survival of primates that have received porcine xenografts, the same animals underwent a splenectomy to prevent humorally mediated immunological damage (Cozzi et al., 2000). In order to save human lives, it is important not only to master the precise surgical technique, but also to recognize all the factors that may affect the rejection or return of physiological functions of organs after transplantation.

The aim of this study was to evaluate the effects of total splenectomy and autologous spleen transplantation in a porcine model on complete blood count and cell morphology. Also, we aimed to determine the functional effectiveness of autotransplanted splenic tissue by its capacity to remove erythrocyte having Howell-Yolly bodies from the blood stream.

2. Materials and methods

2.1 Animals, anaesthesia and surgery

The experimental protocol was approved by the Department of Veterinary Science, Ministry of Agriculture, Republic of Croatia and was conducted in accordance with the guidelines for the treatment of laboratory animals. Nineteen pigs of either sex, aged three months, weighing 19-26 kg were used in the experiment. Food was withheld from all the pigs 12 h and water 2 h before the experiment. All animals were premedicated with 2 mg/kg i.m. of xylazine (Xylapan, Vetoquinol, Bern, Switzerland), and left auricular vein was catheterized percutaneously for continuous infusion of lactated Ringer's solution at a rate of 10 ml/kg/h (Infusion pump BIOF 3000, Biotron CO, Kangwondo, South Corea) during surgical procedures and for the administration of drugs. Anaesthesia was induced with 5 mg/kg i.v.

of ketamine (Ketaminol 10, Intervet, Boxmeer, The Netherlands) and 10 µg/kg i.v. fentanyl (Fentanyl-Jannsen, Jannsen Pharmaceutica, Beerse, Belgium), and animals were intubated, connected to a circle system and maintained on spontaneous ventilation. Anaesthesia was maintained with 1.5% isoflurane (Forane, Abbott, Queenborough, UK) and oxygen and continuous intravenous infusion of fentanyl in a dose of 0.8 µg/kg/min. Supplemental doses of ketamine were applied during surgery to maintain sufficient anaesthesia depth. Preoperative antibiotic prophylaxis was administered using 20 mg/kg ampicillin and sublactam *i.v.* (Penactam, Krka, Novo Mesto, Slovenia).

After anaesthesia induction, animals were randomly divided into three groups: sham-operated pigs with spleens intact (control group, n=6), splenectomized pigs (n=6), and splenectomized pigs with small fragments of 20% mass of the spleen autotransplanted into the greater omentum (n=7).

2.2 Blood sampling and experimental protocol

Two blood samples of each pig were taken from the *v. auricularis lateralis* just before surgery and on the first, fifth, twelfth and twenty sixth day postoperatively. Exceptionally, blood samples for reticulocyte, and differential white blood cell counting were also taken on the fortieth postoperative day. First sample was collected into the Vacutainer® tubes containing K_3EDTA anticoagulant (BD-Vacutainer, Plymouth PL6 7BP UK) and the other was taken without anticoagulant and was used to make blood smears. Hematological parameters: red blood cell count (RBC), white blood cell count (WBC), hemoglobin concentration (Hgb), hematocrit (Htc), mean corpuscular volume (MCV), mean corpuscular hemoglobin (MCH), mean corpuscular hemoglobin concentration (MCHC), red blood cell distribution width (RDW), platelet count (PLT) and mean platelet volume (MPV) were determined using automated blood analyzer (SERONO-9120 Baker System). Reticulocyte counting was done on brilliant cresyl blue stained blood smears, and differential leukocyte count and morphological changes of blood cells were determined by identifying 200 consecutive leukocytes on May Grünwald stained blood smears using immersion objective with 1000x enlargement of the light microscope (Olympus BX 41). The frequency of blood cells immature precursor, degenerative neutrophils or increased reactive lymphocytes is reported as a few (5% to 10%) or moderate (11% to 30%). Similarly, semi quantitative evaluation of red blood cell morphology based on average number of abnormal cells per 1000x microscopic monolayer field was used to assess morphological changes in erythrocyte (Weiss, 1984).

The results were statistically analyzed by calculating mean values, standard deviation, and coefficient of variability, and were presented in tables as the mean values ± standard deviation. The significance of the differences between the results was verified using the Student *t*-test and Statistica 7.1 computer programme.

3. Results

3.1 Red blood cell count (RBC), hemoglobin (Hgb) and hematocrit (Htc)

Total red blood cell count in sham-operated pigs was significantly decreased only on the fifth day postoperatively compared to the value before surgery. In splenectomized pigs red blood cell count was significantly lower on the first, fifth, twelfth and twenty sixth day postoperatively compared to the value before surgery. In pigs with autologous splenic transplants, red blood cell count was significantly decreased on the fifth and twelfth day after surgery compared to the value before surgery. Hemoglobin and hematocrit values in sham-operated pigs were significantly decreased on the fifth day postoperatively compared to the values before surgery. Splenectomized pigs showed significantly lower values of these parameters on the fifth, twelfth and twenty sixth day postoperatively compared to the values before surgery. In pigs with splenic autotransplants, hemoglobin and hematocrit values were significantly decreased on the first, fifth and twelfth day after surgery compared to the values before surgery (Table 1.).

3.2 Mean corpuscular volume (MCV), mean corpuscular hemoglobin (MCH), mean corpuscular hemoglobin concentration (MCHC) and red blood cell distribution width (RDW)

There were no statistical differences of mean corpuscular volume value in sham-operated pigs before and after surgery. Compared to the value before surgery mean corpuscular volume value showed significant raise in splenectomized pigs on the twelfth and twenty sixth day postoperatively, and in contrast autotransplanted pigs showed significantly decreased value of mean corpuscular volume on the first, fifth and twelfth day postoperatively. There were no statistical differences of mean corpuscular hemoglobin value in sham-operated pigs before and after surgery while mean corpuscular hemoglobin concentration value was significantly higher on the twelfth day after surgery compared to preoperative value. In splenectomized pigs significant raise in values of both parameters was noted on the fifth day postoperatively when compared to the values of these parameters before surgery. In pigs with splenic autotransplants mean corpuscular hemoglobin value was significantly decreased on the first and twelfth day after surgery, but the mean corpuscular hemoglobin concentration value was significantly raised on the fifth day after surgery when compared to preoperative values. There were no noted significant changes of red blood cell distribution width values except in sham-operated pigs on the twenty sixth day postoperatively when compared to the same value before surgery (Table 1.).

3.3 Total and differential white blood cell count

In group with autotransplanted splenic tissue on the fifth postoperative day total white blood cell count dropped significantly in comparison with the preoperative value as well as in comparison with the value measured in the control group on the same day of experiment. After this, on the twelfth and twenty sixth day of the experiment, significant increase of white blood cell count in comparison with the preoperative value was noted in all experimental groups of pigs (Table 1.). Changes in absolute differential count of segmented neutrophils followed the same pattern as those in the total white blood cell count during whole experimental period in each of the groups of pigs.

Compared to the value right before surgery, rise in absolute count of unsegmented neutrophils was noted, with significant increase on the first and twelfth day in the control group, first and fifth day in splenectomized group and first, twelfth and twenty sixth day in group with autotransplanted splenic tissue (Table 2.).

Although absolute number of lymphocytes was decreasing postoperatively in all experimental groups of pigs, it was significantly decreased only on the fifth day in splenectomized group and in this group it remained at low values until the end of experimental period. In contrast, on the twelfth postoperative day absolute number of lymphocytes in control and autotransplanted group started to rise, even exceeding preoperative levels.

Relative differential number of monocytes ranged from one to eight percent in all blood smears. Still, statistical analysis showed significant decrease of absolute number of monocytes on the fifth day after the surgery in control group compared to the value before operation and twelfth day after splenectomy compared to the control group of the same day. Relative differential number of eosinophils on blood smears ranged from zero to twelve percent in all groups. Only statistically significant shift in the absolute number of eosinophils occurred on the first day after the surgery in control group compared to values before the surgery. Relative number of basophils in all groups ranged from one and three percent and statistically significant increase in number was found on the fifth day in the group with autotransplanted tissue compared to the values before surgery and control group of the same day (Table 2.).

3.4 Ratio of absolute differential number of neutrophils and lymphocytes (N/L)

Compared with the preoperative values, significantly elevated neutrophil/lymphocyte ratio was recorded in the control group on the first, fifth and twelfth postoperative day. In splenectomized pigs significant elevation of neutrophil/lymphocyte ratio in respect to preoperative value, as well as in respect to the value of control group on the same day of the experiment, appeared on the fifth day postoperatively and it remained on the significantly higher values till the end of experimental period. On the twelfth day of the experiment significant decrease of neutrophil/lymphocyte ratio in comparison with the sham-operated pigs on the same day was reported in group with autotransplanted splenic tissue (Table 3.).

		Before surgery	Days after surgery			
			1st	5th	12th	26th
WBC 10^9/L	Sham-operation		27.33±9.26	24.94±11.60	**38.95±5.88	**28.14±0.42
	Splenectomy	22.26±3.82	20.26±3.32	26.37±9.01	*39.23±12.09	*27.13±7.57
	Autotransplantation		23.87±0.21	*18.13±4.53+	***34.9±6.75	**28.91±3.18
RBC E*10^{12}/L	Sham-operation		7.22±0,52	***5.85±0.55	6.84±0.16	5.09±1.79
	Splenectomy	6.89±0.11	*6.33±0.42^{+}	***5.19±0.44^{+}	**3.01±1.49^{+}	*4.73±0.97
	Autotransplantation		6.35±0.29^{+}	**5.20±1.12	*5.92±0.94^{+}	4.55±1.18
Hgb g/L	Sham-operation		134.5±14.14	**109.4±9.19	125.75±4.27	99.5±29.44
	Splenectomy	126.71±5.66	120.6±10.61^{+}	***101.83±7.22	**69.75± 18.53^{++}	*106.33±8.96
	Autotransplantation		*112.57±4.95^{++}	**93.57±19.61^{+}	**106.57± 16.29^{++}	85.5±13.28

		Before surgery	Days after surgery			
			1st	5th	12th	26th
Htc L/L	Sham-operation		0.42±0.05	***0.33±0.03	0.38±0.01	0.30±0.09
	Splenectomy	0.39±0.01	0.37±0.03^{+}	***0.30±0.03^{+}	*0.21±0.07^{+}	*0.32±0.04
	Autotransplantation		*0.35±0.02^{+}	**0.28±0.07	**0.33±0.05^{+}	0.26±0.04
MCV fL	Sham-operation		57.87±2.33	56.56±1.13	55.7±1.3	59.8±2.66
	Splenectomy	56.92±0.78	59.04±1.48	58.57±2.54	*69.7±8.58^{+}	*68.67±6.22
	Autotransplantation		*54.6±1.34^{++}	**53.84±1.93^{+}	*54.57±1.58	57.25±3.14
MCH pg	Sham-operation		18.63±0.49	18.74±0.28	18.4±0.65	19.85±1.21
	Splenectomy	18.41±0.57	19.1±0.42	***19.65±0.57^{+}	22.13±2.81	23±3.01
	Autotransplantation		*17.74±0.26^{+}	17.99±0.62	*17.81±0.59	19.2±2.08
MCHC g/L	Sham-operation		322.67±2.83	330.8±1.41	*330.25±4.11	331.5±5.19
	Splenectomy	323.57±4.95	323.6±1.41	**335.5±8.19	344.48±13.08	333.33±6.59
	Autotransplantation		324.86±8.49	*334.71±12.45	326.29±5.5	335.5±6.35
RDW %	Sham-operation		23.2±3.39	22.54±2.83	22.7±2.14	*21.85±0.17
	Splenectomy	23.01±0.07	23.08±3.54	23.62±3.5	24.48±4.43	23.4±1.17
	Autotransplantation		23.87±2.69	23.43±1.32	22.93±1.11	22.15±0.87
PLT E*10^{9}/L	Sham-operation		509.33±16.26	554±46.67	389.33±19.43	272±125.73
	Splenectomy	551.92±359.72	400±147.35	534.25±381.81	***96±25.94^{+++}	286.33±219.21
	Autotransplantation		587.67±326.51	690±431.74	445.53±405.88	223±114.28
MPV fL	Sham-operation		10.8±2.12	10.5±0.21	11.4±1.08	12.6±1.42
	Splenectomy	10.49±1.2	11.33±0.79	***11.65±0.87^{+}	*12.63±1.08	10.97±1.37
	Autotransplantation		***12.43±0.42^{+}	***12.5±0.57^{++}	12.45±0.92	12.7±1.63

All values are presented as mean values ± standard deviation.
Statistical difference with respect to the value before surgery:*P<0.05; **P<0.01; ***P<0.001.
Statistical difference with respect to the value in sham operated pigs on the same day of experiment: $^{+}$P<0.05; $^{++}$P<0.01; $^{+++}$P<0.001.

Table 1. White blood cell count (WBC), red blood cell count (RBC), blood hemoglobin concentration (Hgb), hematocrit (Htc), mean corpuscular volume (MCV), mean corpuscular hemoglobin (MCH), mean corpuscular hemoglobin concentration (MCHC), platelet count (PLT), mean platelet volume (MPV) and red blood cell distribution width (RDW) in the peripheral blood of observed pigs during the experiment

		Before surgery	Days after surgery			
			1st	5th	12th	26th
Segmented neutrophils	Sham-operation	7.52±3.93 31.3% (6-50%)	13.12±6.85 44.7% (7-64%)	12.15±9.85 47.2% (39-63%)	**19.10±3.80 48.5% (41-54%)	**10.99±3.21 39.17% (31-49)
	Splenectomy		5.67±7.08 27.4% (14-61%)	11.32±10.00 41.3% (22-54%)	**24.38±13.99 61.75% (55-68%)	*14,00±3.28 48.5% (40-60%)
	Auto-transplantation		8.34±4.27 34.3% (18-56%)	*4.20±0.74++ 22.1% (8-36%)	*14.07±5.08 38.9% (11-55%)	*11.77±4.51 39.9% (18-57%)
Band neutrophils	Sham-operation	0.58±0.40 2.6% (1-5%)	*1.57±0.19 5.5% (4-8%)	0.63±0.13 2.8% (0-8%)	**1.53±0.05 4.0% (3-6%)	0.32±0.22 1.2% (0-3%)
	Splenectomy		**1.85±0.80 9.8% (5-15%)	**3.67±2.83++ 14.5% (5-28%)	1.58±2.18 4.5% (0-10%)	0.67±0.40 2.25% (0-4%)
	Auto-transplantation		**1.84±0.21 7.9% (4-18%)	1.00±0.39 5.7% (1-14%)	*1.41±0.06 3.9% (2-8%)	*1.64±0.08+ 5.43% (0-12%)
Lymphocytes	Sham-operation	13.06±2.88 61.2% (43-86%)	11.94±2.04 47.2% (28-85%)	11.61±2.29 47.6% (37-54%)	*16.81±2.67 43.7% (36-51%)	*15.54±3.82 55.2% (45-63%)
	Splenectomy		11.62±3.44 57.0% (29-70%)	**9.39±4.88 36.3% (29-49%)	12.52±6.33 31.5% (28-36%)	12.50±0.63+ 45.0% (36-56%)
	Auto-transplantation		12.93±3.51 54.3% (36-69%)	11.96±1.77 66.7% (51-86%)	**17.86±6.51 52.6% (36-79%)	14.22±1.50 50.1% (29-70%)
Monocytes	Sham-operation	0.33±0.27 1.4% (0-3%)	0.36±0.03 1.3% (1-2%)	**0.09±0.13 0.4% (0-1%)	0.48±0.06 1.2% (1-2%)	0.56±0.43 1.8% (0-7%)
	Splenectomy		0.36±0.03 2.2% (0-8%)	0.57±0.75 2.0% (1-3%)	0.18±0.22+ 0.5% (0-1%)	0.49±0.20 1.7% (0-5%)
	Auto-transplantation		0.28±0.38 1.3% (0-3%)	0.36±0.12 2.0% (0-5%)	0.53±0.51 1.6% (0-4%)	0.28±0.32 1.0% (0-3%)
Eozynophils	Sham-operation	0.75±0.60 3.3% (0-9%)	**0.21±0.18 1.0% (0-3%)	0.41±0.27 1.8% (0-4%)	0.95±0.45 2.2% (0-6%)	0.63±1.05 2.3% (0-5%)
	Splenectomy		0.71±0.31 3.4% (1-5%)	1.29±0.22 5.3% (1-12%)	0.48±0.66 1.5% (0-3%)	0.58±0.48 2.3% (0-4%)
	Auto-transplantation		0.48±0.38 2.3% (0-5%)	0.44±0.24 2.3% (0-3%)	0.83±0.06 2.6% (1-5%)	0.85±0.72 3.0% (1-6%)
Basophyls	Sham-operation	0.03±0.07 (0-1%)	0.10±0.02 (0-1%)	0.04±0.02 (0-1%)	0.08±0.23 (0-1%)	0.10±0.21 (0-1%)
	Splenectomy		0.04±0.14 (0-1%)	0.13±0.03 (0-2%)	0.08±0.21 (0-1%)	0.07±0.02 (0-1%)
	Auto-transplantation		0.00±0 (0%)	*0.18±0.14+ (0-3%)	0.20±0.22 (0-2%)	0.15±0.14 (0-2%)

Absolute differential values (10^9/L) are presented as mean values ± standard deviation
Relative differential values (%) are presented as mean value, and minimum and maximum values in the brackets
Statistical difference with respect to the value before surgery:*P<0.05; **P<0.01; ***P<0.001.
Statistical difference with respect to the value in sham operated pigs on the same day of experiment: $^{+}$P<0.05; $^{++}$P<0.01; $^{+++}$P<0.001.

Table 2. Absolute and relative white blood cell differential count in the peripheral blood of observed pigs during the experiment

	N/L ratio				
	Day 0	Day 1	Day 5	Day 12	Day 26
Sham-operation	0.61	*1.39	*1.09	*1.25	0.76
Splenectomy	0.61	0.83	**1.62+	***2.13++	*1.18
Autotransplantation	0.61	0.89	0.45++	0.93	1.09

Statistical difference with respect to the value before surgery: *P<0.05; **P<0.01; ***P<0.001.
Statistical difference with respect to the value in sham operated pigs on the same day of experiment: +P<0.05; ++P<0.01; +++P<0.001.

Table 3. Ratio of absolute differential number of neutrophils and lymphocytes (N/L) in the peripheral blood of observed pigs during the experiment

3.5 Platelet number (PLT) and mean platelet volume (MPV)

There were no statistical differences in platelet count in sham-operated and autotransplanted pigs, while on the twelfth postoperative day platelet count in splenectomized pigs was significantly lower in comparison with the platelet count before surgery, and to the value in the control group at the same experimental day. There were no statistical differences of mean platelet volume value in sham-operated pigs before surgery and the value of mean platelet volume on days after surgery. In splenectomized pigs significantly higher mean platelet volume value was noted on the fifth and twelfth day postoperatively. In autotransplanted pigs statistical differences were noted on the first and fifth day after the surgery in comparison with the value before surgery (Table 1.).

3.6 Reticulocyte count (RTC)

Prior to surgeries, reticulocyte count in all experimental pigs ranged within 0.5 to 1.5 %. On the first postoperative day reticulocyte count was significantly increased (2 to 4 %) when compared to the value before surgeries and it continued to grow simultaneously in all experimental groups on the fifth (4 to 8 %), twelfth (6 to 8 %) and twenty sixth (6 to 9 %) postoperative day. On the fortieth day after the surgery, reticulocyte count continued to increase in splenectomized (7 to 16 %) and autotransplanted pigs (7 to 18 %), while at the same time it began to decrease in sham-operated pigs (2 to 3 %), although was still significantly higher when compared to the preoperative value. Corrected reticulocyte count (reticulocyte production index - RPI) is shown in Table 4., and was extremely high on twenty sixth experimental day in splenectomized and autotransplanted pigs (Table 4.).

	RPI				
	Day 0	Day 1	Day 5	Day 12	Day 26
Sham-operation	0.5	1.2	2.3	3.3	1.1
Splenectomy	0.5	1.0	2.0	1.8	4.5
Autotransplantation	0.5	1.0	2.0	1.9	4.0

Table 4. Reticulocyte production index (RPI) in experimental pigs

3.7 Morphological changes of red blood cells

Polychromasia (the heterogeneous staining of red blood cells), as well as increased number of Howell-Jolly bodies (nuclear remnants found in red cells) were present on the blood films of all experimental groups, regardless of the surgical procedures, although both of these morphological changes were more manifested and frequent in pigs with total splenectomy. Five to seven erythrocytes containing Howell-Jolly bodies were found per 1000x microscopic monolayer field on the blood smears of splenectomized pigs. Erythroblasts (immature, nucleated red cells) sporadically appeared on the blood films of splenectomized pigs and pigs with transplanted autologous splenic tissue on all postoperative days. Abnormally shaped erythrocytes, such as leptocytes and codocytes, were found only on the blood smears of splenectomized pigs from the twelfth to the fortieth postoperative day.

3.8 Morphological changes of white blood cells

Neither morphological changes nor precursor cells were found on the blood films of experimental pigs prior to surgeries. On the first postoperative day a few (one to three %) reactive lymphocytes and a few (two to five %) metamyelocytes were found on each smear of control pigs. Similar results were found in the splenectomized group, but number of metamyelocytes was higher than in the control group (three to five %). Results found in group with autotransplanted tissue were almost identical to those in splenectomized group of pigs.

On the fifth day after the surgery reactive lymphocytes were found at only one blood smear from the control group, but blood smears of other two groups contained averagely three to four reactive lymphocytes. Splenectomized group had the largest number of metamyelocytes (four to six %), and also contained dividing cells, while in the group with autotransplanted tissue number of metamyelocytes was smaller (two to five %).

On the twelfth day after the surgery reactive lymphocytes became rarer, and were found only on one smear of splenectomized group, but still on almost all smears (one to two %) in the group with autotransplanted tissue. Metamyelocytes appeared sporadically on the blood smears of each experimental group. Twenty-six days after surgeries reactive lymphocytes were no longer noted on blood smears, and number of found metamyelocytes was decreasing until the fortieth postoperative day when they completely disappeared.

4. Discussion

4.1 Hematocrit, hemoglobin and erythrocyte count

Sham operated pigs exhibited the fastest recovery of hematologic values after surgery. Although red blood cell values of autotransplanted group were significantly lower when compared to sham operated pigs, postoperative blood regeneration took less time than in splenectomized pigs. In contrast to other two surgical procedures, total splenectomy resulted in a greater decrease of red blood cell values, even below physiological values (according to Jain (1993)), which persisted for a longer period (Diagram 1.). Hemoglobin and hematocrit values changed codependently with the changes of red blood cell count in all experimental groups on all postoperative days (Diagram 2., 3.). Postoperative oligocythemia, followed by decrease of hemoglobin and hematocrit, as the result of blood loss is a very well known founding. Durance of postoperative blood regeneration depends on many factors (e.g. degree of tissue lesion and trauma, blood loss and availability of hematopoiesis activating substances). The significant decrease of erythrocyte values and long postoperative recovery after total splenectomy and autotransplantation of splenic tissue have been documented in mice (Sipka et al., 2006), dogs (Lorber, 1958) and humans (Knežević et al., 2002). Results of this study suggest that observed decrease of erythrocyte values and postoperative recovery in each experimental group were in accordance with severity of surgical traumas (sham-operation, splenectomy and transplantation of autologous splenic tissue).

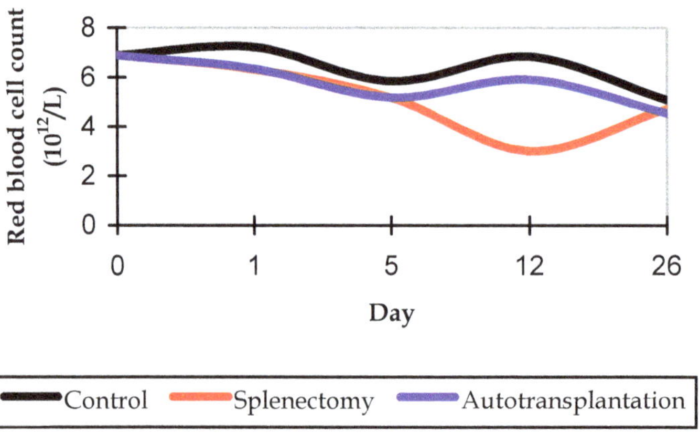

Diagram 1. Changes in red blood cell count in the blood of experimental pigs during the experiment

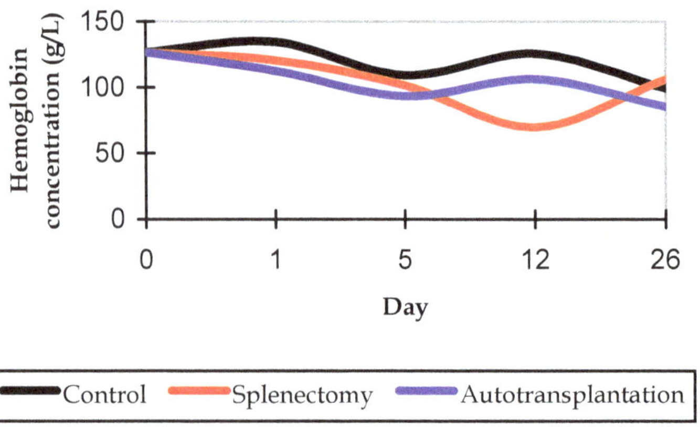

Diagram 2. Changes in blood hemoglobin concentration of experimental pigs during the experiment

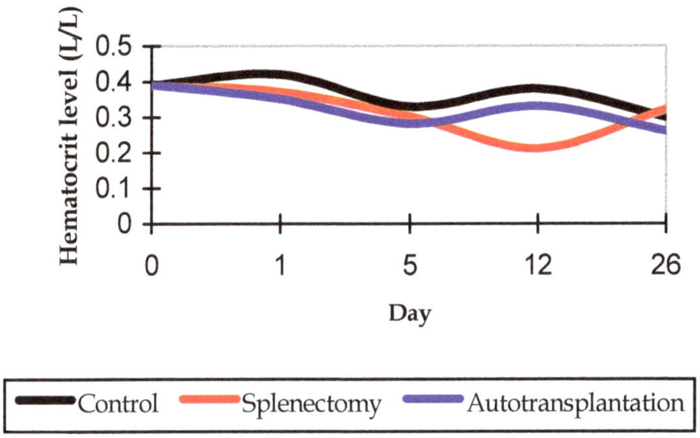

Diagram 3. Changes in hematocrit level in the blood of experimental pigs during the experiment

4.2 Mean corpuscular volume, mean corpuscular hemoglobin and mean corpuscular hemoglobin concentration

As previous experiments report, splenectomized patients of different species have higher mean corpuscular volume values than autotransplanted and sham-operated patients (Knežević at al., 2002, Lorber, 1958). The aging erythrocytes undergo changes in their plasma membrane which make them retain the fluid inside the cell, thus aged erythrocytes have higher mean corpuscular volume values. Total splenectomy leads to increased number of circulating old red blood cells. This, combined with significant reticulocytosis, led to high mean corpuscular volume values of splenectomized pigs in this study (Diagram 4.). Lower postoperative value of mean corpuscular volume in autotransplanted pigs was expected as the result of significantly lower concentration of hemoglobin. Surgical trauma and blood loss led to inadequate iron supply for the developing erythroblasts and consequently to limited hemoglobin synthesis. The red blood cell membrane shrinks to fit its hemoglobin content, thus volume of the cell decreases.

4.3 Total and differential white blood cell count

Leukocytosis, characterized by neutrophilia, initial lymphocytopenia and later recovery of lymphocyte count, was recorded postoperatively in all experimental groups (Diagram 5., 6., 7.). Increase in total leukocyte count after splenectomy and autotransplantation of splenic tissue as well as persistent leukocytosis are main characteristics of white blood cell count in mice (Bessler et al., 2004), rabbits (Karagülle et al., 2007) and humans (Zhang et al., 2002). However, in present study the differences in the degree of leukocytosis among the groups were not detected, except on the fifth postoperative day when a significant decline in the total number of leukocytes in pigs with a transplanted tissue was established compared to the control group at the same day of the experiment. Therefore, present leukocytosis has not been regarded as a change specific for splenectomy or autotransplantation rather than a post-injury inflammatory response due to tissue lesions during operation.

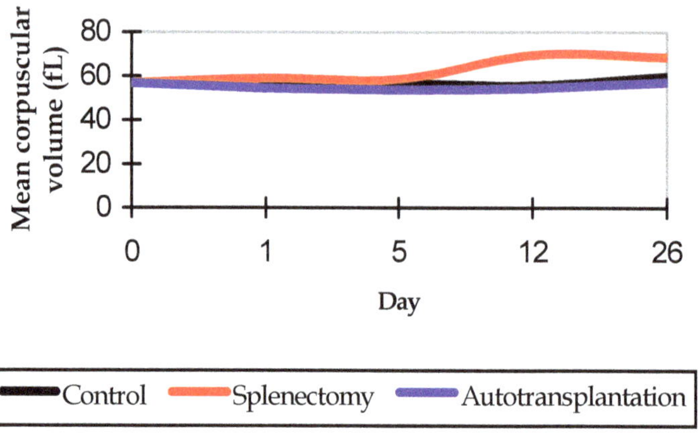

Diagram 4. Changes in erythrocyte mean corpuscular level of experimental pigs during the experiment

Due to differential leukocyte count in various species following splenectomy diverse reports were published. Some authors find an increase neutrophil and lymphocyte count Tarnuzi & Smiley (1967), other significantly higher lymphocyte count while neutrophil count remained unchanged (Bessler at al., 2004). Opposite to that, Sipka at al. (2006) found a significant increase in neutrophil count while lymphocyte count remained unchanged. However, some researches found none significant changes in differential neutrophil and lymphocyte count in blood after splenectomy or autotransplantation of splenic tissue (Resende & Petroianu, 2003; Shokouh-Amiri at al., 1990). In present study there does not seem to be a unique form of changes in differential blood count after splenectomy and autotransplantation of the spleen so we can conclude that the pattern of recorded changes in each experimental group corresponded with the degree of immune response of circulating white blood cells and stress caused by the surgical procedure.

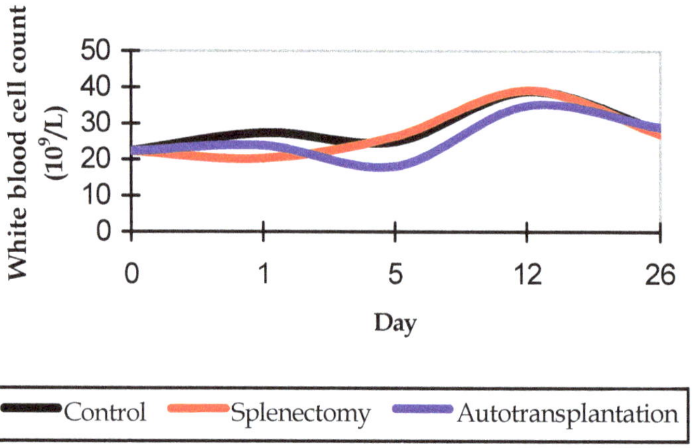

Diagram 5. Changes in total leukocyte count in the blood of experimental pigs during the experiment

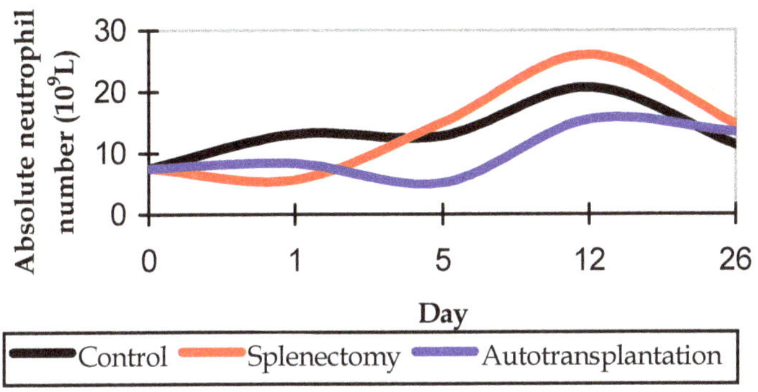

Diagram 6. Changes in absolute neutrophil number in the blood of experimental pigs during the experiment

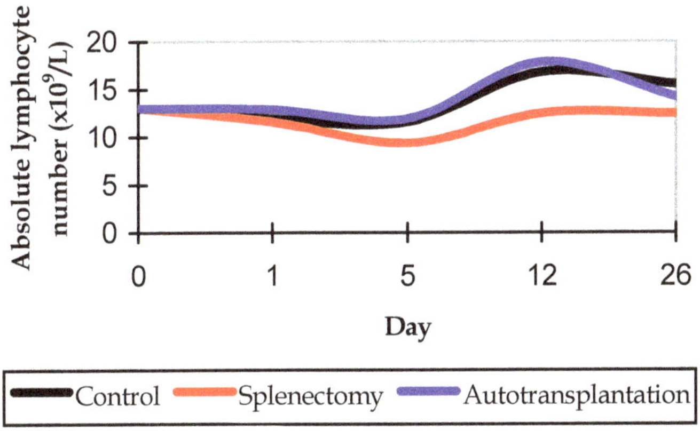

Diagram 7. Changes in absolute lymphocyte number in the blood of experimental pigs during the experiment

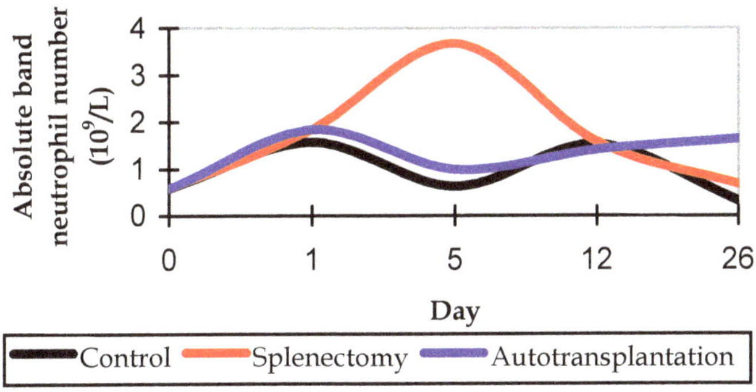

Diagram 8. Changes in absolute band neutrophil number in the blood of experimental pigs during the experiment

Apart from changes found in absolute neutrophil count, there were also changes in number of band neutrophils. Before the surgeries, relative band neutrophil count found on blood smears was 2.6 % in average. Compared to that value, it was evident that amount of band neutrophil increased during postoperative period in all groups. The largest increase was found in group of splenectomized pigs, where up to 28 % band neutrophils per smear were found (Diagram 8.). Increased number of band neutrophils, subsequent with findings of granulocyte precursors and dividing cells, suggest an increased bone marrow activity and release of immature cells, as well as their mobilization from the marginal pool.

4.4 Ratio of absolute differential number of neutrophils and lymphocytes

As it is well known, significant neutrophilia and lymphocytopenia occur as an immediate immune response following multiple traumas, surgical procedures, endotoxemia and sepsis. Since duration, pattern and degree of this immune response highly depend on the extensiveness and severity of surgical procedure, ratio of neutrophils and lymphocytes (N/L) can be considered as a reliable indicator of the immune response progress (Zahorec, 2001). Although both, sham-operated and splenectomized group of pigs in our study had significant postoperative increases in neutrophil/lymphocyte ratio (Diagram 9.), the change was more pronounced in splenectomized group indicating that splenectomy imposed greater stress on the organism than sham operation. The lowest value of neutrophil/lymphocyte ratio during the research was recorded on the fifth postoperative day in the group of autotransplanted piglets. Described decrease came as a result of concurrent lymphocytopenia and neutropenia on the fifth day of the experiment in the blood of piglets with splenic autotransplants.

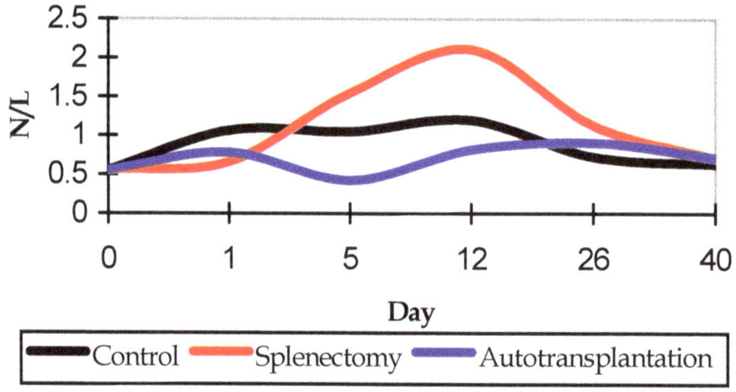

Diagram 9. Changes in ratio of absolute number of segmented neutrophils and lymphocytes (N/L) in the blood of experimental pigs during the experiment

4.5 Platelets

Diverse reports on the platelet level in various species following splenectomy have been published. The response has been reported to be either unchanged (Resende & Petroianu,

2003; Resende et al., 2002) or increased (Karagülle et al., 2007; Knežević et al., 2002; Miko et al., 2003). As one third of total platelets is physiologically sequestered in the spleen, and spleen is also the site of platelet destruction, it is expected, that after their removal, thrombocytosis will develop. In contrast, this study demonstrates significant decrease of platelet number in splenectomized animals (Diagram 10.). As documented, total splenectomy leads to decreased number of T-lymphocytes (Smith et al., 1999; Westermann & Pabst, 1986) which are essential factors in the production of platelets (Mazur, 1987), so we can conclude that this could be the reason of thrombocytopenia that has shortly occurred in splenectomized group of this study.

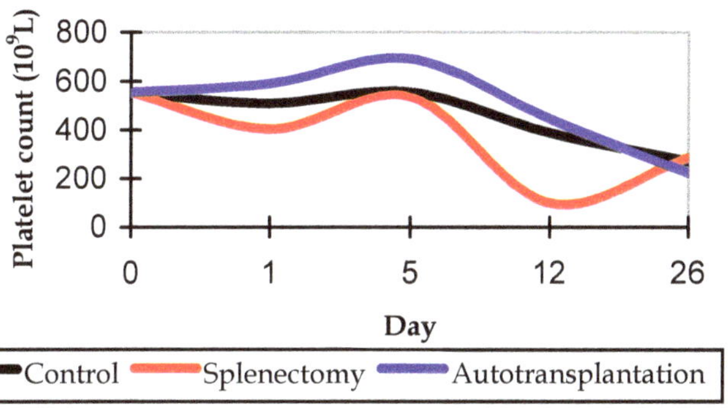

Diagram 10. Changes in platelet count in the blood of experimental pigs during the experiment

4.6 Reticulocytes

Usually, the degree of reticulocytosis is related to the magnitude of hemorrhage during the surgery. Also, many studies report that reticulocytosis following splenectomy is more significant than following other surgical procedures (Knežević et al., 2002; Miko et al., 2003). All experimental groups in this study had the same rate of reticulocytosis growth until twenty sixth day after surgeries when accelerated recovery from acute postoperative anemia was observed in the control group of pigs, suggesting that the least blood loss and surgical trauma occurred during the sham operation (Diagram 11.). In contrast, number of reticulocytes in the pheripheral blood of splenectomized and autotransplanted pigs continued to grow on the twenty sixth and fortieth postoperative day as the result of inadequate blood filtration and prolonged life span of reticulocytes, as well as the loss of splenic humoral control mechanism responsible for releasing young red blood cells into the blood stream. Because of the different intensity of anemia determined in the experimental pig groups, the reticulocyte production index was calculated to avoid erroneously elevated reticulocyte count (Table 4.). On the first postoperative day reticulocyte production index 1 in all three groups of pigs showed insufficient response of bone marrow to compensate postoperative anemia. From fifth to twelfth postoperative day reticulocyte production index in splenectomized and autotransplanted pigs was increased, but still insufficient for compensation of anemia. At the same time, higher reticulocyte production index (over 3) in control group was matched with recovery of red blood cell count. On the twenty sixth postoperative day, data indicates extremely high values of reticulocyte production index in splenectomized and autotransplanted pigs, but that was probably due to increased reticulocyte production in bone marrow, and inadequate blood filtration and prolonged life span of reticulocytes, as well as the loss of splenic humoral control, as mentioned before.

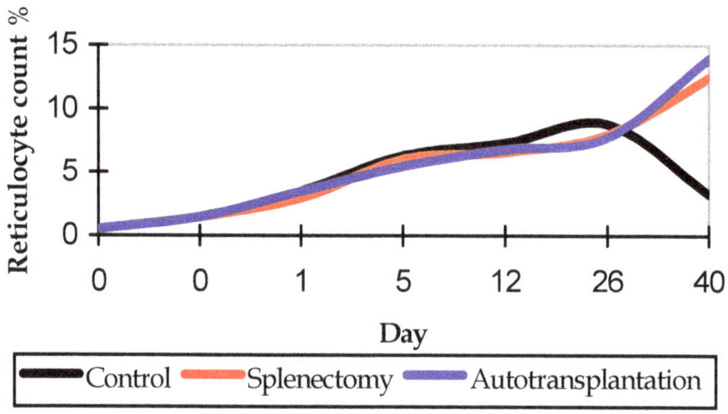

Diagram 11. Average percentage of reticulocytes in the peripheral blood of observed pigs during the experiment

4.7 Erythrocyte morphology

The main developments found in this study were the creation of leptocytes and codocytes and increased number of Howell-Jolly bodies in the peripheral blood of splenectomized pigs (Picture 1.). This founding is in accordance with the results of previous studies on various species, so we can conclude these changes were specific for splenectomized patients. Some authors use the number of erythrocytes containing Howell-Jolly bodies to assess preservation of spleen's blood filtering function (Patel et al., 1981; Resende & Petroianu, 2003; Resende et al., 2002), but number of oxidatively modified erythrocytes containing Heinz bodies can also be used for that purpose (Haklar et al., 1997). Polychromasia and increased number of circulating erythroblasts (Picture 2.) came as a side effect of significant reticulocytosis in all experimental groups. More frequent occurance of morphologically abnormal red blood cells on the blood films of autotransplanted pigs when compared with sham-operated pigs suggests that the autologous splenic tissue was not able to filtrate the blood effectively.

There is still controversy about the effectiveness of regenerated splenic tissue, but the one conclusion of all researches done is common, that functionality and histological restitution of the transplanted splenic tissue depends on the amount of successfully transplanted mass of spleen (Haklar et al., 1997; Sipka, et al., 2006; Tang et al., 2003). In the present research the implant in overall amount of 20 % has not been enough for keeping filtration function of healthy spleen, which correlates with researches from Tang et al. (2003), who find that architecture of red and white pulp, as well as restitution of cardiovascular system is not sufficient for another seven months after transplantation.

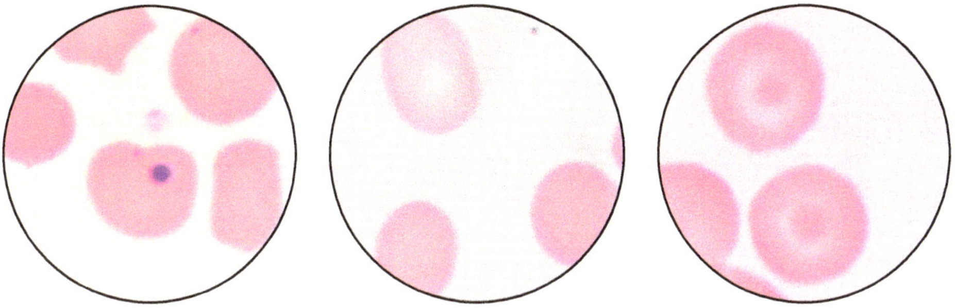

Picture 1. Erythrocyte containing Howell-Jolly bodies, leptocyte and codocytes

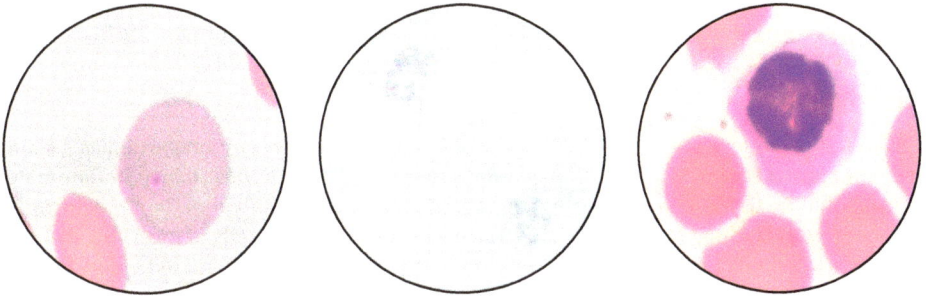

Picture 2. Polychromatophyl, reticulocyte and acydofile erythroblast

4.8 Morphological changes of white blood cells

On the first and fifth day of the experiment morphological evaluation of white blood cells revealed the presence of reactive, granulated and cytotoxic lymphocytes on the blood films of all experimental groups (Picture 3.). After this, morphologically altered lymphocytes appeared only on the twelfth postoperative day on the blood smears of pigs with autotransplanted splenic tissue. Most likely, in this case, inflammatory cascade and production of cytokines were triggered as a response to extensive tissue lesions following autotransplantation, thus leading to the greater number of morphologically altered lymphocytes in the peripheral blood. Metamyelocytes, and dividing cells appeared

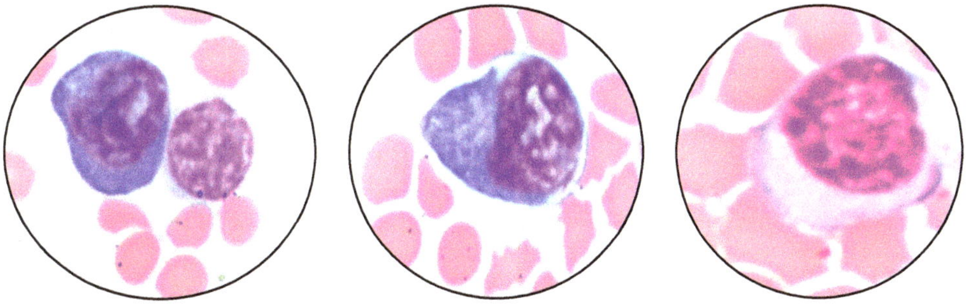

Picture 3. Reactive lymphocytes

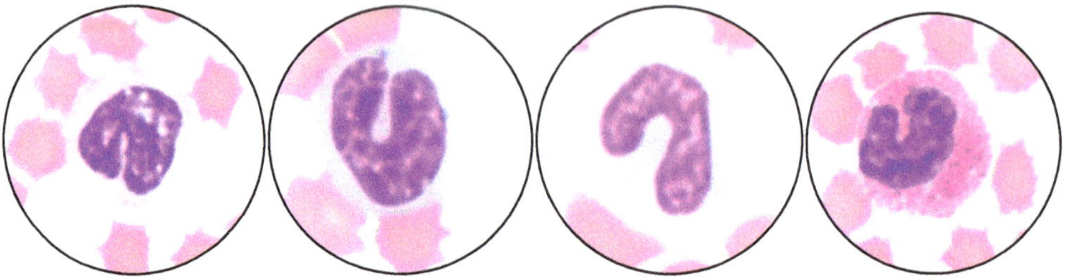

Picture 4. Metamyelocyte, band neutrophils and band eozynophil

sporadically in the peripheral blood of all experimental animals until the twelfth day, but they were most commonly found on the blood smears of splenectomized piglets, with the highest frequency on the fifth day of the experiment (Picture 4.). These results correspond with those reported in splenectomized human patients (Labar & Hauptman, 1998).

5. Conclusion

All groups showed leukocytosis following the operation but this was not regarded as a change specific for splenectomy or autotransplantation, rather than a post-injury inflammatory response due to tissue lesions during operation. Increased number of band neutrophils, subsequent with findings of granulocyte precursors and dividing cells, suggest an increased bone marrow activity and release of immature cells, as well as their mobilization from the marginal pool. Anemia and reticulocytosis found in blood samples of all three groups of pigs may have been physiological results showing the classical postoperative organism reaction to blood loss and surgical trauma. On the other side, frequenter appearance of variations in red blood cell morphology such as appearance of leptocytes, codocytes and Howell-Jolly bodies on the blood smears of splenectomized pigs when compared with other two experimental groups suggests that this was a change specific for splenectomy. More frequent occurance of morphologically abnormal red blood cells on the blood films of autotransplanted pigs compared with sham-operated pigs suggests that the autologous spleen tissue was not able to filtrate the blood effectively. The mass of implant in overall amount of 20% has not been sufficient for keeping filtration function of healthy spleen, therefore should the amount of transplanted mass of spleen be increased.

6. References

Bessler, H., Bergman, M., Salman, H., Beilin, B. & Djaldetti, M. (2004). The relationship between partial splenectomy and peripheral leukocyte count. *Journal of Surgical Research*, 122, No. 1, (November 2004), pp. (49-53). ISSN 0022-4804

Cozzi, E., Bhatti, F., Schmoeckel, M., Chavez, G., Smith, K. G. C., Zaidi, A., Bradley, J., Thiru, S., Goddard, M., Vial, C., Ostilie, D., Wallwork, J., White, D.J.G. & Friend, P. (2000). Long-term survival of nonhuman primates receiving life-supporting transgenic porcine kidney xenografts. *Transplantation*, 70, No.1, (July 2000), pp. (15-21). ISSN 0041-1337

Dyce, K.M., Sack, W.O. & Wensing C.J.G. (2002). *Textbook of veterinary anatomy*. (3rd ed.) Saunders Ltd, ISBN 721689663, Philadelphia, London, New York, St. Louis, Sydney, Toronto.

Haklar, G., Demirel, M., Peker, O., Eskitürk, A., Işgör, A., Söyletir, G. & Yalçin, A.S. (1997). The functional assessment of autotransplanted splenic tissue by its capacity to remove oxidatively modified erythrocytes. *Clinica Chimica Acta,* 258, No. 2, (February 1997), pp. (201-208). ISSN 0009-8981

Jain, N.C. (1993). *Essentials of Veterinary Hematology.* Williams and Wilkins, ISBN 0-8121-1437, USA.

Karagülle, E., Hoşcoşkun, Z., Kutlu, A.K., Kaya, M. & Baydar, S. (2007). The effectiveness of splenic autotransplantation: an external study. *Turkish Journal of Trauma & Emergency Surgery,* 13, No. 1, (October 2007), pp. (13-19). ISSN 1306-696

Khan, P.N., Nair, R.J., Olivares, J., Tingle, L.E. & Li, Z. (2009). Postsplenectomy reactive thombocytosis. *Baylor University Medical Center Proceedings,* 22, No.1, (January 2009), pp. (9-12). Available from: http://www.ncbi.nlm.nih.gov/pmc/articles/PMC2626351/?tool=pubmed

Knežević, S., Stefanović, D., Petrović, M., Djordjević, Z., Matić, S., Artiko, V., Milovanović, A. & Popović, M. (2002). Autotransplantation of the spleen. *Acta Chirurgica Jugoslavica,* 49, No. 3, pp. (101-106). ISSN 0354-950X

Labar, B. & Hauptmann, E. (1998). *Hematologija.* Školska knjiga, ISBN 953-0-30598-2, Zagreb.

Lorber, M. (1958). The Effects of Splenectomy on the Red Blood Cells of the Dog with Particular Emphasis on the Reticulocyte Response. *Blood,* 13, No 10, (October 1958), pp. (972-985). ISSN 0006-4971

Marques, R.G., Petroianu, A. & Coelho, J.M.C.O. (2003). Bacterial phagocytosis by macrophage of autogenous splenic implant. *Brazilian Journal of Biology,* 63, No. 3, (August 2003), pp. (491-495). ISSN 1519-6984 Available from: http://www.scielo.br/scielo.php?pid=S1519-69842003000300015&script=sci_arttext&tlng=es

Mazur, E.M. (1987). Megakaryocytopoiesis and platelet production. *Experimental Hematology,* 15, No. 4, (May 1987), pp. (340-350). ISSN 0301-472X

Miko, I., Brath, E., Nemeth, N., Toth, F.F., Sipka, S., Kovacs, J., Sipka S., Fachet, J., Furka, A., Furka, I. & Zhong, R. (2003). Hematological, hemorheological, immunological, and morphological studies of spleen autotransplantation in mice: preliminary results. *Microsurgery,* 23, No. 5, (October 2003), pp. (483-488). ISSN 0974-3227

Patel, J., Williams, J.S., Shmigel, B. & Hinshaw, J.R. (1981). Preservation of splenic function by autotransplantation of traumatized spleen in man. *Surgery,* 90, No. 4, (October 1981), pp. (683-688). ISSN 0039-6060

Resende, V., Petroianu, A. & Junior, W. C. T. (2002). Autotransplantation for treatment of severe splenic lesions. *Emergency Radiology,* 9, No. 4, (August 2002) pp. (208-212). ISSN 1438-1435

Resende, V. & Petroianu, A. (2003). Functions of the splenic remnant after subtotal splenectomy for treatment of severe splenic injuries. *The American Journal of Surgery,* 185, No. 4, (April 2003), pp. (311-315). ISSN 0002-9610

Sipka, S. Jr., Bráth, E., Tòth, F. F., Fabian, A., Krizsan, C., Barath, S., Sipka, S., Nemeth, N., Balint, A., Furka, I. & Mikò, I. (2006). Distribution of peripheral blood cells in mice after splenectomy or autotransplantation. *Microsurgery,* 26, No. 1, (January 2006), pp. (43-49). ISSN 0033-8419.

Smith, E., DeYoung, N.J. & Drew, P.A. (1999). Immune cell subpopulations in regenerated splenic tissue in rats. *ANZ. Journal of Surgery,* 69, No. 7, (July 1999), pp. (522-525). ISSN 1445-2197.

Shokouh-Amiri, M. H., Kharazmi, A., Rahimi-Saber, S., Hansen, C. P. & Jensen, S. L. (1990). Phagocyte function after splenic autotransplantation. *Archives of Surgery*, 125, No. 5, (May 1990), pp. (595–597). ISSN 0004-0010

Tarnuzi,A. & Smiley, R.K.(1967). Hematologic effects of splenic implants. Blood. 29. No. 3, (August 1966), pp. (373-384). ISSN 0006-4971

Tang, W.H, Wu, F.L., Huang, M.K. & Friess, H. (2003). Splenic tissue autotransplantation in rabbits: no restoration of host defense. *Langenbecks Archives of Surgery*, 387, No. 9-10, (January 2003), pp. (379-385). ISSN 1435-2443

Teske, E. (2000). Leukocytes - Lymphocytes, In: *Schalm's Veterinary Hematology*, Feldman, B. F., Zinkel, J. G., Jain, N. C. Eds., pp. (223–228). Lippincott Williams & Wilkins, ISBN 0-683-30692-8, Philadelphia, Baltimore, New York, London, Buenos Aires, Hong Kong, Sidney, Tokyo.

Theodorou, G. L., A. Mouzaki, Tsiftsis, D., Apostolopoulou, A., Mougiou, A., Theodori, E., Vagianos, C. & Karakantza M. (2007). Effect of non-operative management (NOM) of splenic rupture versus splenectomy on the distribution of peripheral blood lymphocyte populations and cytokine production by T cells. *Clinical and Experimental Immunology*, 150, No. 3, (October 2007), pp. (429-436). Available from: http://www.ncbi.nlm.nih.gov/pmc/articles/PMC2219385/

Timens, W. & Leemans, R. (1992). Splenic autotransplantation and the immune system. *Annals of Surgery*, 215, No. 3, (March 1992), pp. (256-260). ISSN 0003-4932

Tillson, D.M. (2003). Spleen. In: *Textbook of Small Animal Surgery*, Slatter, D.H, Ed., pp. (1046-1062), Saunders Co. LTd, ISBN 9780721686073, Philadelphia.

Traub, A., Giebnik, G.S., Smith, C., Kuni, C.C., Brekke, M.L., Edlund, D. & Perry, J.F. (1987). Splenic reticuloendothelial function after splenectomy, spleen repair, and spleen autotransplantation. *The New England Journal of Medicine*, 317, No. 25, (December 1987), pp. (1559-1564). ISSN 1533-4406

Weiss, D.J. (1984). Uniform evaluation and semiquantitative reporting of hematologic data in veterinary laboratories. Cited in: *Atlas of veterinary hematology. Blood and Bone Marrow of Domestic animals,* Harvey J.W., pp. (18-19). W.B. Saunders Co., ISBN 0-7216-6334-6, USA

Westermann, J. & Pabst, R. (1986). Autotransplantation of splenic fragments: lymphocyte subsets in blood, lymph nodes and splenic tissue. *Clinical & Experimental Immunol*ogy, 64, No. 1, (April 1986), pp. (188-194). ISSN 1365-2249.

Zahorec, R. (2001). Ratio of neutrophil to lymphocyte counts — rapid and simple parameter of systemic inflammation and stress in critically ill. *Bratislava Medical Journal*, 102, No.1, (January 2001), pp. (5–14). ISSN 0006-9248. Available from: http://www.bmj.sk/2001/10201-01.PDF

Zhang, H., Chen, J., Kaiser, G.M., Mapudengo, O., Zhang, J., Exton, M. S. & Song, E. (2002). The Value of Partial Splenic Autotransplantation in Patients with Portal Hypertension. *Archives of Surgery*, 137, No.1, (January 2002), pp. (89–93). ISSN 0004-0010

Permissions

The contributors of this book come from diverse backgrounds, making this book a truly international effort. This book will bring forth new frontiers with its revolutionizing research information and detailed analysis of the nascent developments around the world.

We would like to thank Charles H. Lawrie, for lending his expertise to make the book truly unique. He has played a crucial role in the development of this book. Without his invaluable contribution this book wouldn't have been possible. He has made vital efforts to compile up to date information on the varied aspects of this subject to make this book a valuable addition to the collection of many professionals and students.

This book was conceptualized with the vision of imparting up-to-date information and advanced data in this field. To ensure the same, a matchless editorial board was set up. Every individual on the board went through rigorous rounds of assessment to prove their worth. After which they invested a large part of their time researching and compiling the most relevant data for our readers. Conferences and sessions were held from time to time between the editorial board and the contributing authors to present the data in the most comprehensible form. The editorial team has worked tirelessly to provide valuable and valid information to help people across the globe.

Every chapter published in this book has been scrutinized by our experts. Their significance has been extensively debated. The topics covered herein carry significant findings which will fuel the growth of the discipline. They may even be implemented as practical applications or may be referred to as a beginning point for another development. Chapters in this book were first published by InTech; hereby published with permission under the Creative Commons Attribution License or equivalent.

The editorial board has been involved in producing this book since its inception. They have spent rigorous hours researching and exploring the diverse topics which have resulted in the successful publishing of this book. They have passed on their knowledge of decades through this book. To expedite this challenging task, the publisher supported the team at every step. A small team of assistant editors was also appointed to further simplify the editing procedure and attain best results for the readers.

Our editorial team has been hand-picked from every corner of the world. Their multi-ethnicity adds dynamic inputs to the discussions which result in innovative outcomes. These outcomes are then further discussed with the researchers and contributors who give their valuable feedback and opinion regarding the same. The feedback is then collaborated with the researches and they are edited in a comprehensive manner to aid the understanding of the subject.

Apart from the editorial board, the designing team has also invested a significant amount of their time in understanding the subject and creating the most relevant covers. They scrutinized every image to scout for the most suitable representation of the subject and create an appropriate cover for the book.

The publishing team has been involved in this book since its early stages. They were actively engaged in every process, be it collecting the data, connecting with the contributors or procuring relevant information. The team has been an ardent support to the editorial, designing and production team. Their endless efforts to recruit the best for this project, has resulted in the accomplishment of this book. They are a veteran in the field of academics and their pool of knowledge is as vast as their experience in printing. Their expertise and guidance has proved useful at every step. Their uncompromising quality standards have made this book an exceptional effort. Their encouragement from time to time has been an inspiration for everyone.

The publisher and the editorial board hope that this book will prove to be a valuable piece of knowledge for researchers, students, practitioners and scholars across the globe.

List of Contributors

Nirmalee Abayasekara and Arati Khanna-Gupta
Brigham and Women's Hospital, Harvard Medical School, Boston, MA, USA

Chiara Vitale
DI.ME.S. Università di Genova, Genova, Italy

Renato Zambello
Padova University School of Medicine, Department of Clinical and Experimental Medicine, Hematology and Clinical Immunology Branch - Padova, Italy

Mirna Balsamo
Istituto G. Gaslini - Genova, Italy

Maria Cristina Mingari
DI.ME.S. Università di Genova, Genova, Italy
IRCCS A.O.U. S.Martino-IST Istituto Nazionale per la Ricerca sul Cancro, S.C. Immunologia - Genova, Italy

Massimo Vitale
IRCCS A.O.U. S.Martino-IST Istituto Nazionale per la Ricerca sul Cancro, S.C. Immunologia - Genova, Italy

Ciro Roberto Rinaldi and Ana Crisan
Department of Haematology - United Lincolnshire Hospital NHS Trust - Boston, UK

Paola Rinaldi
University Federico II and CEINGE Biotecnologie Avanzate - Naples, Italy

Hasan A. Abd El-Ghaffar, Nashwa K. Abosamra, Dalia Salem, Sherin M. Abd El-Aziz and Layla M. Tharwat
Clinical Pathology Department, Faculty of Medicine, Mansoura University, Mansoura, Egypt
Oncology Center, Mansoura University, Mansoura, Egypt

Sameh Shamaa
Internal Medicine Department, Faculty of Medicine, Mansoura University, Mansoura, Egypt
Oncology Center, Mansoura University, Mansoura, Egypt

Nadia Attwan
Pathology Department, Faculty of Medicine, Mansoura University, Mansoura, Egypt

Tarek E. Selim
Clinical Pathology Department, Faculty of Medicine, Mansoura University, Mansoura, Egypt

Charles H. Lawrie
Biodonostia Institute, San Sebastián, Spain
IKERBASQUE, Basque Foundation for Science, Bilbao, Spain
Nuffield Department of Clinical Laboratory Sciences, University of Oxford, UK

Anastasia S. Tsingotjidou
Laboratory of Anatomy and Histology, Faculty of Veterinary Medicine, Aristotle University of Thessaloniki, Greece

Jun Lu and Ai Kotani
Tokai University Institute of Innovative Science and Technology, Japan

Bidisha Chanda
University of Tokyo Institute of Medical Science, Japan

Antonia Rotolo, Paolo Nicoli, Daniela Cilloni, Giuseppe Saglio and Angelo Guerrasio
M.D., Division of Hematology and Internal Medicine, Italy

Ubaldo Familiari
M.D., Pathology Department, Department of Clinical and Biological Sciences, San Luigi Gonzaga Hospital, University of Turin, Turin, Italy

Kazuo Nakamura
Nihon Pharmaceutical University, Japan

Xinliang Mao and Biyin Cao
Cyrus Tang Hematology Center, Soochow University, P.R.China

Sarah Parisi and Antonio Curti
Department of Hematology and Oncological Sciences "L. and A. Seràgnoli", University of Bologna, Bologna, Italy

Larry H. Bernstein
Triplex, USA

Gil David and Ronald R. Coifman
Yale University Department of Mathematics, Program in Applied Mathematics, New Haven, CT, USA

James Rucinski
New York Methodist Hospital-Weill-Cornell, Brooklyn, NY, USA

K. Satué and A. Hernández
Department of Animal Medicine and Surgery, School of Veterinary Medicine, Cardenal Herrera-CEU University, Valencia

A. Muñoz
Department of Animal Medicine and Surgery, Equine Sport Medicine Centre, School of Veterinary Medicine, University of Córdoba, Spain

Nina Poljičak-Milas and Matko Kardum
Faculty of Veterinary Medicine, Department of Pathophysiology, University of Zagreb, Croatia

Anja Vujnović
Croatian Veterinary Institute, Croatia

Josipa Migić
Pliva d.o.o., Croatia

Dražen Vnuk
Faculty of Veterinary Medicine, Surgery, Orthopedics and Ophthalmology Clinic, University of Zagreb, Croatia

www.ingramcontent.com/pod-product-compliance
Lightning Source LLC
Chambersburg PA
CBHW070730190326
41458CB00004B/1111
* 9 7 8 1 6 3 2 4 2 3 1 3 9 *